GENDER IN HISTORY

Series editors:
Pam Sharpe, Patricia Skinner and Penny Summerfield

The expansion of research into the history of women and gender since the 1970s has changed the face of history. Using the insights of feminist theory and of historians of women, gender historians have explored the configuration in the past of gender identities and relations between the sexes. They have also investigated the history of sexuality and family relations, and analysed ideas and ideals of masculinity and femininity. Yet gender history has not abandoned the original, inspirational project of women's history: to recover and reveal the lived experience of women in the past and the present.

The series Gender in History provides a forum for these developments. Its historical coverage extends from the medieval to the modern periods, and its geographical scope encompasses not only Europe and North America but all corners of the globe. The series aims to investigate the social and cultural constructions of gender in historical sources, as well as the gendering of historical discourse itself. It embraces both detailed case studies of specific regions or periods, and broader treatments of major themes. Gender in History titles are designed to meet the needs of both scholars and students working in this dynamic area of historical research.

Women's medical work in early modern France

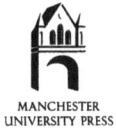

MANCHESTER
UNIVERSITY PRESS

Also available

*'The truest form of patriotism':
feminist pacifism in Britain, 1870–1902*
Heloise Brown

Masculinity in politics and war: gendering modern history
Stefan Dudink, Karen Hagemann
and John Tosh (eds)

*Noblewomen, aristocracy and power
in the twelfth-century Anglo-Norman realm*
Susan Johns

WOMEN'S MEDICAL WORK IN EARLY MODERN FRANCE

⇥ Susan Broomhall ⇤

Manchester University Press
Manchester and New York

distributed exclusively in the USA by Palgrave

Copyright © Susan Broomhall 2004

The right of Susan Broomhall to be identified as the author of this work has been asserted by her in accordance with the Copyright, Designs and Patents Act 1988.

Published by Manchester University Press
Oxford Road, Manchester M13 9NR, UK
and Room 400, 175 Fifth Avenue, New York, NY 10010, USA
www.manchesteruniversitypress.co.uk

Distributed exclusively in the USA by
Palgrave, 175 Fifth Avenue, New York NY 10010, USA

Distributed exclusively in Canada by
UBC Press, University of British Columbia, 2029 West Mall, Vancouver, BC, Canada V6T 1Z2

British Library Cataloguing-in-Publication Data
A catalogue record for this book is available from the British Library

Library of Congress Cataloging-in-Publication Data
A catalog record for this book is available from the Library of Congress

ISBN 13: 978 0 7190 6287 2

First published by Manchester University Press 2004

First digital paperback edition published 2011

Printed by Lightning Source

Contents

ACKNOWLEDGEMENTS		*page* vi
NOTES ON TEXT		viii
	INTRODUCTION	1
1	Women and the medical guilds	16
2	The university: women and the Faculty of Medicine in Paris	44
3	Hospital nursing by women religious: the Hôtel-Dieu in Paris	71
4	Female healing before the law	96
5	The book trades: female medical practice in print	127
6	Nursing, caring, curing: women's work in municipal child care	156
7	The world of the court: women serving the royal family	186
8	French women and reproductive knowledge at the Spanish court	214
9	Elite women and reproductive knowledge: the Nassau sisters	232
	AFTERWORD	257
	SELECT BIBLIOGRAPHY	261
	INDEX	281

Acknowledgements

Many people have contributed to this work in different ways, and I would like to thank them here. This project would not have been possible without the financial support of a French Government postgraduate scholarship, and an Australian Research Council fellowship. Chapter 8 (originally published as "Women's little secrets": defining the boundaries of women's reproductive knowledge in sixteenth-century France', *Social History of Medicine*, 15:1, 2002, pp. 1–15) is reproduced in amended form by permission of Oxford University Press. The staff of the Bibliothèque Nationale, the Bibliothèque Mazarine and the Archives Nationales have always been most helpful at every opportunity. The staff at the Bibliothèque Municipale de Reims helped me to pursue a thread that led to Isabelle Estevent. In Tours, I am grateful for the cheerful assistance of the staff of the Bibliothèque Municipale, the Archives Départementales d'Indre-et-Loire, and the Archives Municipales de Tours.

I would also like to thank the Centre d'Etudes Supérieures de la Renaissance at Tours for their lively community of scholars. Professor Jean-Paul Pittion provided encouragement and support for this project in its early stages. Professor Pierre Aquilon helped me to discover a whole new world in the archives through his advice and paleographical assistance. Dr Jacqueline Vons has continued to support the project from its origins to the present text. The staff of the CESR library were always ready to assist in the course of my research. My French family, les Viout, gave us a warm and memorable welcome into their home in Corrèze and to France generally. I am also grateful to Anne Filiol for her unfailing patience in reading drafts of the early manuscript.

In Australia, the School of Humanities at The University of Western Australia has provided an animated and important forum for the production of the final text, particularly staff and postgraduates in the History, and Medieval and Early Modern Studies discipline groups. The staff of the Scholars' Centre at the Reid Library have been ever willing to assist with enquiries for obscure texts. Judy Berman, Toby Burrows, Patricia Crawford, Philippa Maddern, Pam Sharpe and Stephanie Tarbin have all provided specialist advice, acted at times as a sounding board for various ideas, offered suggestions on chapters or readings, and been there for coffee when inspiration failed me.

Elsewhere, too, friends and colleagues have encouraged me to continue this text, providing advice, comments, suggestions for further reading and introductions to other scholars: I would particularly like to thank Natalie Zemon Davis, Sarah Ferber, Lyndal Roper, Lisa Wynne Smith and Hilary Marland. I feel privileged to have received such careful and valuable advice on earlier drafts of this text from a wonderfully supportive group of scholars who were so willing to critically engage with the work: I am very grateful to Alison Klairmont

Lingo, Cathy McClive, Lianne McTavish, Trish Skinner, Stephanie Tarbin and Colette H. Winn.

My parents, Margaret and Andrew Broomhall, have always been ready to lend support when needed, whether phone calls and food supplies from home, or comments on drafts of the work (even if I couldn't always answer the 'what happened to her in the end?' question). Finally, this work belongs to Tim, with all my love. For sacrificing his career, the English language, his family, friends and the Jags, to be with me in Tours. If he hadn't made me post the application letter, this work might not exist at all.

Notes on text

Although this study concerns women and medical work in early modern France, its arguments may be of interest to researchers examining other European environments. For greater accessibility to these readers, all foreign-language quotations have been translated into English. All translations are my own, except where otherwise indicated. Scholars are welcome to contact me for the original text of works cited.

All book titles are referred to in their original language. As titles of early modern texts tend to be lengthy, I have used short titles in the main body of the text, but full details in the notes and bibliography. Square brackets indicate publication details that are uncertain.

Introduction

For a majority of the French population during the period known as the Renaissance, most medical care would come at the hands of women. Most of the population was poor, illiterate and lived outside of urban areas. When children were born, they would generally be nursed by their mothers. The elite child would be cared for by a wetnurse and governess, while the orphaned or abandoned child would typically be placed in the care of a townswoman, under the supervision of the local Hôtel-Dieu. It was mothers and wives who tended colds or minor ailments. A broken arm was as likely to be treated by the local bonesetter as by doctors or surgeons. The poor and grievously ill would seek medical treatment from their local Hôtel-Dieu where much of their care would be undertaken by women, often nuns. Most women, when pregnant, would seek advice from other women in their family or surrounds. They prayed for a safe birth to female saints, such as Margaret and Mary, as well as to God. They would be delivered almost always by a midwife or women in their family or village. Finally, it would be family members, or a paid female sicknurse, who nursed the dying in their last days.

Women have been crucial to medical service provision in the European past. Increasingly historians acknowledge the presence of women in the broader medical spectrum, although there are very few studies which document who such women were, what their specific medical practices and theories were, and how their medical work was perceived by contemporary communities. Yet, as Monica H. Green has argued, 'documenting the historical experience of women practitioners must be the concern of all social historians of medicine, not simply those who specialize in women's history'.[1] In this study, I hope to address these issues in relation to women's medical work in France between approximately 1460 and 1630.

Women's medical work, like that of other providers, needs to be situated in specific historical and social contexts. There has been a general supposition in histories of medicine that much of women's contribution to the field has continued unchanged for many hundreds of years. However, with increasing study of the particular female medical practices of midwifery, for example, we know that historical, political, religious, guild and local community contexts, to name a few, have been crucial to how women practised and how they were perceived by contemporaries. Yet for many other areas of female practice, such as their care-giving labour, where techniques passed from mother to daughter in an oral and kinaesthetic tradition, there is a kind of resigned acceptance that these practices were somehow unchanging and cannot be documented in any detail. Although women have been the dominant providers of medical care in the household for many centuries until the present day, it does not follow (and indeed it seems highly unlikely) that what women did, how they understood their form of domestic medicine, and how contemporaries perceived it, have remained unchanged over the same time. We need studies of female medical practice that demonstrate how these activities were structured, influenced by, and engaged with, historically specific events, trends and mentalities.

The period between 1460 and 1630 was a time of great change in France: in society generally and in medical practices and thought specifically. The new print medium for publication influenced the production and communication of new ideas, often by new authors, and how they were understood by new groups of readers.[2] For a certain group of the literate elite, the effect of humanism on the development and dissemination of medical ideas was significant.[3] The upheaval of the reforming religious movements divided France and caused civil war in the second half of the sixteenth century. For Catholics, the decrees of the Council of Trent altered some spiritual beliefs, including healing practices, and modified the daily lives of those in religious communities.[4] The growing authority and control imposed by the crown affected a range of activities, including how, and by whom, hospitals were administered. The trend towards incorporation of occupational activities in guilds, colleges and confraternities led to new forms of recognition for some medical practices. Exploration to new lands introduced new drugs to Europe, as well as what appeared to contemporaries to be previously unknown diseases. Women's medical practices interacted with contemporary debates and situations, and need to be analysed in such contexts. It may be the case that some of the ways in which women practised or were perceived were not unique to this period, but pre-dated it and/or continued afterwards. However, we need to nuance our understanding of female medical work by knowing where and why such continuities or differences occurred.

This study adopts a number of methodological approaches which will help to highlight and understand women's medical practices, and may provide new ways to perceive their contribution to the history of medicine more generally.

INTRODUCTION

Historians of medicine in France have traditionally emphasised the progression towards professionalisation that occurred as one of the defining characteristics of the period known as the Renaissance. They have highlighted the internal controversy and debate between medical professionals in studies of their manuscript and printed texts.[5] Their works depict the medical world as one marked by great men and their discoveries leading ever forward in linear progression towards acknowledged 'scientific truths'. Increasingly, however, this history of linear progression and a clear epistemology has been debated by philosophers of science. Alexandre Koyré focused on the relationship between scientific theories and the philosophy of the time which produced them, emphasising the importance of contextualising scientific thought.[6] Gaston Bachelard's ideas about epistemological obstacles and epistemological ruptures explored the meanings behind the differentiation between 'sanctioned science' and 'marginalised science'.[7] Steven Shapin and Simon Schaffer have encouraged analysis of moments of scientific controversy because of the opportunities they offer to see opposing points of view: the rejected and accepted scientific knowledge.[8] As Thomas Kuhn argued, 'historians confront growing difficulties in distinguishing the "scientific" component of past observation and belief from what their predecessors had readily labelled "error" and "superstition"'.[9] Such arguments have given rise to examination of the theories and practices of a wider pool of practitioners in a more inclusive history of scientific practices and epistemologies.

More recently, the historian Jacques Roger has argued that modern knowledge 'must not either serve as the organising principle of a historical reconstruction nor as the criteria of judgement, indeed of condemnation, of science of the past'.[10] David Bloor proposes a more extreme view, whereby the historian must treat truth as error, in a system of symmetry, so as not to privilege theories that were later accepted as scientific truth over those that were not.[11] Both Roger and Bloor's methodology demand that a variety of epistemologies be considered alongside those of the scientific 'canon'. Yet one of the most striking elements of histories of medicine in France has been the pre-dominant position, until very recently, of the text, almost to the detriment of all other historical source materials. University-trained and university-recognised practitioners, physicians, surgeons and apothecaries are probably the best documented and most historically visible medical communities, through their scientific and popular vernacular publications, but we cannot assume from this that they were the most important, relevant, accessible and authoritative to all people living in sixteenth-century France. In what sense did the university-trained or university-approved medical practitioners constitute the medical 'paradigm', the 'normal science', if most of the population did not access their knowledge – either because they were illiterate (certainly in Latin and largely in French) or because they did not use their medical services and thus were not exposed to these theories?[12] To privilege texts written by university-trained or university-approved medical personnel would seem to over-represent their power and influence in sixteenth-century medical practice and epistemologies. Other contemporary primary sources, men and women's letters, archives of Hôtels-Dieu, trials and legal documents, and literature among them, all suggest other practices were also important, perhaps even more important and influential to the majority of the population.

Some recent French texts have been more accommodating of a wider view of the medical spectrum, taking in more than elite, university-educated men. François Lebrun broadens the range of participants in medical care in the early modern past and envisages a division between official practices and the alternative medicine of empirics, conjurors and holy healers, but does not include women in his work.[13] Matthew Ramsey has recently produced an important and influential study of eighteenth- and nineteenth-century medicine which inverts the medical hierarchy and examines medical practices from 'the bottom up'.[14] Ramsey's study develops a new and important perspective, seeking to understand the history of popular medicine from the point of view of its practitioners.[15] Using a synchronic approach, Ramsey's taxonomy reveals the great variety of medical practitioners in France at that time.[16]

The most recent and comprehensive addition to the history of early modern France medicine, Laurence Brockliss and Colin Jones' influential 1997 *The Medical World of Early Modern France*, highlights many of the changes that have occurred in the current historiography of medicine. The authors seek to re-define the boundaries of the 'medical world' employing a more open framework to conceptualise medical epistemologies and practices, in order to include 'the whole set of practitioners of health services, trained and untrained, educated and non-educated, male and female, working in France between the sixteenth century and the French Revolution'.[17] Yet, despite their claimed receptivity to the influence of what they term 'the medical penumbra', their framework for understanding the field of medicine privileges the 'trained and legally authorised corporative medical community' at the centre of the field and pushes outside that core, 'the plethora of different types of "popular" medical practitioner, male and female, rich and poor, educated and uneducated, and so on'.[18]

Given Brockliss and Jones' acknowledgement that, from a patient's perspective, 'trained and untrained practitioners were largely viewed as offering an *à la carte* range of services, from which a choice was made according to a hierarchy of resort which was subject to constraints such as relative accessibility, geographical remoteness, size of personal income, religious disposition, the nature, circumstances, or phase of an illness or medical conditions, and so on',[19] what then justifies the placement of the elite corporative medical community at the core of Brockliss and Jones' schema? Even they argue in their introduction that '"history from below" plus research centring on popular culture [have] both demonstrated the irrelevance of most of the activity of most trained medical practitioners for most of the population and for most of the time prior to 1850 at least'.[20] In what sense can we possibly argue, then, that elite professional science was mainstream, if the majority of people most frequently used other medical practices, whether by choice or by practical constraints? Brockliss and Jones' text is a detailed and valuable work of overarching changes and transitions in early modern medicine across a wide-ranging number of disciplines and specialties, but there is nonetheless room to produce further studies of specific groups of early modern medical practitioners, as I do here for women.

Beyond France itself, there has been a growing emphasis placed on re-thinking medical practices and on the social history of early modern medicine more generally. In a key essay in 1979, Margaret Pelling and Charles Webster already warned against 'undervaluing the activities of arbitrarily defined sections of the medical community'.[21] For early modern Bologna, Gianna Pomata has emphasised the power of patients in choosing their healer. Importantly, she has also argued that the corpus of healers and their organisation was in part shaped by notions of the body.[22] David Gentilcore incorporates the practices of a wide range of medical service providers in his studies of health and healing practices in seventeenth- and eighteenth-century Italy.[23] The idea of medical pluralism in the early modern world seems in such texts as these a well-established concept. Physicians, empirics, surgeons, apothecaries, folk healers, and religious personalities all vied with each other (as well as worked together) for medical legitimacy and patients, and together formed a composite picture of healers and healing in early modern Europe.

Rather than adopting a top-down or bottom-up approach, in this study I wish to focus on women because, as practitioners, they cut across most sectors of medical practice. By examining women, I do not wish to create simplistic dichotomies between official university medicine and the traditional, popular practices of women, as some historians perceive them. Firstly, women's medical work was not merely 'popular', it could also be official, authorised by university and guild medical communities, ecclesiastical and municipal bodies, as well as the crown, to name just a few. Secondly, women were not a unified group of medical practitioners: as we shall see, they participated in medical practice in many diverse ways, with varied degrees of authority and recognition from different communities. Because women's medical work cut across learned, rural, university, royal, religious, popular, elite, guild, domestic and local communities, all of whom had an interest in health and medicine, a study of female practitioners provides a means to see a cross-section of sixteenth-century medical practices and theories. This framework may help us rethink what we mean by such terms as 'medical' and 'practitioner' and where we look, as historians, to find such terms expressed and enacted in the past.

There are of course already a number of studies concerned to highlight the participation of women in medicine. Some of the earliest studies sought to provide an overview of women's practices and to demonstrate the continuity of their participation in medicine.[24] More recently, Monica H. Green has produced an important initial survey of women's medical practices and care across medieval Europe. As she has argued, 'if we choose to ignore women's medical practice we simultaneously choose to ignore the health care received by a significant portion of the medieval population, male and female'.[25] Specific groups of women have also been studied for certain historical periods. The work of midwives has been the subject of much recent study.[26] There has also been some attention given to the work of women as nursing sisters in hospital organisations.[27] Women's care-giving work is beginning to be recognised as needing historicisation, but there are few studies as yet which elaborate how this might be undertaken.[28] In this study, I will pay particular attention to how women's work as medical practitioners across a range of medical domains and different environments was perceived by contemporaries, both in and outside medical communities. It is not my intention to proclaim that women's participation was wholly beneficial by any means,[29] or indeed to judge the efficacy of their work by modern standards more generally. I want to understand here how contemporaries responded to female medical practice, what opinions they formed of the utility of women's medical work, and how women interacted with such bodies about their medical participation.[30]

As regards source materials, this project decentralises university medical texts and employs a range of sources produced by a variety of situations, positions, authors and discourses. Sources such as manuscript and early printed works, personal correspondence, hospital and poor relief ledgers, hagiography and legal commentaries can all contribute to an understanding of women's medical work. I use a combination of detailed case studies, diachronic, textual and comparative analyses, in order to use the available resources to best effect. In doing so, I hope to demonstrate both the range of medical practices in which women were involved as well as explore their work, and perceptions of it, in some depth. The materials provide breadth not only of the medical domains in which women worked, but also of social and economic levels, urban and rural environments, formal and informal practice, paid and unpaid medical care, varied political and religious contexts, individual circumstances and networks, and cover different regions of France.

Gender has rarely featured in histories of medicine as the category of historical analysis in the way that Joan Scott has convincingly argued is possible.[31] In a study particularly focused on women, it is essential here to recognise the role of gender as a factor, like class and religion, which greatly influenced the lives of those in sixteenth-century France. In this study, it will be key to examine how gender affected women's work status and opportunities,[32] as well as knowledge creation and transmission, and corporeal knowledge. My use of 'gender' borrows from Toril Moi's appropriation of Pierre Bourdieu's theories. Moi argues cogently that 'one of the advantages of Bourdieu's theory is that it not only insists on the social construction of gender, but that it permits us to seize the immense *variability* of gender as a social factor'.[33] There need be no fixed hierarchy of class over gender, or the reverse, but rather such factors are fluid and changeable according to specific contexts.[34] Indeed, as my study demonstrates, for some women in particular contexts, elite social status could override their gender so that they could contribute to medical discussion, but the same women were unable to contribute to other medical fields (or even the same fields) in other situations. Gender as a 'socially *variable* entity . . . carries different amounts of symbolic capital in different contexts'.[35]

A key subject of my investigation will be to understand reproductive theories and practices. Understanding and debate on women's bodies and corporeal knowledge are central aspects in both gender historiography and theorising within gender studies itself.[36] The importance of the lived experience of the body cannot be understated in particular areas of female medical authority during the early modern period, such as pregnancy and childbirth. For early modern Germany, Barbara Duden has emphasised the importance of understanding early modern perceptions of the body, and distinguishing them from our own, as well as the gendering of such perceptions.[37] My project is inflected by important international feminist scholarship both on science and medicine, and their critiques of the influential work of Michel Foucault on the construction of power systems through knowledge.[38]

Feminist historians and philosophers such as Londa Schiebinger, Sandra Harding and Lorraine Code have drawn attention to the gendered nature of contemporary and past scientific production and axiology, and increasingly emphasised its Eurocentrism, mostly drawing on sources from the eighteenth century onwards.[39] In the field of medical history in particular, Ludmilla Jordanova has emphasised the gendered process of the construction of both medical knowledge and its historiography.[40] While embracing many of these scholars' arguments, my study pushes back the boundaries of their conclusions to an earlier era. In particular, it seeks to reject any notion of a past 'golden age' of equal scientific participation suggested by the heavy focus on the gendered development of 'modern' (eighteenth-century and onwards) modes of scientific scholarship.

Finally, it is necessary to define medical terms and concepts in this text in ways which are inclusive of women's experiences. For instance, non-university-trained or guild-trained practitioners are often referred to as 'untrained'. In the present study, I would argue that we need to re-define in what sense we use such terms as 'trained' and 'educated', and employ them more flexibly and clearly, in order to understand medical practices and epistemologies that do not fit the traditional models that historians have created for the elite university-educated 'canon'. A term such as 'qualified' could mean different things to different contemporary groups, but is commonly used by historians to mean university or guild-qualified. The use of such terminology has implications for how we recognise and value certain skills, practices and knowledge as medical even today. I have tried to use such words as regulated, trained, patronised, educated and authorised, with reference to the specific body concerned in that context, so as to be explicit as to which of the diverse communities in France is meant. The designation of an appropriate practitioner could be influenced by many community interests, often beyond the control of the patients themselves.[41] Some women's spiritual healing, for instance, might be Church-approved and regulated, and patronised by a local community, but such practitioners were likely to be seen as untrained in the university medical context. When discussing medical work as approved by various communities, I intend the word community as a group of people with shared interests, as stakeholders in a specific context. Thus people are members simultaneously of many different types of physical and abstract communities that define their identity in particular environments. Louise Bourgeois, for instance, is part of the professional medical community recognised by the university, a community of Catholic medical practitioners, a community of female midwives in Paris, and a community of mothers, to name just a few.

Moreover, the key terms 'medicine' and 'medical' are used in this work to define activities that contemporaries perceived as medical: that is, actions which were concerned with the maintenance of health and treatment of illness. As Green has argued for the medieval period, 'we need to challenge our comfortable assumption that we know what these terms meant and look instead at precisely what significance medieval people themselves attached to them and what kind of medical practice they implied'.[42] Including the maintenance of health as medical practice – for which university-trained physicians were employed at the court, a domain on which they wrote abundant printed texts, and advised and supported municipal councils in their public health measures – may help to expose and historicise the preventative and primary health care work that many women performed. As Sue Fisher notes, 'the medical profession as a whole has a longstanding commitment to high-technology specialty care and a much poorer record with regard to primary and preventive care'.[43] In the same way, histories of medicine have tended to focus on the interventionist practices of medicine and rarely analysed primary and preventative care: even though contemporaries did see these as medical. Even today, the word medicine is defined by the *Oxford English Dictionary* to incorporate all these aspects of medical work as 'that department of knowledge and practice which is concerned with the cure, alleviation, and prevention of disease in human beings, and with the restoration and preservation of health'.[44] Women's medical work performed both in the treatment of sickness and in maintaining health will be examined here. The medical care contributed by women will include such domains as child health, primary emergency treatment, palliative care, culinary therapy, and hospital nursing to name a few.

The following study is structured in such a way as to demonstrate how different contexts and communities responded to women's medical work in varied and sometimes contrasting ways. My first two chapters are situated in the world of the two major institutions examined by most previous studies of French medicine: the university medical faculties and the medical guilds. By using these privileged sites of medical work, I hope to show how it is both possible and instructive to analyse the interaction and work of female practitioners with these bodies. Neither group, inasmuch as they can be considered internally unified bodies, excluded the medical work of women solely on the grounds that they were women, but instead demonstrated much more ambivalent attitudes towards female practitioners. The first chapter, examining the late fifteenth-century guild medical community, explores how some female medical practices could be inhibited by guild incorporation, and others given legal, university and royal recognition. In the second chapter, the perceptions of the university medical faculties are explored by analysing the early sixteenth-century prosecutions of female practitioners. It seems that the faculty was concerned with eradicating the competition of only a small number of women, and left many more to practise unhindered.

The following two chapters explore religious understandings of female healing work as lay and religious women. Chapter 3 examines how religious women interacted in the management and daily activities in early sixteenth-century hospitals, in a period when their governing body changed from ecclesiastical to lay administrators. The fourth chapter focuses on the position of women's healing in the mid-sixteenth century under ecclesiastical and secular law, particularly in relation to contemporary understandings of charity, sanctity and witchcraft.

The fifth chapter continues the study of women's domestic and charitable medical labour, by exploring the impact of print in the context of women as readers and patrons of medical literature, with a focus on the publication of manuals contributing to the domestic care discourse. Chapter 6 completes the focus on regulatory frameworks for women's medical work, by examining the role of women in the municipally-organised systems of poor relief and child care for foundlings and orphans.

The last three chapters follow women's gynaecological and reproductive knowledge, particularly in the contexts of elite and royal court life. Chapter 7 analyses the changing relationship of women as medical service providers to the French royal family, in particular focusing on how women practised as child carers to the royal children. In the following chapter, an international context to women's reproductive knowledge is explored in relation to women's knowledge of menstruation and pregnancy, demonstrating how notions about authority in medicine could be flexible in the interplay of international politics between France and Spain. Creation and transmission of reproductive knowledge among elite women is the subject of the final chapter, which explores correspondence as a continuing key resource of health care knowledge for literate women into the early seventeenth century. The examples of each chapter demonstrate how adaptable the extent and nature of women's contribution to medical practice, and contemporary perceptions about it, could be. By placing the chapters in an approximate chronological order, I wish to be clear about the sequence of sixteenth-century events but not to suggest a wider historical narrative of change to the perceptions of women's medical participation in the sixteenth century. These studies will rather demonstrate just how important a variety of immediate and local contexts continued to be to women's (and men's) medical work.

I have not included a conclusion to this study, but rather a brief afterword. The book does not seek to conclude current debate about women's participation in medical practice but rather to provide points of departure for future studies. I hope it will demonstrate that medicine in sixteenth-century France was not perceived as an exclusively male activity by any means, by either men or women at the time, nor even by those who formed the university and guild medical communities. On the contrary, the masculinisation of medical history appears to be a modern phenomenon – one that recent studies are now beginning to address by incorporating women into medicine, just as their contemporaries did.

Notes

1 Monica H. Green, 'Documenting medieval women's medical practice', in Luis Garcia-Ballester, Roger French, Jon Arrizabalaga and Andrew Cunningham (eds), *Practical Medicine from Salerno to the Black Death* (Cambridge: Cambridge University Press, 1994), p. 351. See collected essays by Green in her *Women's Healthcare in the Medieval West* (Aldershot: Ashgate, 2000).

2 See Elizabeth L. Eisenstein, *The Printing Press as an Agent of Change: Communications and Cultural Transformations in Early Modern Europe* (Cambridge: Cambridge University Press, 1979); for the experiences of women specifically, see my *Women and the Book Trade in Sixteenth-Century France* (Aldershot: Ashgate, 2002).

3 For changes to university medicine, see A. Wear, R. K. French and I. M. Lonie (eds), *The Medical Renaissance of the Sixteenth Century* (Cambridge: Cambridge University Press, 1985).

4 Ole Peter Grell and Andrew Cunningham (eds), *Medicine and the Reformation* (London and New York: Routledge, 1993).

5 For two examples of this trend, see C. A. Ernest Wickersheimer, *La Médecine et les médecins en France à l'époque de la Renaissance* (Paris: A. Maloine, 1906); H. Brabant,

Médecins, malades et maladies de la Renaissance (Brussels: La Renaissance du livre, 1966).

6 See G. Jorland, *La Science dans la philosophie*. Les recherches épistemologiques d'Alexandre Koyré (Paris: Gallimard, 1981).

7 See D. Lecourt, *L'Epistémologie historique de G. Bachelard* (Paris: Vrin, 1969).

8 Steven Shapin and Simon Schaffer, *Leviathan and the Air-Pump: Hobbes, Boyle, and the Experimental Life* (Princeton: Princeton University Press, 1985), pp. 7 and 11.

9 Thomas S. Kuhn, *The Structure of Scientific Revolutions* (3rd edn) (Chicago: The University of Chicago Press, 1996), pp. 2–3.

10 Jacques Roger, *Pour une histoire des sciences à part entière* (Paris: Albin Michel, 1995), p. 54.

11 David Bloor, *Knowledge and Social Inquiry* (London: Routledge and Kegan Paul, 1976), p. 5.

12 From signatures of marriage registers between 1686 and 1690, it seems that 29 per cent of men and 14 per cent of women were able to sign their names. M. Fleury and P. Valmary, 'Les progrès de l'instruction élémentaire de Louis XIV à Napoléon III d'après l'enquête de Louis Maggiolo (1877–1879)', *Population*, 12 (1957), pp. 71–93, in R. Chartier (ed.), *A History of Private Life*, vol. 3: *Passions of the Renaissance*, trans. A. Goldhammer (Cambridge, Mass.: The Belknap Press of the Harvard University Press, 1989), p. 113.

13 François Lebrun, *Se soigner autrefois: Médecins, saints et sorciers aux XVIIe et XVIIIe siècles* (Paris: Temps Actuel, 1983).

14 Matthew Ramsey, *Professional and Popular Medicine in France, 1770–1830: The Social World of Medical Practice* (Cambridge: Cambridge University Press, 1988).

15 *Ibid.*, pp. 9–10.

16 *Ibid.*, pp. 11 and 129.

17 Laurence Brockliss and Colin Jones, *The Medical World of Early Modern France* (Oxford: Clarendon Press, 1997), p. 8.

18 *Ibid.*, p. 14.

19 *Ibid.*, p. 19.

20 *Ibid.*, p. 3.

21 Margaret Pelling and Charles Webster, 'Medical practitioners', in C. Webster (ed.), *Health, Medicine and Mortality in the Sixteenth Century* (Cambridge: Cambridge University Press, 1979), p. 166.

22 Pomata's works include her recent English translation *Contracting a Cure: Patients, Healers and the Law in Early Modern Bologna* (Baltimore: The Johns Hopkins University Press, 1998).

23 David Gentilcore, *From Bishop to Witch: The System of the Sacred in Early Modern Terra d'Otranto* (Manchester: Manchester University Press, 1992); *Healers and Healing in Early Modern Italy* (Manchester: Manchester University Press, 1998).

24 Melinda Lipinska, *Des femmes médecins depuis l'antiquité jusqu'à nos jours* (Paris: G. Jacques, 1900); *Les Femmes et le progrès des sciences médicales* (Paris: Masson, 1930); Kate Campbell Hurd-Mead, *A History of Women in Medicine from the Earliest Times to the Beginning of the Nineteenth Century* (Haddam: The Haddam Press, 1938); Muriel Joy Hughes, *Women Healers in Medieval Life and Literature* [1943] (Freeport: Books for Libraries Press, 1968); Lilian R. Furst (ed.), *Women Healers*

and Physicians: Climbing a Long Hill (Lexington: The University Press of Kentucky, 1997).
25 Green, 'Documenting medieval women's medical practice', p. 352. See also her 'Women's medical practice and health care in medieval Europe', in Judith M. Bennett *et al.* (eds), *Sisters and Workers in the Middle Ages* (Chicago: The University of Chicago Press, 1989), pp. 39–78, and *Women's Healthcare in the Medieval West*.
26 Two recent monographs include Hilary Marland (ed.), *The Art of Midwifery: Early Modern Midwives in Europe* (London: Routledge, 1993); Doreen Evenden, *The Midwives of Seventeenth-Century London* (Cambridge: Cambridge University Press, 2000). Specific literature on the French midwife Louise Bourgeois will be discussed in later chapters.
27 Carol Rawcliffe, *Medicine and Society in Later Medieval England* (Stroud: Sutton, 1997); 'Hospital nurses and their work', in R. Britnell (ed.), *Daily Life in the Late Middle Ages* (Stroud: Sutton, 1998), pp. 43–64; Colin Jones, *The Charitable Imperative: Hospitals and Nursing in Ancien Regime and Revolutionary France* (London: Routledge, 1989); Marie-Claude Dinet-Lecomte, 'Les Sœurs hospitalières au service des pauvres malades aux XVIIe et XVIIIe siècles', *Annales de démographie historique* (1994), pp. 277–92.
28 Some examples include Marie-Françoise Collière, *Promouvoir la vie* (Paris: Inter-Editions, 1982); John Carmi Parsons and Bonnie Wheeler (eds), *Medieval Mothering* (New York: Garland Publishing, 1996); Naomi J. Miller and Naomi Yavneh (eds), *Maternal Measures: Figuring Caregiving in the Early Modern Period* (Aldershot: Ashgate, 2000).
29 Brockliss and Jones, for example, are somewhat dismissive of histories of medicine which expound the 'idea that so-called medical charlatans were in fact indigenous healers whose wholly beneficial influence was cut short by the progress of the nefarious medical professions. This line of argument has been posed most starkly by feminist scholars who have highlighted the gendered nature of the elite attack on charlatans.' Brockliss and Jones, *The Medical World of Early Modern France*, p. 15.
30 Ludmilla Jordanova, 'The social construction of medical knowledge', *Social History of Medicine*, 8:3 (1995), pp. 361–81. My approach is also informed by anthropological studies of medicine, particularly in relation to selection, evaluation and validation of medical services, including Charles John Erasmus, 'Changing folk beliefs and the relativity of empirical knowledge', *Southwestern Journal of Anthropology*, 8 (1952), pp. 411–28; Carolyn Fishel Sargent, *The Cultural Context of Therapeutic Choice: Obstetrical Care Decisions Among the Bariba of Benin* (Dordrecht: D. Reidel, 1982); Byron J. Good, *Medicine, Rationality, and Experience: An Anthropological Perspective* (Cambridge: Cambridge University Press, 1994).
31 See Joan Scott, 'Gender: a useful category of historical analysis', *American Historical Review*, 91 (1986), pp. 1053–75. Joan Cadden's work provides one example of how gender analysis can be fruitful to histories of medicine: *The Meanings of Sex Difference in the Middle Ages: Medicine, Science, and Culture* (Cambridge: Cambridge University Press, 1993).
32 For comparative studies, B. A. Hanawalt (ed.) *Women and Work in Preindustrial Europe* (Bloomington: Indiana University Press, 1986); Merry Wiesner-Hanks, *Working Women in Renaissance Germany* (New Brunswick: Rutgers University Press, 1986);

Judith M. Bennett, '"History that stands still": women's work in the European past', *Feminist Studies*, 14:2 (1988), pp. 269–83; and anthropological studies, Hilary Graham, 'Providers, negotiators, and mediators: women as the hidden carers', in Ellen Lewin and Virginia Olsen (eds), *Women, Health and Healing: Toward a New Perspective*, (New York: Tavistock, 1985), pp. 25–52; Hilary Rose, 'Women's work: women's knowledge', in Juliet Mitchell and Ann Oakley (eds), *What is Feminism?* (Oxford: Basil Blackwell, 1986), pp. 161–83; Agnes Miles, *Women, Health and Medicine* (Milton Keynes: Open University Press, 1991); Margaret A. Perkinson, 'Socialization to the family caregiving role within a continuing care retirement community', *Medical Anthropology*, 16 (1995), pp. 249–67; Rosemary Pringle, *Sex and Medicine: Gender, Power and Authority in the Medical Profession* (Cambridge: Cambridge University Press, 1998).

33 Emphasis in the original. Toril Moi, *What is a Woman? And Other Essays* (Oxford: Oxford University Press, 1999), p. 288. I would like to thank Lianne McTavish for drawing my attention to Moi's work on Bourdieu and encouraging me to understand my work in this way.

34 *Ibid.*, p. 289.

35 *Ibid.*, p. 291.

36 See Moira Gatens, 'Towards a feminist philosophy of the body', in B. Caine, E. Grosz and M. de Lepervanche (eds), *Crossing Boundaries: Feminism and the Critique of Knowledge* (Sydney: Allen and Unwin, 1988), pp. 59–70; Elizabeth Grosz, *Volatile Bodies: Toward a Corporeal Feminism* (Sydney: Allen and Unwin, 1994).

37 Barbara Duden, *The Woman Beneath the Skin: A Doctor's Patients in Eighteenth-Century Germany*, trans. Thomas Dunlap (Cambridge, Mass.: Harvard University Press, 1991).

38 M. Foucault, *The Archaeology of Knowledge*, trans. A. M. Sheridan (New York: Harper, 1972); Colin Jones and Roy Porter (eds), *Reassessing Foucault: Power, Medicine and the Body* (London: Routledge, 1994); Don Bates (ed.) *Knowledge and the Scholarly Medical Traditions* (Cambridge: Cambridge University Press, 1995).

39 Londa Schiebinger, *The Mind Has No Sex? Women and the Origins of Modern Science* (Cambridge: Harvard University Press, 1989); *Nature's Body: Gender in the Making of Modern Science* (Boston: Beacon Press, 1993); *Has Feminism Changed Science?* (Cambridge, Mass.: Harvard University Press, 1999); Sandra Harding, *Whose Science? Whose Knowledge? Thinking From Women's Lives* (Milton Keynes: Open University Press, 1991); *Is Science Multicultural? Postcolonialisms, Feminisms, and Epistemologies* (Bloomington: Indiana University Press, 1998); Lorraine Code, *What Can She Know? Feminist Theory and the Construction of Knowledge* (Ithaca: Cornell University Press, 1991); *Rhetorical Spaces: Essays on Gendered Locations* (New York: Routledge, 1995).

40 Ludmilla Jordanova, *Sexual Visions: Images of Gender in Science and Medicine between the Eighteenth and the Twentieth Centuries* (London: Harvester Wheatsheaf, 1989); 'Gender and the historiography of science', *British Journal for the History of Science*, 26 (1993), pp. 469–83; 'The social construction of medical knowledge', pp. 361–81.

41 Lisa W. Smith's work, on the importance of family relationships to women's medical decisions in eighteenth-century England, is one example of how the medical

marketplace model of complete patient choice in selecting a practitioner is in need of review. 'Reassessing the role of the family: women's health care in eighteenth-century England', *Social History of Medicine*, forthcoming.

42 Green, 'Documenting medieval women's medical practice', pp. 341–2.
43 Sue Fisher, *Nursing Wounds: Nurse Practitioners, Doctors, Women Patients and the Negotiation of Meaning* (New Brunswick: Rutgers University Press, 1995), p. 224.
44 *Oxford English Dictionary* (2nd edn), vol. 9 (Oxford: Clarendon Press, 1989), p. 549.

1

Women and the medical guilds

IN THE SIXTEENTH CENTURY, guild organisations ordered practice and knowledge in a number of medical fields. Some health-care workers – such as barbers, surgeons and apothecaries – had corporate structures to regulate their medical knowledge and practice established in the middle ages. Other workers such as midwives only began to form a licensed representative body during the sixteenth century. How did women work in medical fields that were regulated by the medical guilds? What opportunities did they have to work as participants in the medical guild structures, and to understand guild medical knowledge?

Understanding the participation of women in medical guilds necessitates an examination of the medieval medical world in which many of these corporations were formed, and from which those instituted in the sixteenth century developed. In this chapter, we will first focus on women's interaction with the guild organisation of the barbers, surgeons and apothecaries in the medieval and early modern eras, and then examine how these structures influenced the creation of a new licensed group in the sixteenth century and women's participation within it.

Isabelle Estevent and the barbers' guild in Reims

The unusual case and circumstances of one particular female barber in conflict with the barbers' guild in Reims provide an opportunity to examine the perceptions held by barbers of their own medical knowledge and practices. Understanding their interpretations of medical expertise helps us to explore contemporary notions of the authority to practise the medical arts, and how female practice was understood within that.

In 1462 in Reims, the 70-year-old master barber Jehan Estevent, declared his intention to retire from his profession in order to become a hermit. His wife, Isabelle, 52,[1] 'has been divorced and separated from the said Jehan Estevent by the authority of justice and the church because this Estevent wished to enter into religion in the profession of a hermit'.[2] In September of the same year, Estevent prepared a notarial act in which, 'in consideration of the great love and natural affection which he had and has towards Isabelle his wife' he gave over to her in the form of a gift his profession.[3] Estevent gave henceforth:

> to the said Isabelle his wife for the rest of her life all the trade, tools and workshop of barbering, and all such rights and powers that the said donor has and could have in the said town of Reims because of the trade and workshop of barbering. He places and transmits them to the said Isabelle his wife to enjoy and possess.[4]

Had Estevent died, Isabelle could have assumed his profession as the widow of a master barber. However, Estevent's circumstances were somewhat unusual. Isabelle would be left as though widowed, but her husband was still alive, and furthermore he was leaving the profession of his own free will. Through the notarial act, Estevent hoped to put his ex-wife in the position of a widow in the eyes of the barbers' corporation in Reims.

However, by February of 1463, Jehan Biguet and Pierre Gravelle, master barbers of Reims, took action against Isabelle Estevent on the grounds that she was practising surgery without approval: 'those who wish to be involved in the trade of a barber must be approved and she has not been'.[5] The barbers did not specifically refer to Isabelle's sex as the bar to her authority to exercise surgery, though presumably the reason for their claim was that she did not fit the usual reasons for which a woman could exercise the occupation: she was not the widow of a barber but his ex-wife. Isabelle was stripped 'of several of her goods, furniture and tools of the said trade, to which she was opposed' and the two parties brought forth a case before the bailiff and magistrates of Reims.[6]

Isabelle appealed to the *Parlement* of Paris against the guild's ban on her practice, but her appeal was dismissed. The trade of barbery was forbidden to her and her tools confiscated, and the appeal dismissal reported: 'the said supplicant by fault or inadvertency is on the wrong track in her opinion'.[7] As a result, Isabelle decided to bypass the court procedure and appeal directly to the King, Louis XI. The king had the power to intercede through the legal mechanism of *justice personnelle*. This enabled him to issue *lettres de grâce*, *d'évocation* or *cassation*, where he granted privilege from a certain law, altered a judgement rendered, or reversed a decision of a supreme court. By this mechanism, the king could override a particular ruling on the grounds of compassion, though it was usually clearly indicated as an exception to the law.[8] In August 1464, Isabelle received her answer. Louis XI found her particular circumstances such that he resolved the matter in her favour by special grace, though significantly he noted that it was an exceptional case and recognised the normal validity of the barbers' claims.[9] Louis XI affirmed that typically the occupation could not be passed on through such means, as a gift from husband to wife, nor the guild's authority circumvented. Louis's 'extraordinary' grace to Isabelle clarified the typical situation for other women.

However, the barbers persisted in their refusal to accept Isabelle Estevent into the guild, doubting her claims made in the appeal to the king. In October 1464 they again went to the courts. This time, the barbers claimed that Isabelle had lied about her circumstances in order to obtain the king's grace.[10] In June 1465, over two full years since the original protests against her, Isabelle provided all of the documentary evidence before the court for all to see. This included the letter of grace, her divorce from Jehan Estevent, and also the notarial act of his gift of the profession to her: 'in response she said that the royal letters obtained by her are good and valid . . . [as is also] the divorce by letters made under the seal of the court of Reims, said also that her husband gave to her his right and tools of barbery as he was able to do.'[11] She persisted in her conviction about her rights to practise and declared of the barbers' latest case against her, 'and by all this [evidence that she produced in her favour], the said case is null and void'.[12] To appreciate fully the arguments for and against women's participation made by Estevent and the barbers of Reims, we need to understand the relation of barbers' work to that of other medical practitioners, as well as the functions of medical guilds both in regional centres such as Reims and in the capital Paris, which was the seat of the one of the most powerful university faculties of medicine.

Barbers in the medical world

A barber was responsible for the majority of practical aspects of treatment that a physician might prescribe to the patient. Those of more modest social classes probably bypassed the prescription of the physician altogether and went directly to the barber for both diagnosis and then treatment. Barbers performed phlebotomy and minor surgery, as well as cutting hair and beards.[13] To cite the 1473 regulations of the barbers in Reims, a qualified barber was required to know how to:

comb, trim and tidy a beard, which is a thing sometimes necessary to both healthy and sick people, to make blades used for bleeding, and to have knowledge of all the veins which are in the human body, and the causes for which one should bleed them, and with this the knowledge to know if one bleeds an artery instead of a vein, the bleeding of an artery is most perilous to the human body, to know also the convenient times for bleeding, and which veins should be bled by the advice of the physician, and which not, and which people are able to be bled, and which not.[14]

At the end of their apprenticeship, barbers could hang the sign of the three basins, the symbol of the guild, above their workshops. Since 1366, barbers in Paris had been dispensed from the night watch, 'those who are concerned with the facts of surgery, are sent for in the night at great need, for lack of *mires* and surgeons of the said town, and if they cannot be found in their houses, several great perils and inconveniences could ensue.'[15] Such *lettres patentes* encouraged a very positive public perception of the medical work performed by barbers.

Women did work as barbers in the medieval past. Women who reported their occupation as barbers can be found in the tax rolls of late thirteenth-century and early fourteenth-century Paris.[16] Regulations of barbers' guilds made provisions in their wording for the possibility of both male and female members. In Rouen, the 1407 regulations of the barbers talked of '*aucun* or *aucune* of the said trade of barbery'.[17] The 1465 statutes of the Parisian barbers described both 'masters and mistresses of the said trade'.[18]

However, it would be unrealistic to assume from such evidence that women participated as full and equal members of the barbers' guilds. Monica H. Green has drawn attention to the fact that already, in the early fourteenth century, the percentage of women described as barbers in the 1313 tax rolls was lower than that of the 1297 rolls, and both numbers were smaller than that of the 1292 rolls. Although Green notes that each *taille* targeted slightly different members of the Parisian community, she notes too that over the same period the number of women working in medicine outside the guild structure, as *miresses*, remained relatively steady.[19] Other sources appear to support the idea that the guilds began to decrease the possibilities for female participation. In many guild-regulated professions, women's opportunities to participate had become increasingly limited towards the end of the medieval period. Cécile Béghin's study of women's work in medieval Languedoc has indicated that female apprenticeships generally were rare by 1360 and had practically disappeared from the sources in the fifteenth century.[20]

Increasingly, women's participation was restricted to widowhood and was highly conditional. According to the statutes of many barbers' guilds at the end of the fifteenth century, the widow could only continue a business while she remained a widow. Then, in 1484, the right of women to practise surgery in their own right was dissolved by Charles VIII, although widows were allowed to continue the workshop of their husband.[21]

What pushed certain medical guilds to exclude women progressively from their work during the later middle ages and into the sixteenth century? One reason lies in the relationship of these guilds to the university faculties of medicine, and how the latter group perceived corporative practitioners. Within the medical community, there were deep divisions and hierarchy. Physicians distinguished themselves from apothecaries, barbers and other healers as the elite medical corps by their induction into the university education system. In practical terms, they prevented 'unqualified' non-physicians from attending their classes and from sharing in their learned medical knowledge by transmitting it in Latin and, until the advent of print, through manuscript circulation. They perpetuated beliefs in the superiority of their practices and textual epistemology through such texts. Sixteenth-century physicians bore witness to the pride of their profession in their written works. The royal physician Jean Fernel claimed that, since medicine was studied after first taking a broad arts degree, and 'as medicine discusses and explains the admirable structure or fabrication and nature of man, as she researches and recognises the birth and the decay of all things, the properties and virtues of animals and plants . . . it is suitable to name it the universal art'.[22] Like many others, Laurent Joubert, Chancellor of the medical faculty in Montpellier, was similarly convinced of the eminence of his profession. He dedicated the first chapter of his *Erreurs populaires* to reinforcing the public's impression of the 'excellence of the art of medicine above all the human arts.'[23]

Physicians also created a hierarchy of medical practices differentiating between those to be seen as 'higher' and 'lower', privileging theoretical over manual activities. Those activities considered by physicians to be superior were those they undertook themselves, including diagnosis of illness, which (in their view) required an understanding of, and familiarity with, learned medical literature. By contrast, physicians disdained to intervene manually in the treatment of the patient (unless the patient was of the highest social classes) by actually carrying out bleedings, clysters, and operations themselves. On the whole, the early modern physician was, Emile Forgue has argued, disdainful of all manual actions.[24] Among the medical practices relegated by the faculty to the bottom of the scale by this logic were those of barbers. In his description of a dissection at the Montpellier medical faculty, the medical student Thomas Platter recalled the hierarchy of medical and corporeal practice within the university. While the presiding doctor gave the lecture, it was a surgeon who actually held the blade and dissected the body.[25]

Despite the views of physicians, barbers enjoyed an important role in the eyes of the general public, and were perhaps more visible medical workers than the more elusive university-trained physicians. Most frequently, administrators of the poor relief such as that in Tours employed barber-surgeons and bonesetters, rather than the more expensive physicians, to treat the complaints of patients. In 1581, they covered the costs of Bertherand Boutroye, a poor beggar with a wife and three children, to be 'medicated by the surgeon of the poor in this town of a cold and a flux of humours which had struck him in one of his arms'.[26] Barbers also established control over practitioners whose skills bordered on their domains of medical expertise, such as those who performed fistula, cataract, hernia and stone removal. In Amiens, lithotomists, 'master incisors of the stone or hernia', who did not number sufficiently to form their own guild, were required to pay the barbers' guild a fee of 5 sol tournois 'for each incision'.[27] However, in so far as it was the faculties of medicine and physicians who held power and authority in the greater medical community (power and authority accorded them by the king and legal system), the guilds strove to imitate them and to gain their esteem.

Within the hierarchy of medical practices and epistemology created and sustained with royal support by the medical faculties, barbers had little esteem or medical authority. In Paris, where the powerful and influential presence of the medical faculty was more evident than in the countryside, barbers felt keenly their lower status allotted by the faculty and accredited by the king. As early as 1268, a breakaway group of barbers there sought to re-define their corporative identity, creating a confraternity under the auspices of St Damien and St Cosme. From now on, in Paris at least, a distinction was to be made between barber–artisans and the new barber–surgeons. By the fourteenth century, this latter group, the (barber–)surgeons, began to copy more closely the faculty, stipulating that confraternity members know Latin and wear the bonnet and long robe of physicians.[28] They now refused to bleed and shave patients, leaving these manual tasks to the barber(–artisans),[29] but more often the division was created by the social status of their clients. While surgeons were employed by private patrons (whom they condescended to bleed) barbers treated a broader public. Bypassing the faculty of medicine, surgeons sought to gain the recognition of the king for their medical work. For example, in 1360, the regent Charles bestowed letters on the corporation of surgeons, recognising its continued status as a separate entity from the medical faculty.[30]

Surgeons of the long robe (a distinguishing term for the surgeons of the St Damien and St Cosme confraternity: since now barber–artisans not wanting to be demoted in prestige in relation to this new group preferred to call themselves surgeons as well) used the crown to protect their medical skills and training procedures from those 'below' who might claim similar expertise. In 1470, Louis XI, like monarchs before him, passed letters preventing any from performing the 'art of surgery' if they had not been licensed. Surgery was no longer presented as a manual skill but a learned art and science.[31] In passing regulations for surgeons in Rouen in 1452, Charles VII spoke of the 'praiseworthy science of surgery'.[32] The regulations made by the lieutenant of the bailiff in Rouen in 1502 also distinguished between the work of 'sworn masters of the science and art of surgery, and custodians of barbery and phlebotomy'.[33]

By the sixteenth century, the more surgeons attempted to augment their prestige, the more the faculty in Paris supported the position of the modest barbers. The latter accepted and recognised the authority of the faculty and physicians. Surgeons did not recognise the superiority of physicians: they claimed equal training and quality. In 1493, the faculty permitted barbers to attend courses in Latin and to have a skeleton for anatomy lessons. By the end of the fifteenth century, the faculty charged one of its doctors to regulate the knowledge of barbers by offering to explain anatomical texts 'in the familiar French language'.[34] In 1505, the faculty opened its doors to barbers as students of the university and offered them protection as students under the university's special legal status. In exchange, the barbers accepted to undertake only simple surgical acts and to submit to examination by two physicians to become master barbers. Unlike the surgeons, the student barbers also consented to pay fees to the faculty.[35]

While the university continued to promote the status of barbers over surgeons within the boundaries of its authority, surgeons continued to seek recognition from the crown. In 1544, François I accorded professors, students and masters in surgery the same privileges as students, regents and graduates of the university.[36] In 1577, Henri III recognised that the master surgeons and professors of the 'art and science of surgery' in Paris were authorised to continue their instruction and work in Paris and elsewhere, and forbade the university to cause trouble or prevent them from doing so.[37] In riposte to this move, only two months later, the barbers renewed their contract with the faculty, recognising physicians as their superiors and masters, and promising to treat them with honour and reverence.[38] Thus throughout the fifteenth and sixteenth centuries, the rivalry for medical superiority between the physicians, surgeons and barbers continued unabated, with the crown as arbiter between the rights of the university, as the foremost medical training organisation, and those of other providers.

In Montpellier, the other great university town in France, the situation was somewhat less complicated but echoed the same ongoing struggles for medical recognition between guild and university. The surgeons' guild remained entirely independent of the medical faculty until 1496, when the crown reinforced the power of the university over the guild corporations by insisting that university staff witness the examination procedures of journeyman surgeons. In return, the crown ordered in 1514 that the faculty was to offer special courses for surgeons to be taught in French.[39] In contrast to the complex local politics in Paris, elsewhere, as the crown increasingly bestowed superiority on the university medical system, it expected that the university would open up its learning to other medical groups in return. Surgeons thus gained increasing access to university training.[40]

As barbers sought to align themselves ever more closely with the university faculties, another means by which to assimilate their guilds to the university medical system was to reduce the participation of female barbers. Firstly, women were not permitted to attend university classes generally, could not be students of the university, nor practise the medical work of physicians. So to exclude women as members from the barbers' guild would make the study of barbers' medical practices more similar to the male-only knowledge disseminated by the universities. Moreover, since female work in all its forms was poorly remunerated and less prestigious in the wider community, precisely because it was the work of women,[41] by removing women from their numbers barbers could raise their esteem and approach the status of physicians.

Finally, women could not have the same commitment to medical work as a career as could male guild members. As Natalie Zemon Davis has argued, women's working lives were less stable than men's.[42] Many married more than once, and they were likely to assist in the occupation of their husband. Thus flexibility to different working environments was more important than was commitment to a single craft or set of skills. Their activities were frequently interrupted by pregnancies, the care of children and household work. From the perspective of the guild, female barbers could not have the same lifelong commitment to the craft and the corporation as did men, in a culture which valued a life consecrated to medical study and practice, and glorified it as a noble male goal.

Women as wives and widows of barbers

If women's opportunities to practise as full members of barbers' guilds decreased over the middle ages and were forbidden after 1484 as a result of the battle for status in the medical marketplace, what do we make then of this unusual case in which a master barber, and member of the guild structure, perceived of his professional knowledge and the authority to which it accredited him as tangible entities that he could give to his wife? It is not impossible, of course, that Isabelle had learnt the skills and knowledge by observing her husband at work, and possibly by his instruction to her. However, at no point was such a claim made, either by Jehan Estevent in giving his profession to her, or by Isabelle in defending her right to practise before the guild. Indeed, the guild itself apparently made no comment on Isabelle's competency to practise surgery. If no one evaluated her skills and manual dexterity necessary to conduct surgical manoeuvres, if the guild of barbers in Reims never examined her knowledge or practices, it was in part because their own system seemed to permit some women to perform surgical work as widows.

How then did contemporaries such as the barbers' guild understand surgical competence? For men, surgical epistemology derived from apprenticeship with a master barber and the transmission of his practical experience. However, for women, it was sufficient to be the wife of a barber to gain access to exercise the profession. Their capacity to perform surgical work seemed to be taken as implicit. The guild's own statutes allowed for the possibility that widows would step into the breach left by their husband, to continue to use his tools and maintain his clientele and to pass them on to their children as an inheritance. Cécile Béghin has called this practice a measure of charity and implicit recognition of the competence of widows. It was a likely reality that wives observed their husbands at work in the boutique and indirectly had transmitted to them the same practical experience. As she argued, the 1255 statutes of the barbers' guild in Montpellier specified that all the members of the barber's *familia*: that is, his wife, sons, daughters, apprentices and servants 'having power to clip and shave' had to submit to the same rules as the barber himself, although they did not enjoy the same benefits and privileges as did the barber himself within the guild system.[43] Although the guild could not limit the spread of the arts of surgery, it could attempt to monopolise its practice and to identify authoritative practitioners.

The statutes of the barbers' guilds thus created familial dynasties which managed a heritage of surgical knowledge. Women were important in the creation and transmission of skills within these dynasties. In 1452, Dame Léonard Pachaude, the widow of a barber in Avignon, willed the entire workshop of her late husband, including basins, pots, mirrors, sharpening stones, phials, braziers, chests, chairs, razors, scissors, and books of surgery, to one Pierre Theurot, a barber in Châlons-sur-Saone, who lived in Avignon and had cared for her while she was sick.[44] The official regulations of the Parisian barbers in 1438 stipulated that 'that no barber or barberess, of whatever condition they be, can or should suffer to allow a woman or girl to work at the said trade, nor have either in the workshop, unless she be the wife or daughter of a master of the trade.'[45] This control of the very sight that women might have of the work of barbers had two implications. On the one hand, it showed that wives and daughters of masters already knew what went on in the workshop of the barber, and that they were allowed to observe (and perhaps practise) the work. It further implied that it was more likely that barbers would marry daughters of master barbers, in a practice Judith Brown has termed 'occupational endogamy'.[46] They had many more opportunities to meet each other in the places where they passed most of their time. In doing so, the guild encouraged the development of family traditions of surgical knowledge.

The evidence of guild regulations seems to suggest that women as wives and widows could practise surgery in some measure through a kind of unofficial apprenticeship to their husbands and fathers. Alison Klairmont Lingo cites a 1551 case with many parallels to that of Isabelle Estevent, where a woman in Lyon went to court to demand her right to practise her husband's profession as a surgeon after his death, as an expression of her property rights. The court having upheld her rights, she paid 9 livres tournois for the licence to practise as a surgeon.[47] Klairmont Lingo argues that such women had a 'shared work identity' with their husbands. In another case in Lyon, when they were forbidden from practising barbery and surgery by the guild, a husband and wife appealed to the king in 1537, thereby circumventing the authority of the local guilds.[48] As Estevent's and these cases demonstrate, women were prepared to go to court to defend their rights to practise. Moreover, their actions in pursuing a ruling through legal bodies beyond the jurisdiction of the guild mirror Estevent's conduct in bypassing local guild authority to appeal to the king.

But were most women really practising, and were they even defending their rights to do so? Some regulations were more explicit about what guilds envisaged in permitting widows to practise surgery. In Avignon, the town statutes of 1558 allowed the widow of a surgeon, 'as long as she remained under his name, to keep open his boutique having it run by an able and approved servant'.[49] Apart from continuing a source of income for families, guilds may have authorised this practice particularly because boutiques and their clientele could be maintained until a master's son could take over the business. This explains too the mention of her keeping the master's name: it could act as an important 'trademark' of medical quality. Perhaps the favourability of courts and crown to the pleas of widows in such cases such as the 1551 case in Lyon and Isabelle Estevent's rested more on the recognition that businesses should be protected for sons, rather than recognition or approval of women's surgical practice.

Wives and widows could be indeed recognised by the wider community as having the skills to conduct medical work. When Benoist du Cluzel, the barber at the Hôtel-Dieu in Lyon, died in 1538, he (and the Hôtel-Dieu) left his daughter to continue his work for a short time, before a new barber was employed.[50] Françoise Page, the wife then widow of a master surgeon, was paid by the same Hôtel-Dieu to perform medical work for twenty years, most commonly treating the pox and herpes.[51] But was this because she was the wife of a surgeon? Treating the pox was not necessarily surgical work, and elsewhere too women were paid to nurse its victims, without necessarily having connections to surgeons or barbers as husbands.[52] It seems more likely that Page was recognised as a medical practitioner, but not specifically as a surgical practitioner. The Hôtel-Dieu in Lyon certainly recognised the valuable contribution of female medical labour. When one of its nursing staff, Laurence Demey, requested permission to leave the hospital in order to marry the barber–surgeon Pierre Chevellu, the hospital gave a form of dowry to Demey: it was Chevellu who replaced Françoise Page in 1599 as the hospital's new practitioner in cases of pox, for which he received about 50 écus a year depending on the number of cases he treated. Yet when Chevellu died and Demey asked to take over his trade and revenue, the hospital refused, employing another surgeon to continue the work.[53] It is clear that some women did perform surgical work, and may have continued the work of their husbands or fathers, even without sons to take over the business, often because they were employed by external bodies such as the hospitals who disregarded the guilds' regulations. But even here, the hospital progressively fell into line with the guild's position and employed guild-recognised practitioners.

Returning to the case of Estevent and the barbers of Reims, to understand their position, we can examine the regulations which the barber-surgeons composed in 1473, some ten years after Estevent's case, through which their concerns become more clear. At this date Pierre Gravelle and Jehan Biguet were still the elected representatives of the corporation, so the policies pursued by them in the case against Estevent are likely to mirror those found in the regulations confirmed under their leadership. Their regulations state that all those who wished to open a barber's shop in Reims must be examined and approved by the corporation. Any barber who opened a shop without going through this process would be fined 100 sol tournois and his instruments confiscated. This point also made clear that any debate on the matter would be resolved by them or their lieutenant 'in full, without the possibility of a long trial'.[54] It seems likely that this inclusion elucidating the jurisdiction of the guild in this matter was added to prevent a repeat of incidences like Isabelle Estevent's appeal to the king.

Moreover, the guild clarified its position on business transfers: 'no master worker of the said trade can give his workshop to some worker or servant of the trade, whoever he may be, if the said master worker does not hold or occupy it personally, and is its head, or if it is not by necessity and debt of illness or old age, which is known and demonstrated to the masters of the trade'.[55] Finally, the regulations clarified the guild's position on widows' surgical work: they could keep workshops open, as long as they remained widows, 'provided they have in their workshops expert valets, who the masters of the trade will supervise'.[56]

Such evidence suggests that as long as the guild's regulations were respected, women were not barred from continuing businesses, though it seems unlikely barbers in Reims envisaged women actually carrying out surgical procedures themselves. Their concerns with Isabelle Estevent may have been twofold. Perhaps she was indeed working as a barber: though her surgical knowledge and expertise were never discussed by the guild. What seems more of a concern to the guild was what it perceived as the Estevents' usurpation of its power to regulate and control the profession and authoritative practitioners, through the notarial act of the gift. Had Jehan Estevent died, the guild would have no doubt permitted his widow's continuation of his business. Guilds recognised that women's involvement could indeed be beneficial to the smooth transmission of medical skills from one generation to the next. However, the practice of surgery was conditioned by submission to the power of the corporation and by the respect of their regulations, which the Estevents had tried to circumvent.[57]

As a conclusion to the story of Isabelle Estevent, the 1473 regulations of the Reims barbers include the names of no women among its 18 members. Yet in this list of the master barbers are included 'Jehan Estevent the elder' as well as one 'Jehan Estevent the younger'.[58] This suggests that part of the Estevent family's actions were indeed to protect the rights of a son not yet of age to take over the business in 1462. The elder Jehan Estevent may have intended Isabelle's participation in the guild to have been a stopgap to maintain a business and clientele until their son could practise as a master in his own right.[59]

Women and apothecaries' guilds

Were the conditions on women's surgical practice particular to the barbers' work or a feature of guild-regulated medical practices such as pharmacy more generally? An apothecary prepared the script composed by a physician, which required a knowledge of powders, plants and other pharmaceutical drugs. Apothecaries enjoyed public esteem for their medical services as did barbers and surgeons. The *lettres patentes* of François II stipulated that, like members of the Faculty of Medicine, apothecaries were exempt from the Paris watch for they 'are subject day and night and at all hours, to public service'.[60] However, although apothecaries did not suffer from quite the same stigma of manual labour as did barbers, they too had insecurities about the status of their medical work for other reasons.

The most pressing problem for apothecaries was to clarify their status as medical, rather than mercantile, professionals, and to distinguish themselves from the grocers and spicers with whom they were often grouped in the same guild. The *lettres patentes* of Charles VIII drawn up in 1484 had grouped together the Parisian trades concerned with 'works and merchandise of spicery, apothecary, works of wax and confections of sugar'.[61] In Rouen, at the beginning of the sixteenth century, the apothecaries were also part of the same corporation as the chandlers, confectioners and spicers, whose 1502 regulations were drawn up by three physicians and three members of the corporation.[62] In Abbeville, the apothecaries were joined to the haberdashers, chandlers and spicers.[63] The Parisian apothecaries sought recognition of their particular expertise and accused the grocers of usurping their medical arts through the amalgamation. Because 'several questions and debates have since arisen between the members of one estate and the other', the new statutes of 1514 attempted to clarify the situation: 'simple spicers ... are of a distinct and separate state and merchandise from apothecary spicers, because those who are spicers are not apothecaries, but those who are apothecaries are spicers'.[64] In 1560, in the *lettres patentes* of François II, the apothecaries attempted to exclude practitioners unlicensed by the guild masters, and this restriction applied equally to other professions:

> there are some merchants among others, barbers and surgeons and others, usurping the said state of apothecary and spicer, under the colour and word of merchant, interpreting it as they desire, who sell drugs, spices, merchandise entering the human body ... as if the town of Paris were a village and not guild regulated.[65]

This last phrase suggests that contemporaries were aware of the existence of practitioners in the country and their relative liberty. Indeed even distillers who produced eaux-de-vie claimed to accomplish a medical task. Their statutes authorised the possession of furnaces to master distillers 'who have need of them for several operations of medicine, as is permitted according to the ordonnances of the Court, to have permission to conduct the said operations.'[66]

Like barbers, apothecaries also had an ambiguous relationship with the university from which they sought recognition without wanting to position themselves as inferior in the medical hierarchy. Throughout the sixteenth century, the *Parlement* and provost of Paris favoured the rights of physicians to inspect apothecaries' workshops and to examine the quality of their pharmaceutical merchandise.[67] As early as 1496, apothecaries in Montpellier had been forced to accept a yearly inspection from the faculty's physicians, as the crown argued it was in the public interest.[68] In return, the university slowly accepted a counterpart obligation to provide medical instruction. After 1550, the university permitted apothecaries to take some classes with medical students.[69] The College of Apothecaries founded in Montpellier in 1572 separated spicers from apothecaries, and brought the latter, now required to know Latin, into an ordered corporation under the supervision of the university.[70] Like barbers, apothecaries signed similar contracts which acknowledged the superior authority of the physicians whose presence was required for examinations and inspection of apothecaries' shops. After a six-year apprenticeship, the Parisian candidate of 1610 'will be firstly interrogated, and examined by the said master apothecaries in the presence of a doctor of medicine who will be delegated by the dean of the said faculty'.[71] Each corporation struggled to balance recognition and position with the medical faculties.

Despite the similarities between apothecaries' and barbers' concerns for status, their guilds developed different opportunities for women to practise. From the beginning of the sixteenth century, corporations of apothecaries had emphasised a textual basis to their knowledge that was not commonly present in barbers' guilds where the skills were largely learnt through observation and hands-on practice. The 1502 statutes of the apothecaries, chandlers, confectioners and spicers of Rouen stipulated that apothecaries possess 'the remedies of the antidotary of Nicolas and of Mesué'.[72] The twelfth-century Antidotary of Nicolas of Salerno was frequently cited as the key text in apothecaries' regulations. In Amiens in 1576, new candidates were required to know Latin as were members of the 1572 established College of Apothecaries in Montpellier. Although there has been little study of the literacy of apothecaries' wives, if a few might be literate in French, most were unlikely to understand Latin. Therefore, textual transmission excluded women from understanding pharmaceutical knowledge.

Moreover, guilds began to gender-segregate the transmission of pharmaceutical knowledge. Wives of apothecaries in Paris and Montpellier where apothecaries and surgeons could take some classes with students at the medical faculties, were thus barred from one form of their knowledge. Guilds mirrored the universities' practice of excluding women from the physical location of knowledge transmission. In the 1576 statutes regulating the admission of apothecaries in Amiens, it was stipulated that wives and widows of masters could attend the guild dinner, but they were to leave when, after dinner, the candidate had to demonstrate in a garden or field that he knew the important herbs and plants.[73]

However, it is possible to find cases where apothecaries prepared for wives to assume their businesses as their widows. When Pierre Braillier, master apothecary in Lyon, wrote his will in July 1564, he arranged for his wife Jeanne Dabaron to assume his practice at one of the city's largest municipal institutions, the *Aumône Générale*.[74] As with barbers, widows could maintain a husband's workshop, but under constrained conditions. Most guilds obliged a widow to have an approved journeyman to perform the daily tasks of the workshop. In 1484, the regulations of the apothecaries of Paris stipulated that widows could maintain the business of their husbands on the condition that they employed 'a good servant, expert and knowledgeable, able and sufficient, who will be examined and approved by the masters of the trade'.[75] In Rouen in 1502, widows were to have a learned master valet to manage and maintain their boutiques.[76] Clearly widows were not considered by the guild as capable in their own right. In Bordeaux, if a widow had children, the four beadles imposed an expert journeyman upon her, whose choice was approved by them, until her eldest son reach his sixteenth year and could be trained in turn.[77] In the Parisian statutes of 1514, women's incapacities were emphasised further. She could maintain the workshop, but 'she cannot take apprentices herself, because she cannot call herself expert'.[78] Thus even if widows had the opportunity to continue the trade of their husband, they were rarely accorded the same privileges as their male counterparts.

The guild regulated the behaviour of widows. In Bordeaux, the regulations of the apothecaries' corporation in 1693, mostly unchanged since 1542, specified that 'a wife of a deceased master, without children, can keep the workshop of her husband, on the condition that she live honestly'.[79] What constituted honest behaviour was the judgement of the guild. Such a clause could potentially be used to oppose female practice of the occupation.

A guild of their own? Licensing Parisian midwives

If in the sixteenth century women's access to medical work through the guilds of their husbands was increasingly limited, and their ability to practise as independent providers completely abolished, what effects might stricter licensing have on a domain of medical practice that was largely the preserve of female practitioners: midwives? As with barbers and apothecaries, to understand the reasons for accreditation of midwives we must first understand its status as a medical discipline.

At the beginning of the sixteenth century, midwives were usually experienced older women whose activities were supervised by the Church, rather than the university medical corps. The Church's emphasis on regulating their activities rested more on their moral reputation and ability to administer baptismal sacraments if necessary than on examining their medical capacity and knowledge. Gabrielle de Bourbon paid several women as midwives to assist at the birth of her grandchild in 1505, suggesting that rather than one specialised expert, several women with skills and knowledge assisted each other at the birth.[80]

Although obstetrics had long been a subject of theoretical study in the medical faculties, it was only towards the sixteenth century that such interest translated into a wider practical interest, with ramifications for women's work in the field. In 1536, Paul Bienassis stimulated new university interest in France when he translated Eucharius Roeslin's key text into French, *Des divers travaulx et enfantements des femmes et par quel moyen l'on doit survenir aux accidens qui peuvent eschoir devant et apres iceulx travaux. Item, quel lait et quelle nourrisse on doit eslire aux enfans.* Alison Klairmont Lingo estimates that in the next 100 years some 22 texts appeared (14 original and 8 translations) concerning female health issues.[81]

Most formally trained medical practitioners who published in this field had both good and bad to report about midwives. Most wrote disparagingly of the midwife, as a generality, but could cite one or two who were worthy of special regard for their skills, practices or learned knowledge. Laurent Joubert, the chancellor of the Faculty of Medicine in Montpelliet, commented on midwives' lack of learned medical knowledge (even though women were unable to attend university and unlikely to be taught Latin to access such knowledge). He claimed he was 'not ignorant of the uterine anatomy as they are for the most part. But I want to exempt at least good Gervaise, a matron of Montpellier, truly a wise woman and well advised who does not fail to attend public anatomies when we have a female to hand'.[82] Such accounts that designated one midwife worthy of special regard whose practices and knowledge were beyond those of other women, only succeeded in condemning the competence of the profession in general.

In particular, physicians and surgeons reproached midwives for rushing births. According to Jacques Guillemeau, 'Some midwives either by ignorance or impatience, or to rush to the delivery of other women, rip the membranes and pierce the waters with their nails.'[83] Still more critical was Jacques du Val,

> often by their ignorance, ... they send a great many straight to their graves, or mutilate their tender and malleable bodies, which cannot endure violence without encountering problems. Such that instead of helping women and children, sadly they trouble them.[84]

One of the areas of conflict, claimed physicians, was midwives' unwillingness to call in doctors when problems arose during a birth, arriving 'often too late, through the obstinacy of relatives and midwives'.[85] Physicians and surgeons often attributed their unsuccessful intervention on being called too late to help. In Tours in November 1583, the surgeon Guillaume Herpin refused to treat the wife of a silk worker Pierre Bonnadventure, who was suffering in childbirth. He claimed that when he had done so previously in a similar situation, 'after a matron had destroyed everything', the family had taken him to court for misconduct. Herpin certified in the notarial act that he prepared in his defence that 'he was maddened for the great labour that several other women had suffered and endured since he had been troubled, even that there had been five dead for lack of being helped' but that he would not take responsibility for further deaths which were not his fault.[86] It seems likely that some midwives did hesitate too long before calling for the assistance of others, but such criticisms could also be used to hide the incompetency of physicians and surgeons when women and children died from their intervention.

University-trained practitioners also complained that midwives hid their knowledge: a criticism of which the medical faculties could equally be accused. Jacques du Val claimed that his text would reveal their secret knowledge, even hidden from each other. 'For rarely do they want to communicate their secrets and experiences one to the other: and by this means the young are constrained to learn and make their tests to the great detriment of several honourable women and families'.[87] Laurent Joubert went further. The interest that gynaecology aroused, and the confusion on the subject, led Joubert to bring together the data that he possessed, publishing what he presented as authentic depositions of midwives across France to give readers knowledge of their special terms and understanding of the female body.[88] Joubert saw these depositions as 'more inept than lewd (given that they are unknown terms)' because the terms were not known to him.[89] Yet his own evidence (whether authentic or not) was used to show that there were common practices, understandings and terminology among midwives from diverse and distant regions of France (Carcassonne, Paris and Béarn).[90] Joubert himself accredited these understandings, albeit unknowingly, because he argued that uniformity among midwives' knowledge denoted authority, which he then used to support his own arguments.

The most vicious attack against midwives was the curious and, it should be added, exceptional view of the Poitevin gentleman, Gervais de la Tousche. La Tousche produced an extraordinary attack on 'this idiot and incompetent race that we call midwives who to speak plainly and truthfully, we should rather call executioners and murderers of innocent blood, by their perverse incompetence'.[91] La Tousche critiqued the lack of learned knowledge of the midwife and saw her modest social position as a fault: 'they are a heap of poor deprived little women, not only in mind and understanding but also in all means to live'.[92] He advised women to ask their midwife:

> in which books and under which teachers they have learned their trade and science, ... they will tell you that it is fifty, indeed sixty years and more that they have exercised this trade, and that they know it very well, ... such that if you want to believe their babble, they will prove to you that by such that millions of women and children who die miserably by their ignorance at birth and in their hands, do not die by their fault or incompetence, but that it is the will of God.[93]

La Tousche ridiculed the experience of midwives; experience that conferred upon them authority, and which was generally recognised by even most university-trained physicians and surgeons as an advantage.

Instead, La Tousche offered a unique solution: women should care for themselves in childbirth with the help of neighbours. This answer was likely to find even less favour with the medical faculties than employing midwives over whom they at least had some control. La Tousche suggested that childbirth was not a medical issue at all, exposing an alternative contemporary view to that presented by both elite physicians and most midwives. He argued that women could 'give birth naturally without trouble, as do all the other female animals on the earth, and without the help of another'.[94] He likened women to pear trees, when the fruit was ready it would simply fall from the tree.[95] Thus La Tousche recommended to his prospective female audience that, rather than employ midwives: 'you be wise women to each other, neighbour to neighbour, not waiting any more for any foreign midwives: but only for yourselves, and your neighbours and friends.'[96] In fact, La Tousche was arguing that women had natural alternative knowledge about their bodies, and needed no medical theories at all. La Tousche represents the only layman to enter publicly the female health debate. His views suggest that there was a range of ways to perceive obstetrical issues, and that although increasing medical literature included obstetrics among its discussion, it was still possible for contemporaries to privilege such notions as an 'innate' female practice and understanding of their body over that derived from either learned medicine or experience.

Interest in midwives' work was not restricted to medical debates, however. Sixteenth-century legal authorities too began to look more closely at the power of midwives. The midwife's role did not pertain only to childbirth in the medical world of the Renaissance. In some ways, she was considered the specialist in all that concerned the female body, and particularly pregnancy. When a notary examined the remains of a prematurely born child in a broken pot for a court case in 1526, he particularly noted for the court record the presence of 'Jehanne Pailhera, expert and deliverer of children'.[97] It was the midwife (or often a group of them) who had the power in legal cases to decide if a girl or woman was a virgin, raped or capable of having children. She was often called upon to give her opinion in rape trials, after examination of the girl in question. This was a power contested by physicians for a question sprang to their minds: were midwives helping other women to enjoy their sexuality while attesting to their virginity?

After 1550, the midwife had to be assisted by at least a physician or a master surgeon. However, it seems that the real application of these statutes took some time to take effect. Anne Robert, a lawyer at the Parisian *parlement*, complained that judicial power continued to be accorded to ignorant midwives who 'write, alone, the report of virginity, corruption of pregnancy of girls or women, without a physician, or two surgeons of Châtelet, or one of them, . . . Added to that, it is necessary to write and sign the said reports and few of them know how to write'.[98] It was also the task of the midwife, after 1550 in conjunction with a physician or surgeon, to determine the fate of unions. A husband wishing to annul his marriage on the grounds of his wife's sterility had to await the examination by a midwife who would decide whether his request was valid. The surgeon Jacques Guillemeau attested in his works that he had been required to visit a woman with the midwife, Germaine Hassart, to determine for the courts whether she was capable of having children.[99]

The rising vernacular literature about women's health and the public attention towards its practice throughout the sixteenth century had implications for women's obstetrical work. The thorough research of Annie Saulnier for the later fifteenth century suggests that parish midwives were often nominated by local women.[100] The elected *ventrière* took up her office by swearing an oath before the local courts which gave her authority to practise. Saulnier found, however, that the length of practice of half the midwives recorded by the officials was only one year. Only 15 per cent (18 of 116) worked for more than five years. Saulnier noted changing trends in the work of midwives even over the twelve-year period of her study. Towards the end of the period, authorities increasingly required practising midwives to register their medical work. Furthermore, not only was there a trend for communities to have an approved midwife, but increasingly the same women were re-elected as midwives. Such evidence suggests that the notion of a recognised individual with particular obstetrical expertise began to take precedence over the idea that all women who had given birth might act as a birthing expert for a year or two.

Public attention to the powers of midwives to proclaim virgins, or procure abortions, resulted in increased regulation to the field. In 1556, a royal edict concerning criminal acts linked to maternity, in particular infanticide and abortion, tacitly proposed the notion of collusion between the midwife and the pregnant woman, since it contained rules regarding the regularisation of midwifery as an occupation. It stipulated that midwives could no longer work without being enrolled on the bailiff's register and without the provincial medical superintendent verifying the quality of the applicant's apprenticeship.[101] This prompted the drawing up of the statutes of the corporation of midwives in Paris which were officially recognised in 1560. Henceforth, in theory, as well as the usual apprenticeship with an experienced midwife, theoretical training was to be given by a master surgeon. She would still need a certificate of morality but she now also needed to undergo an examination by a jury composed of a doctor, two experienced midwives and two master surgeons. If she was successful, the candidate had to swear an oath to the provost of Paris or the *lieutenant criminel* of her region. Once her diploma was signed by the clerk of Châtelet and sealed by the *prévoté*, she was permitted to hang from her house the sign of the licensed midwife: a woman carrying an infant, a child with a candle, or a cradle with a fleur-de-lys.

The midwife swore to reveal the identity of anyone she knew practising illegally, to treat both the rich and poor, to remove her rings, to wash her hands before a birth and to call a doctor if the delivery presented difficulties.[102] She would receive the death penalty for procuring an abortion and was required to recommend to women that the child be baptised or perform this herself if she thought death was imminent. Midwives were not to provoke fights or gossip about other women but to 'comport themselves wisely and as prudent women'.[103] Each midwife was required to have a printed copy of the statutes. But although the 1560 regulations have been much cited as a sign of a renewed vision of midwifery, its impact, even in Paris, was slow. Legal action was taken against several women who were practising without licences as late as 1587 and 1595.[104] Indeed the statutes of 1560 were not published until 1600.[105] Although midwifery became increasingly accredited and controlled by the medical faculties, university-trained physicians made clear that they considered it at the lower end of the medical spectrum. It was enough that midwives be trained by a master surgeon, not a doctor. The university's minor interest in protecting the field was demonstrated by the fact that only one physician was required on the panel who examined the apprentice midwife.

In the countryside, there were moves to bring in more stringent statutes but the application of regulations was more difficult to enforce. Even after the introduction of the midwives' statutes in Paris, in other areas midwives continued to be regulated more by the Church than by local university-trained physicians, especially in towns that had no medical faculty. In Tours, if a woman, married or widowed, wished to become a midwife, she was required to notify the local curé who would verify whether she was of good reputation, and interrogate her on the sacraments of baptism, so as to assure himself that she knew what to pronounce and how it was to be administered. She was to swear an oath on the Bible that she would treat both rich and poor and declare all illegitimate children.[106] In some towns such as Loches, Chinon, Tours and Amboise, a physician also witnessed this oath, and signed a *procès-verbal*.[107] In other towns, the mayor might search out an experienced midwife who had trained in a large city, especially Paris. The Hôtel-Dieu in Paris provided one location where women from both the town and country could gain recognised experience in midwifery. Indeed, it was there that the royal midwife Louise Bourgeois sent her daughter, when the latter declared her intention to follow in her mother's footsteps:

> I thought it was necessary for her to see a large number of women give birth in a small space of time, to make sure of her resolution and not to be astonished by various deliveries: so I asked the midwife of that place and the nun who was the *dame des accouchées* to send for her when women were to give birth, she was there many times in six or seven months, she saw a great number give birth and had delivered more than fifty before she was yet sixteen.[108]

The midwife Tareau, after having obtained her professional training in Paris, established her practice in her home town of Tours in 1586. She exercised her occupation in the parish of Saint-Pierre-le-Puellier and was still working there in 1596.[109]

Regulation of midwifery was not initially motivated in any sense by a medical faculty seeking to promote better practice by women. Indeed it appears that guild incorporation for midwives meant little more than licensing and examination by surgeons. By linking an edict on infanticide to a push for better regulation of midwives, the crown saw midwives as collaborators protecting women from prosecution for bastard-bearing, by delivering their illegitimate children secretly. Unwilling to support mother or child in their poor relief systems, urban centres increasingly instructed midwives to withhold their medical expertise until a mother declared the name of the child's father. To the north of

France, in Lille, the city magistrates directed midwives in 1590 'when they deliver illegitimate infants of old or young women, to inquire of them who is the father, and afterwards to inform these women that they must report this to the said messieurs, following which [the midwife] will make the said report in order to avoid having many abandoned infants dependent upon the public finances of this town'.[110] As Hilary Marland has argued, such a directive brought midwives into conflict: their status and income depended on trust and respect from groups with differing interests, such as town authorities, law courts and the clients whom they delivered. In complying with the magistrates' order, midwives were forced to betray the trust of one of the interest groups they served.[111]

In summary then, unlike barbery, surgery and pharmacy, licensing of midwives did not come about as the result of women seeking recognition for the value and public good of their medical work: instead, it was imposed upon midwives as a result of legal, royal and medical bodies' fears over midwives' powers as authorities to proclaim virginity and their capacity to procure abortions. Tighter regulation of their practice allowed recognised medical authorities such as surgeons and physicians to supervise their work, and religious and legal authorities to use the midwife as an instrument of moral and social welfare regulation. Accreditation – that is, the command for midwives to be licensed and supervised – did not constitute the conventional bonds and advantages of sorority and support of other guild-incorporated trades. Of course, the effects of licensing were not necessarily all negative. Even if the motives for regulation of midwives were not recognition of their skills, those women who trained and practised under this system might still command greater authority and standing, in both the wider and medical community. Some women then sought out accreditation of their skills through the licensing system because of the opportunities it provided them for status, some financial security and guild positions.

Guild regulation of certain medical work had a profound effect on female practice even before the sixteenth century. As barbers and apothecaries sought closer ties with the university medical faculties, they structured the sites and methods of transmission of their skills in ways that increasingly excluded women. Women could no longer be practitioners in their own rights. By the sixteenth century, the medical guilds' adoption of an increasingly textual basis to their knowledge, and on instruction from the medical faculties, barred many wives from understanding the theory of their partners' work. Widows' rights to take over a husband's business may have permitted some women to practise, but the guilds' intentions seem to have been that women were in charge only in name. The early modern trend towards licensing of midwives was a double-edged sword. While it brought greater recognition and status to midwifery as a legitimate medical field from the universities, midwives paid a price in greater supervision of their practice and in pressure to forego the rights of their patients in order to uphold the religious and moral programmes of legal, municipal and religious authorities.

Notes

1 Bibliothèque municipale de Reims (BM de Reims), MS 1081, liasse 4, fols 10v–11r. I have standardised the spelling of names throughout.
2 *Ibid.*, fol. 8v.
3 *Ibid.*, fol. 12r. For further details on the idea of *entre vifs* donations, see Natalie Zemon Davis, *The Gift in Sixteenth-Century France* (Madison: The University of Wisconsin Press, 2000), pp. 32–3.
4 BM de Reims, MS 1081, liasse 4, fol. 12v.
5 *Ibid.*, fol. 7r.
6 *Ibid.*, fol. 8v.
7 *Ibid.*, fol. 9r.
8 For further explanation of these procedures, see Jean Brissaud, *A History of French Public Law*, trans. James W. Garner (London: John Murray, 1915); François Olivier-Martin, *Précis d'histoire du droit français*, 3rd edn (Paris: Librairie Dalloz, 1938); R. Doucet, *Les Institutions de la France au XVIe siècle*, vol. 2 (Paris: A et J. Picard, 1948).
9 BM de Reims, MS 1081, liasse 4, fol. 9v.
10 *Ibid.*, fol. 10r.
11 *Ibid.*, fol. 10v.
12 *Ibid.*, fol. 10v.
13 Emile Forgue, 'Histoire de la chirurgie', *Histoire générale de la médecine, de la pharmacie, de l'art dentaire et de l'art vétérinaire*, ed. M. Laignel-Lavastine, vol. 2 (Paris: Albin Michel, 1938), p. 402.
14 *Archives législatives de la ville de Reims, Seconde Partie: Statuts*, ed. Pierre Varin, vol. 1 (Paris: Imprimerie de Crapelet, 1844), p. 982.
15 René de Lespinasse (ed.), *Les Métiers et corporations de la ville de Paris XIVe–XVIIIe siècles*, vol. 3 (Paris: Imprimerie Nationale, 1898), p. 643.
16 Based on analysis of work by Herlihy, *Opera Muliebra: Women and Work in Medieval Europe* (New York: McGraw-Hill, 1990) and Beatrice Coucy, 'Contribution à l'histoire sociale des praticiens parisiens à la fin du moyen âge: aspects méthodologiques', *Sources: Travaux Historiques*, 5 (1986), 13–28, in Monica H. Green, 'Documenting medieval women's medical practice', in Luis Garcia-Ballester, Roger French, Jon Arrizabalaga and Andrew Cunningham (eds), *Practical Medicine from Salerno to the Black Death* (Cambridge: Cambridge University Press, 1994), p. 345.
17 Ch. Ouin-LaCroix, *Histoire des anciennes corporations d'arts et métiers et des confréries religieuses de la capitale de la Normandie* (Rouen: Lacointe Freres, 1850), p. 322.

18 Alfred Franklin, *Les Corporations ouvrières de Paris du XIIe au XVIIIe siècle* (1884) (New York: Burt Franklin, 1971), p. 12.
19 Green, 'Documenting medieval women's medical practice', p. 345.
20 Cécile Béghin, 'Donneuses d'ouvrages, apprenties et salariées aux XIVe et XVe siècles dans les sociétés urbaines languedociennes', *Clio. Histoire, Femmes et Sociétés*, 3 (1996), p. 44.
21 C. A. Ernest Wickersheimer, *La Médecine et les médecins en France à l'époque de la Renaissance* (Paris: A. Maloine, 1906), p. 17.
22 Jean Fernel, *Physiologie*, translation of 1655, cited in Jean-Charles Sournia, *Histoire de la médecine* (Paris: La Découverte, 1992), p. 150.
23 Laurent Joubert, *La Médecine et le régime de santé, des erreurs populaires et propos vulgaires* (Bordeaux: Simon Millanges, 1578) ed. Madeleine Tiollais, vols 1 and 2 (Paris: L'Harmattan, 1997).
24 Forgue, 'Histoire de la chirurgie', p. 404.
25 *Journal of a Younger Brother: The Life of Thomas Platter as a Medical Student in Montpellier at the Close of the Sixteenth Century*, ed. Sean Jennett (London: Frederick Muller, 1963), p. 36.
26 Archives municipales de Tours, GG 3, document 835.
27 *Recueil des monuments inédits de l'histoire du tiers état: première série, chartes, coutumes, actes municipaux, statuts des corporations d'arts et metiers des villes et communes de France, region du nord*, ed. Augustin Thierry, vol. 2 (Paris: Firmin-Didot, 1853), p. 569.
28 Forgue, 'Histoire de la chirurgie', p. 404.
29 Alison Klairmont Lingo, 'Print's role in the politics of women's health care in early modern France', in Barbara B. Diefendorf and Carla Hesse (eds), *Culture and Identity in Early Modern Europe (1500–1800): Essays in Honor of Natalie Zemon Davis* (Ann Arbor: The University of Michigan Press, 1993), p. 204.
30 DCLXXVII, *Index Chronologicus Chartarum pertinentium ad historiam Universitatis Parisiensis ad ejus originibus ad finem decimi sexti sæculi*, ed. C. Jourdain (Paris, 1862) (Brussels: Culture et Civilisation, 1966), p. 155.
31 MCCCLXXVI, *Ibid.*, p. 295.
32 Ouin-LaCroix, *Histoire des anciennes corporations*, p. 306.
33 *Ibid.*, p. 305.
34 Forgue, 'Histoire de la chirurgie', p. 402.
35 MDXLIII, *Index Chronologicus Chartarum*, p. 318.
36 MDCCLXXXIII, *Ibid.*, p. 355.
37 MMLXXVI, *Ibid.*, p. 395.
38 MMLXXVII, *Ibid.*, p. 395; Lespinasse, *Les Métiers et corporations*, vol. 3, p. 639.
39 Alison Klairmont Lingo, *The Rise of Medical Practitioners in Sixteenth-Century France: The Case of Lyon and Montpellier* (PhD, University of California-Berkeley, 1980), p. 151.
40 *Ibid.*, p. 153.
41 See Natalie Zemon Davis, 'Women in the crafts in sixteenth-century Lyon', *Feminist Studies*, 8:1 (1982), pp. 47–80, and Judith M. Bennett, '"History that stands still": women's work in the European past', *Feminist Studies*, 14:2 (1988), pp. 269–83.
42 Davis, 'Women in the crafts in sixteenth-century Lyon', pp. 47–80.

43 A. Germain, *Histoire de la commune de Montpellier depuis ses origines jusqu'à son incorporation définitive à la monarchie française*, 3 vols (Montpellier: Jean Martel aîné, 1851), pp. 456–8 cited in Béghin, 'Donneuses d'ouvrages, apprenties et salariées', p. 38.
44 Victorin Laval, *Histoire de la Faculté de Médecine d'Avignon: ses origines, son organisation et son enseignement (1303–1791)*, vol. 1 (Paris: E. Lechevalier, 1889), p. 36.
45 Lespinasse, *Les Métiers et corporations*, vol. 3, p. 654.
46 Green, 'Documenting medieval women's medical practice', p. 332 and Judith C. Brown, 'A women's place was in the home: women's work in Renaissance Tuscany', in Margaret W. Ferguson, Maureen Quilligan and Nancy J. Vickers (eds), *Rewriting the Renaissance: The Discourses of Sexual Difference in Early Modern Europe* (Chicago: The University of Chicago Press, 1986), pp. 206–24.
47 Klairmont Lingo, 'Women healers and the medical marketplace of sixteenth-century Lyon', *Dynamis*, 19 (1999), pp. 79–94, p. 91.
48 *Ibid.*, p. 90.
49 Laval, *Histoire de la Faculté de Médecine d'Avignon*, vol. 1, p. 77.
50 J. Drivon, *Miscellanées médicales et historiques: notes pour servir à l'histoire de la médecine à Lyon* (Lyon: Association Typographique, 1908), p. 12.
51 Klairmont Lingo, 'Women healers and the medical marketplace', p. 89.
52 See also Chapter 6 for further details.
53 Drivon, *Miscellanées médicales et historiques*, pp. 36–7.
54 *Archives législatives de la ville de Reims*, p. 982.
55 *Ibid.*, pp. 985–6.
56 *Ibid.*, p. 986.
57 For another earlier prosecution of a female widow barber, Jeanne Pouquelin, in Paris in 1422, see Geneviève Dumas, 'Les femmes et les pratiques de la santé dans le "Registre de plaidoiries du Parlement de Paris, 1364–1427"', *Canadian Bulletin of Medicine*, 13 (1996), pp. 13–27, especially pp. 11–12.
58 *Archives législatives de la ville de Reims*, p. 980.
59 The fact that the elder Jehan Estevent's name appears also on the list of master surgeons raises more questions though. Had he simply returned from life as a hermit to resume his profession, or did his name represent the participation of Isabelle Estevent? From these documents, we cannot be sure.
60 Lespinasse, *Les Métiers et corporations*, vol. 1, p. 518.
61 *Ibid.*, p. 508.
62 Ouin-LaCroix, *Histoire des anciennes corporations*, p. 307.
63 *Recueil des monuments inédits de l'histoire du tiers état*, vol. 4 (1870), p. 375.
64 Lespinasse, *Les Métiers et corporations*, vol. 1, p. 512.
65 *Ibid.*, p. 515.
66 *Ibid.*, p. 598.
67 See *Index Chronologicus Chartarum*, pp. 341, 386, 408.
68 Klairmont Lingo, *The Rise of Medical Practitioners*, p. 137.
69 *Ibid.*, p. 138.
70 *Ibid.*, p. 139.
71 Lespinasse, *Les Métiers et corporations*, vol. 1, p. 521.
72 Ouin-LaCroix, *Histoire des anciennes corporations*, p. 558.

73 *Recueil des monuments inédits de l'histoire du tiers état*, vol. 2 (1853), p. 847.
74 H. and J. Baudrier, *Bibliographie lyonnaise: recherches sur les imprimeurs, libraires, relieurs et fondeurs de lettres de Lyon au XVIe siècle*, vol. 2 (Paris: F. de Nobele, 1964), p. 92.
75 Lespinasse, *Les Métiers et corporations*, vol. 1, p. 509.
76 Ouin-LaCroix, *Histoire des anciennes corporations*, p. 558.
77 L. Reutter de Rosemont, *Histoire de la pharmacie à travers les âges*, vol. 1 (Paris: Peyronnet, 1931), pp. 295–6.
78 Lespinasse, *Les Métiers et corporations*, vol. 1, p. 512.
79 Reutter de Rosemont, *Histoire de la pharmacie*, p. 295.
80 *Les la Trémoille pendant cinq siècles*. vol. 2, *Louis I, Louis II, Jean et Jacques, 1431–1525* (Nantes: E. Grimaud, 1892), p. 58.
81 Klairmont Lingo, 'Print's role in the politics of women's health care', p. 203.
82 Joubert, *La Médecine et le régime de santé*, vol. 2, p. 234.
83 Jacques Guillemeau, *De l'heureux accouchement des femmes où il est traicté du gouvernement de leur grossesse, de leur travail naturel et contre nature, du traictement estant accouchées et de leurs maladies* (Paris: Nicolas Buon, 1609), p. 169.
84 Jacques du Val, *Des Hermaphrodits, accouchemens des femmes, et traitement qui est requis pour les relever en santé, & bien élever leurs enfans* (Rouen: David Geuffroy, 1612), pp. 50–1.
85 Guillemeau, *De l'heureux accouchement des femmes*, n.p.
86 Louis Dubreuil-Chambardel, 'L'Enseignement des sages-femmes en Touraine', *Bulletin et mémoires de la société archéologique de Touraine*, 48 (1909), p. 45.
87 Du Val, *Des Hermaphrodits, accouchemens des femmes*, pp. 50–1.
88 Joubert, *La Médecine et le régime de santé*, vol. 2, p. 237. Françoise Fery-Hue argues that some of the texts may in fact be bawdy imitations of contemporary medico-legal depositions for rape. See her article, 'Une Expertise pour viol au XVIe siècle: pratique médico-légale et vocabulaire gynécologique', *Violences et contestation au moyen âge, actes du 114e congrès national des sociétés savantes (Paris, 1989)* (Paris: Editions du Comité des travaux historiques et scientifiques, 1990), pp. 321–43.
89 Joubert, *La Médecine et le régime de santé*, vol. 1, p. 58.
90 See also Klairmont Lingo, 'The fate of popular terms for female anatomy in the age of print', *French Historical Studies*, 22:3 (1999), pp. 335–49.
91 Gervais de La Tousche, *La Tres-Haute et Tres-Souveraine Science de l'art et industrie naturelle d'enfanter. Contre la Maudicte et Perverse impericie des femmes que l'on appelle saiges-femmes ou belles meres, lesquelles par leur ignorance font iournellement perir une infinité de femmes & d'enfans à l'enfantement. Adce que desormais toutes femmes enfantent heureusement, & sans aucun peril ny destourbier, tant d'elles que de leurs enfans, estant toutes saiges & perites en icelle science* (Paris: Didier Millot, 1587), fols. Aiir–v.
92 *Ibid.*, fol. 3r.
93 *Ibid.*, fol. Aiiv.
94 *Ibid.*, fol. 5v.
95 *Ibid.*, fol. 11v.
96 *Ibid.*, fol. 3v.
97 Annie Charnay, *Paroles de voleurs: gens de sac et de corde en pays toulousain au début du XVIe siècle* (Paris: Champion, 1998), p. 325.

98 Wickersheimer, *La Médecine et les médecins*, p. 196.
99 Jacques Guillemeau, *Les Oeuvres de chirurgie* (Rouen: Iean Viret, François Vaultier, Clement Malassis, Iacques Besongne, 1649), p. 310. See also Pierre Darmon's study *Le Tribunal de l'impuissance* (1978) (Paris: Seuils, 1985).
100 Annie Saulnier, 'Le visiteur, les femmes et les "obstetrices" des paroisses de l'Archidiaconé de Josas de 1458 à 1470', *Santé, médecine et assistance au moyen âge* (Actes du 110e congrès national des sociétés savantes, Montpellier, 1985) (Paris: Editions du CTHS, 1987), pp. 43–62.
101 René Coursault, *La Médecine en Touraine du moyen-âge à nos jours* (Paris: Maisonneuve & Larose, 1991), p. 49.
102 Wickersheimer, *La Médecine et les médecins*, p. 190.
103 *Ibid.*, p. 191.
104 *Ibid.*, p. 155.
105 *Ibid.*, p. 192.
106 Dubreuil-Chambardel, 'L'Enseignement des sages-femmes en Touraine', p. 49.
107 *Ibid.*, p. 50.
108 Louise Bourgeois, *Observations diverses sur la sterilité, perte de fruicts, foecondité, accouchements, et maladies des femmes et enfants nouveaux naiz* (Paris, Abraham Saugrain, 1617), pp. 74–5.
109 Dubreuil-Chambardel, 'L'Enseignement des sages-femmes en Touraine', p. 52.
110 E. Leclair, *Un chapitre de l'histoire de la chirurgie à Lille* (Lille: 1910), p. 10 cited in Richard L. Petrelli, 'The regulation of French midwifery during the Ancien Régime', *Journal of the History of Medicine* (1971), pp. 276–92, p. 282.
111 Although Marland's point is made in regard to midwives in the eighteenth-century Netherlands, it is equally valid to our study here. Hilary Marland, '"Stately and dignified, kindly and God-fearing": midwives, age and status in the Netherlands in the eighteenth century', in Hilary Marland and Margaret Pelling (eds), *The Task of Healing: Medicine, religion and gender in England and the Netherlands, 1450–1800* (Rotterdam: Erasmus Publishing, 1996), pp. 271–305, p. 296.

2

The university: women and the Faculty of Medicine in Paris

ALONGSIDE GUILD REGULATION, female practice in Paris and other medical centres also faced regulation by their respective medical faculties. In 1322 the Parisian medical faculty pursued a case against a medical practitioner that is perhaps the trial most commonly cited as evidence of the medical faculty's harsh and unrelenting battle against women as medical service providers. Jacqueline Felicie's prosecution can be found in most histories of medicine. The remaining evidence of her trial is rich and exposes a highly competent practitioner of surgery and medicine (as testified by her many witnesses, and a point not debated by her prosecutors), who mounted an eloquent and spirited defence of her practice. Yet despite the evidence of her witnesses, both male and female, and her own justifications of working for the public good, she was fined and forbidden from further practice.[1] This case has come to define, in many histories of medicine, the attitude of the universities, and the learned powers more generally, towards popular medical practices, as aggressive and somewhat misogynistic throughout the middle ages and beyond. As Iain M. Lonie argued for the sixteenth century, as in centuries past, the Paris medical faculty 'waged unremitting war upon outsiders of all kinds'.[2]

I want to ask how representative Felicie's particular case was of the faculty's prosecution of female practitioners, and whether misogyny was at the forefront of the faculty's preoccupation with their practice. More generally, this chapter is concerned to explore how medical faculties perceived women's medical knowledge and practices, and how women responded to these perceptions (if at all) and practised medicine as a result. To do so, I will first concentrate on a study of prosecutions for illegal practice brought before medical faculties. Did the attitude towards women's medical knowledge and practice, and empirical medicine generally, remain constant from the middle ages to the sixteenth century?

Were female practitioners prosecuted at different rates and for different reasons to their male counterparts? What justification did women use to explain their knowledge and practices? Secondly, I will examine what opportunities women had to access university medical knowledge and practice. Could women, as wives and daughters of physicians, learn about university medicine, and through what means?

Illegal practitioners before the medical faculties

My survey of the practitioners whom the Parisian medical faculty chose to pursue (successfully or otherwise) for their medical practice, between 1270 and 1560, is compiled from sources such as the *Commentaires* of the Parisian medical faculty, which record the various expenditure for pursuing such cases,[3] the charters of the university documenting its efforts for legal recognition of its position on medical practice,[4] as well as extant records of specific cases. Analyses of prosecutions are a valuable source for understanding the faculty's activities and concepts of medical practice. Since the interest in this chapter is to understand the views of the university, I will focus here on examining which medical providers the faculty selected to pursue and what justification they provided for these choices, rather than on the outcomes and resolutions of female medical prosecution (dependent on legal perceptions of medical practice), which will be explored in Chapter 4.

If the faculty's own records of its activities are to be believed, it did not pursue a particularly large number of cases for illegal practice: by my survey, 69 cases for the period 1270–1551. For this reason, the focus here will not be limited to the sixteenth century but will examine cases as early as 1270 for the evidence they can provide about continuities and change in the faculty's position on medical practice. The position of the medical faculty of Montpellier will also be analysed for comparison of its policies of prosecution.

Faculty policies on prosecution

The evidence that the university did not pursue a particularly large number of practitioners for their medical work may seem at first glance surprising and contradictory to the claims of many historians. However, it did not mean that the faculty was unconcerned by the issue. To explore the reasons for the small number, we need to summarise how the medical faculty functioned and what its status and preoccupations were.[5]

What I seek to understand as 'the medical faculty' here are specific moments of university life and matter: its minutes of meetings, its interactions with the *Parlement*, and papacy, for example. What it meant to be a student or master in the medieval and early modern faculty would involve different evidence and a different scope, and the experience of individuals would doubtless vary greatly. The historians Cornelius O'Boyle working on the medieval Parisian medical faculty and Françoise Lehoux on Parisian physicians of the sixteenth and seventeenth centuries both emphasise the diversity (economic, social or regional) of Catholic men who received the university's medical education.[6] Nonetheless, in their collective training, such a disparate group was bound to share expectations and preoccupations about its worth, and to join together to achieve common goals. One of these shared ambitions, probably true of all occupational groups, was a desire to see their work recognised as valuable, special and unique (even among rival medical faculties) and to increase their status as practitioners of that skill.

Physicians, like apothecaries, surgeons and barbers in their guilds and corporations, were concerned about their status. As members of the university, physicians emphasised the source of their medical knowledge as learned, rather than practical. Of course, the medical faculty trained its students to practise their knowledge, but it was understood that the *basis* of that knowledge was derived from texts and the intellectual realm, rather than hands-on experimentation. As O'Boyle has argued, the developing 'bookish' culture of university medicine in the middle ages underpinned its status and claims to be a university discipline. Medical students were taught to discern the authoritative texts and logic of their discipline, and to lack this knowledge was a clear sign of non-university medical education. Thus, for the physician, 'to know medicine was to know its authoritative sources.'[7]

Much has been written on the means by which physicians increased their social capital through 'the institutional security of faculty organisation'[8] and 'professionalised' their work,[9] particularly in relation to other medical practitioners. For most of the medieval period, physicians were the only medical providers who trained in the university. For the lay observer, it would be impossible to detect the hidden causes of illness that a university-trained practitioner could discern through rational analysis. Physicians prized their knowledge of Greek and Latin texts, laying claim to the most intellectual basis to their education of all the medical practitioners, to position themselves at the top of a hierarchy of medical service providers.[10] Alison Klairmont Lingo's study of medical practitioners in Lyon and Montpellier during the sixteenth century has emphasised how their claims of specialised learning and status as intellectuals continued to be used by physicians to increase the dignity and nobility of their medical work.[11] The Hellenisation of sixteenth-century university medical education was celebrated by physicians as an exciting break from the Arabic medieval past, a renaissance in textual medical theory,[12] and a further division of their knowledge from those by then encroaching the university domain.

In the light of this constant struggle to maintain supremacy over other medical service providers, it is not surprising that the medical faculties did pursue practitioners whose activities infringed their own areas of interest, just as guilds protected their respective work territory. The faculty sought the protection of ecclesiastical, royal and papal authority to define the legitimacy of the university's product and to limit the role of others in their domain.[13] Threats to those who dared to continue their work ranged from fines and imprisonment to excommunication, depending on the authority concerned. In 1271, the faculty's own statutes encompassed both a range of providers and practices to be banned, declaring 'that no Jew or Jewess presume to operate surgically or medicinally on any person of catholic faith';[14] forbidding 'any male or female surgeon, apothecary or herbalist, by their oaths [to] presume or exceed the limits or bounds of their craft secretly or publicly';[15] and prohibiting providers from composing remedies and from 'every way and method of treatment in which medical skill is called for'.[16] Medical skill then, by the faculty's terminology, was what physicians provided by their specific learned knowledge. We see that the spate of some 31 prosecutions in 1322 included a variety of medical practitioners including a substantial number of practitioners termed surgeons and spicers, who were not pursued later as they fell into guild-regulated groups under the supervision of the faculty. It was a claim that authorities supported. As O'Boyle has argued, papal justifications for protecting physicians' interests stemmed from the logic that only faculty-trained practitioners understood the true science of medicine and how to practise it safely.[17] Many ordinances, *arrêts* and edicts throughout the medieval and early modern era attest to the continuity and repetition of physicians' claims, and also to the continuation of the activities of other medical workers.

By the sixteenth century, the faculty's interests had been distilled but also diversified. The diverse providers under attack were now classified under the generic term 'empirics' as this *arrêt* of the *Parlement* of Paris in 1598 demonstrates, renewing 'the prohibitions made formerly against all empirics, not approved by the Faculty of Medicine, to practise the art of healing'.[18] Bans no longer took the trouble to list out a typology of competitive practitioners of old: Jews, old women, monks for example, for they were all 'other'. In a 1579 *arrêt*, the faculty's claim was simply put: 'None can practise in medicine if he is not a doctor of the said Faculty'.[19] Klairmont Lingo has argued persuasively that the early modern development of the construction of 'the other' – that group of practitioners who were not university-trained or recognised – was a powerful force mobilising physicians into a unified group against the threat of competitors.[20] Now, in the eyes of the physicians, all those whose medical practice was not legitimated by *their* authority (as were for example surgeons and apothecaries who acknowledged the superiority of physicians in their guild regulations) were part of the empirical Other.

Furthermore, apart from the development of the medical Other, the faculty also began to concern itself with the spread of university medical knowledge through printed texts. While the effects of the printing press for women's medical practice will be explored in Chapter 5, it is appropriate to highlight here the impact in the sixteenth century of the printed mode for the increased accessibility of all forms of literature, medical texts included. Although the circulation of authoritative medical texts in manuscripts was by no means a closed system, the university had been able to exert controls over those who had access to its knowledge. It had regulated the work of stationers who produced, organised and hired out medical manuscripts to students. The potential for printing presses to produce medical knowledge *en masse* led the faculty to request restrictions on the circulation of such texts. In 1536, in the famous case against Jean Thibault, a member of the king's own medical retinue who practised without examination from the faculty, the physicians argued to prohibit 'all booksellers to put for sale any unapproved books of medicine'.[21] In 1578, an *arrêt* of the *Parlement* of Paris renewed and extended the physicians' concerns: regulating not only booksellers' activities in the medical domain, but also those of printers. The print trades were banned from 'printing, having printed, or putting for sale any books or treatises concerning medicine or surgery, without them having been first communicated to the Faculty of Medicine'.[22] Thus, the faculty's control over its purview of medicine extended beyond practitioners alone, to the potential learned sources by which they might claim similar dignified scientific knowledge.

Physicians' interest in removing illegal providers cannot be solely attributed to their desire for total economic and status supremacy. Between 1310 and 1329 Jacquart estimates that there were 84 physicians, 26 master surgeons and 97 barbers in the city of Paris for a population of around 200,000.²³ Debus cites the number of physicians from the faculty in 1550s Paris at 70–80, and declining into the 1590s to 40 physicians.²⁴ If such figures reflect the reality, then it seems likely that, on an economic level alone, medical providers of all types could have practised without impacting on each other's 'trade' to any major extent. Could the faculty have other motives then for its prosecutions?

Evidence for the sixteenth century suggests that members of the faculty argued that there was a genuine sense of risk to the community from unchecked medical care, and perhaps too a danger to the medical fraternity as a whole from fraudulent practitioners. In 1516 the dean of the faculty, Louis Braillon, argued that their prosecution was a matter for public safety, when ignorant providers prescribed experimental remedies and treatments that might kill the patient.²⁵ He proceeded to mount the case for the faculty to expend funds for this cause. At the end of the day however, a major issue to the faculty was surely the licensing and regulating of authorised practitioners, because even in cases where medical practitioners provided evidence of successful cures and treatments the faculty did not appear interested in understanding them for the greater good of future medicine.

Although Jean Thibault was a high-profile and educated practitioner, the 'others' that the faculty most commonly described as their targets were clearly poor and illiterate individuals who could not typically have competed for the same clientele as their university counterparts. Michel du Monceau, one dean of the Parisian faculty, described many of the illicit practitioners as of both sexes and of sordid condition.²⁶ Hubert Coquiel, dean in 1531, repeated a similar vision of the practitioners of whose presence they sought to divest Paris.²⁷ Yet the difficulty of prosecuting a practitioner who had gained the confidence of a rich patron (*à la* Thibault) made the faculty cautious about how to proceed.²⁸ When Du Monceau sought to scourge Paris of the physicians' Others, the faculty went about constructing a watertight case for the courts. On legal advice, they presented the *lieutenant criminel* with a copy of the faculty's privileges to demonstrate the legal justification for the prosecution of practitioners overlapping physicians' domains. Then, rather than relying on the force of edicts and ordinances and the local authorities to search out practitioners, physicians identified and reported to the *lieutenant criminel* the names of individual practitioners about whom they could supply solid evidence of unlicensed medical work. To gather this testimony, the faculty drew on its networks of allegiance from the medical guilds. Barbers were made to swear as part of their oath that they would report names of empirics they discovered to the faculty.²⁹ As a result, the faculty tended to focus on individual cases for which they were prepared to spend relatively large sums, in order to guarantee a conviction, which would then serve as an example to other providers. For one practitioner, Laurent le Barbandier, the faculty used entrapment, paying a 'patient' to present herself for Le Barbandier's care, so that members of the faculty could catch him in the act of, and witness to the courts, his medical work.[30]

Medical service providers, however, did not simply bow to the faculty's demands to stop practising. The authority of the faculty was by no means uncontested by other practitioners. Some refused to appear before the faculty to answer charges, thereby rejecting its jurisdiction to regulate their form of medical work. Others mounted a spirited defence of the utility of their work (and often a stinging attack on the efficacy of university medicine) before the faculty. Still others continued to practise even after being fined by the courts, and forced the faculty to re-commence proceedings against them. The case of Jean Thibault, the king's doctor who had even gone into print claiming the faculty was no equal to his skill in treating the plague, had run from 1532 to 1540. Another, Etienne Thiebourg, had first been pursued by the faculty in 1507–8, then again in 1514 and was under renewed investigation in 1520.[31] One unidentified provider attempted to appeal his conviction in 1542.[32] Thus the faculty's prosecution of a provider was no guarantee of its ultimate success. Such evidence of providers' responses to prosecution, more of which I will examine below, makes understandable the faculty's concentration of its effort on a small number of providers for whom it could supply a rock-solid case to the courts.

To return then to the chronology of prosecutions the faculty engaged in, 54 per cent of prosecutions between 1270 and 1551 took place before 1330 (37 of 69 cases). It would seem that after the 31 practitioners, spicers and surgeons pursued in 1322 (including Felicie),[33] the faculty began to select representative cases about whom accurate information could be gathered and for which they would expend large sums, in the hopes of achieving an outcome that would serve to ward off other potential practitioners in their medical domains. After 1322, no more than five practitioners were ever pursued in the same year. After all, cases expended large resources for the faculty, in terms of time and money, and the results were by no means guaranteed. Some deans of the faculty were clearly more concerned with the problems of 'empirics' than others, whether through a personal keenness or because a particular individual's work came to the attention of the faculty to re-ignite the issue. The first half of the sixteenth century marked a renewal of prosecutions, with 35 per cent of total prosecutions from 1270 to 1551 occurring in the period from 1502 to 1551. These deans freshly announced the faculty's long-held intention to eradicate the non-university-trained medical competition, resulting in a rise in the number of practitioners pursued.

Gender in faculty prosecutions

Physicians recognised that female practitioners were one of those 'Other' who were potential competitors in the medical marketplace. In the faculty regulation of 1271, women as well as men were labelled as problematic. In 1352, the royal ordinance of Jean II elaborated on the typology of other medical providers as 'many persons of both sexes, women and old wives, monks, rustics, some apothecaries and numerous herbalists, besides students not yet trained in the faculty of medicine or coming from foreign parts to the town of Paris to practise, ignorant of the science of medicine'.[34] It likewise made clear mention elsewhere of women as providers: 'that no one, of whatever sex or condition, ... shall henceforth make, or advise the making, or dare to administer any medicine alterative, laxative, syrup, electuary, laxative pills, clysters of any sort ... opiate or anything else, or offer medical advice or otherwise exercise the office of a physician in any way'.[35] In the sixteenth century, if the Other was no longer clearly stated in decrees, ordinances and edicts, the typology of providers that physicians saw as competitors were listed elsewhere.

Klairmont Lingo argues that while there had been earlier descriptions of the medical 'underbelly', no one before André du Breil in his 1580 *Police de l'art et science de medecine*, had spent as much time distinguishing between the various sorts of healers.[36] As she demonstrates, when Du Breil's typology was taken up by Thomas Sonnet de Courval in the early seventeenth century, the two authors contributed to the creation of a medical 'Other', differentiating the religious from the secular, rationally trained from the unskilled, and the authentic cures from fraud.[37] Du Breil addressed women's medical work in a number of different fields. He was concerned that women were practising medicine in the guild trades through their privileges as widows: 'as if they were the inheritors of the knowledge of their husbands, like their goods, from which stems an infinite number of errors ... they exercise Medicine contrary to good, according to their whim, without calling or asking for any advice other than their own'.[38] He feared that the processes of guild transmission of skills jeopardised the prestige and practice of the medical arts: 'for it is no more acceptable that a widow of a physician, surgeon, apothecary, and barber practise medicine after the death of their husbands, than a widow of a judge, president, counsellor, lawyer, clerk, court usher or procurer, judge, plead, write, or report causes and trials'.[39] Du Breil lamented women's practice in a range of medical arenas, from religious healing to child care, as will be documented in following chapters. From such sources, we may conclude that physicians did indeed see women as rivals to their medical skills, as well as a threat to the status of their profession, and were as concerned to eradicate their competition as they were male providers.

However, does this attitude constitute misogyny, or simply recognition that people of either sex could be involved in rival medical work? If we examine the list of prosecutions undertaken by the faculty, it seems clear that although women were prosecuted, they were not represented in a proportionately high rate: 19 per cent of prosecutions (13 out of 69 cases) concerned female practitioners, and 10 of these cases (77 per cent of female cases) occurred before 1400.

Were there differences though in the reasons why men and women were prosecuted for medical practice? It is not clear from anything recorded in the *Commentaires* for the female providers named as prosecuted in the sixteenth century (Jeanne Mabille, Marion, and the old woman of Champgaillard), or indeed those in centuries past, that the faculty had any motive against these providers as women. If this was the case, it was not recorded in their minutes. We only know that Jeanne Mabille was brought before the faculty in 1507 for her public medical work providing remedies based on uroscopy.[40] In 1516, when the faculty was paying people to collect evidence and information on the provider Marion, we simply read that she was an old woman who rode a mule.[41] And if the faculty called the old woman of Champgaillard an 'old harpy' in its minutes,[42] it was equally willing to ridicule the expertise of male competitors such as Master Charles, a Spaniard, as the 'cow doctor'.

Did women argue their cases in ways that were specific to their gender? Jacqueline Felicie certainly argued in her trial that part of her practice included treating women's disorders, for which female practitioners were necessary because women were not willing to seek advice from a man.[43] However, I have not seen similar evidence provided by other female practitioners and it does not seem to be the case that any of the women prosecuted in the sixteenth century especially restricted their practice to female clients. Indeed, as Monica H. Green has argued, one of the greatest myths of female practitioners in the middle ages is that they primarily treated female complaints.[44] If anything, I think the evidence of prosecutions through the Paris medical faculty demonstrates the opposite. The faculty was concerned with providers who treated a range of clients, both male and female.

Furthermore, women practitioners were no more apt than men to accept the authority of the faculty in their medical work and found many ways to resist. In 1551, the faculty had to mobilise all its energy to bring to justice the 'old woman of Champgaillard'. She refused to appear before the faculty when summoned by the sergeants and went into hiding for a fortnight. It would take four *gendarmes* and two men wielding swords to lock her safely in prison.[45] After a trial that lasted six months, the courts pronounced a fine of 6 livres parisis, to be divided between king and faculty. The old woman of Champgaillard had the compliance of her husband, who seized control of her goods and distributed his wife's medical supplies, so the dean was never able to exact the fine nor reimbursement for the expense of her pursuit.[46] In this sense, Champgaillard had an advantage over her male counterparts. This course of action, using the legal position of a wife without assets to her own name, was not open to them.

It seems likely that a factor worrying the Parisian medical faculty throughout the middle ages and early modern era more than the gender of medical provider was the influx of foreigners and practitioners who had trained at other institutions than the university in Paris. In the sixteenth century, the faculty pursued several cases against physicians who had trained in other universities. At least 9 of the 24 cases (37.5 per cent) pursued between 1500 and 1551 specifically stated that the practitioners were foreigners to Paris. The case in 1506 against André Charpentier, from Montpellier, and Pierre de Gorris, trained at Ferrara,[47] resulted in an *arrêt* ordering the dean and regents of the faculty to examine incoming practitioners.[48] Not all the foreign practitioners pursued were university-trained. Some, like the Italian Melchior Daast, were recorded in the faculty's minutes in 1527 as unlettered. However, it is clear from an examination of the origins of practitioners pursued by the faculty that concerns about non-Paris-trained providers influenced prosecutions in the sixteenth century, certainly more than the gender of the practitioner appears to have done.

Analysing the prosecutions of the faculty is only one part of the equation; it is important to examine also which practitioners they were *not* pursuing. There were many types of female medical service providers whose work did not interest the faculty at all. We find no sick nurses or child-care workers pursued by the physicians, though in both cases many of their patients (the elderly, the dying and the very young) must have had very high mortality rates, and certainly neither group claimed any university training for their practices. Moreover, no woman whose primary medical work was midwifery was prosecuted by the faculty.

Elsewhere, Monica H. Green has considered whether the activities of midwives were seen as medical at all. Certainly physicians from the medieval to the early modern period wrote, circulated and commented upon childbirth in ways that suggest it was indeed a topic of interest to them. Green suggests that 'midwifery's lack of integration into the medieval medical establishment, I would guess, is due to issues of gender stratification rather than a belief that childbirth has nothing to do with medicine'.[49] From our evidence, one particular case may provide an opportunity to understand the attitude, of the Parisian medical faculty at least, towards midwives and their medical activities.

In 1423, the faculty pursued a case against a practitioner Jean de Dompremi, who, according to the faculty, was a weaver by trade, unable to read either Latin or French, and had no textual basis whatsoever to his practice.[50] His medicine appears to have involved among other things obstetrical work. Dompremi claimed among his medical successes

> a woman of this town who was pregnant, whom he names, the physicians were unhappy about it, because they had visited her for a long time and could see no remedy but to open the said woman to save the child. And yet Dompremi healed her and she is in good health and her child is alive.[51]

The physicians, however, focused their case on the basis that 'a physician should be cleric and expert, but Dompremi ... is a weaver and cannot read French or Latin and has no books ... And even if he has some language and knowledge of *venterie* [obstetrics], it is worthless and he is neither a cleric nor expert'.[52]

In his defence in December 1423, Dompremi claimed that

> there are several and more in Paris, more than one hundred, who practised and practise, men and women not graduates, and we have seen master Salmon who knows Greek but not Latin, and others who practise like La Calabre who has cured illnesses, which the physicians have not known how to, and there are *arrêts* for La Gausse and others whom one has allowed to practise, notwithstanding the contradiction of the physicians. And it is not the prerogative of the *official* to judge this matter which is secular and laic, and proceeds against the public good.[53]

In response, the faculty reiterated its claims that Dompremi lacked the art and science of medicine, accused him of performing abortions and then explained why practitioners such as La Calabre were not prosecuted: 'if Calabre and others concern themselves to visit pregnant women, it is an affair of women to know this, according to the rights of *ventre inspiciendo*, it does not interfere with the facts of medicine principally, and there are prohibitions made by *arrêts* here against those women who would want to intervene in it'.[54] Thus, at first glance, the faculty appeared to promote a position that midwifery was not medicine. While this may seem to contradict Green's suggestions above, I think she is right to point out the gender element involved. For it is clear in the faculty's statements and actions that midwifery was only non-medical when it was performed by women. When midwifery became a licensed enterprise in Paris during the sixteenth century, the medical faculty took no steps to involve themselves in the regulating processes of the women's work nor to offer them instruction as they did for barbers. In the first guild regulations established for the Parisian midwives in 1560, it was the King's chief barber–surgeon who supervised the licensing and oversaw the apprenticeship of new midwives. Examination took place in front of two surgeons, two midwives of the guild and just one doctor.[55]

It appears that women could offer medical help to the elderly, dying, young, and to pregnant women without obstruction by the faculty because these areas of medical work did not compete with their own. So it seems logical that the faculty would be equally unconcerned with women's work in guild-regulated areas. Among the 31 practitioners pursued in 1322 (many of whom appeared to be related), we find several surgeons of both sexes, including 'Johannem cisorem pannorum et Johannam Conversam, ejus uxorem'. 'Margaritam de Ypra cirurgicam Belotam judeam Johannam conversam' are all mentioned as fined in the document confirming Jacqueline Felicie's fine in 1322.[56] Yet after barbers, surgeons and apothecaries formed guilds which were supervised by the faculty through inspections and through the examination procedures of new guild members, thereby acknowledging the superiority of the physicians, the faculty did not continue to pursue these practitioners except in exceptional cases.

One such exceptional case that the faculty did pursue involved a female surgical practitioner, Peretta Peronne. In 1411, the surgeons' confraternity of St Damien and St Cosme, then numbering approximately 11 members,[57] sought the faculty's assistance in pursuing Peronne. She had evidently advertised her surgical expertise very publicly through a sign outside her house 'after the manner of a public surgeon'.[58] This act suggests that women (and men) did not necessarily hide their medical work from public display as a result of the prosecution of similar practitioners by the faculty. It may have seemed that the risk of prosecution was quite small given that faculty prosecutions were representative rather than comprehensive. However, since it was this act which drew the surgeons' attention to Peronne's practice, other providers probably did not commonly advertise their skills in such ways. She was ordered to remove the sign and forbidden further practice until she had been examined. Peretta was to deposit her surgical texts at the office of the provost to be examined by physicians, the examiner and the criminal clerk, and she was herself to be interviewed by the physicians in the presence of the examiner, clerk and two surgeons.[59] In her examinations, she argued that she worked for God and that her prosecution was unjust when other women worked in surgery with no interference from the faculty. She argued that she was a well-established and proven practitioner, not an itinerant and dangerous fake. While the case continued, Peretta even asked to carry on her work 'because she has many sick persons or patients under her care, who required essential remedies and visitation, . . . that permission be granted her to visit these sick persons and patients'.[60] In the end, the masters of medicine concluded that she did not know the letter 'A from a faggot' and critiqued her herbal knowledge. The surgeons' case against Peretta was supported by the faculty for many reasons of which misogyny does not seem prominent: not only did it give them the opportunity to establish their superior authority over the surgeons (who needed their powerful influence), it reinstated that knowledge, of both surgery and medicine, rested on 'correct' understanding of textual sources.

If the conclusions drawn from the evidence of the Faculty of Medicine in Paris suggest that women were generally prosecuted in so far as specific medical activities they performed competed with those of physicians, was this attitude to women practitioners similar in other medical faculties in France? By the sixteenth century, a number of cities in France contained universities providing some medical training, including Montpellier, Toulouse, Cahors, Bordeaux and Perpignan in the south, and Angers, Bourges, Caen, Poitiers and Nantes. However the quality of the education they offered was very variable.

By far the biggest rival to Paris of these institutions was the medical faculty in Montpellier, which was older than Paris and probably better known internationally throughout the medieval and early modern period. If the traditions of the university bestowed on the town of Montpellier a conservative flavour in the early modern period relative to other urban centres, its medical faculty was seen to be far more innovative and responsive to modern developments than that of Paris. It introduced anatomy and botany classes some time before they appeared in the Parisian syllabus, and far more of its students embraced the influences of Paracelsianism as physicians.[61] Apart from its more innovative and open syllabus, the university as a whole had undergone structural reforms that had removed some of its ecclesiastical heritage.[62] Moreover, unlike Paris, it accepted Protestants as students and masters.

Given the differences in its mentalities, were there differences in how Montpellier pursued practitioners? Certainly physicians complained about the role of female practitioners in medical work. Laurent Joubert, the chancellor of the Faculty of Medicine at Montpellier, was strongly disapproving of medical services performed by women: 'There are some people who know nothing at all about medicine, as to discourse or reason, such as ignorant women who know not even to read or write, but who have some observations and rules.'[63] Joubert concurred with the typical university position on medicine: a textual-based logic was more important than empirical observation. Clearly another of Joubert's preoccupations was that a provider's alternative remedies might interfere with those he prescribed, thus rendering his own ineffective and his medical authority questionable in the eyes of the patient. He recalled that a doctor 'considering the nature of the illness and the forces of the patient will prescribe the quality of the nourishment better than the most knowledgeable (or rather) the most vain and presumptuous woman in the world'.[64]

Alison Klairmont Lingo's summary of cases against empirics in Montpellier provides material for comparison.[65] Of the ten cases brought between 1532 and 1583, three involved women. In 1533, the wife of a woodworker was accused of poisoning her patient, one Edmond LaBarbe, who was no less than an aide to the royal surgeon Girard. While the faculty might wish to prohibit competitors, it could not prevent even its own adherents in the 'recognised' medical corporations from using their services. The case, brought forward initially by university students, was pursued as a case of witchcraft but no final result is known.[66] In 1557, Claude Jouve, la Calandre, 'a woman empiric and meddling with the art of medicine and surgery',[67] was condemned by the court of the governor of Montpellier in May. The case went on appeal to the *Parlement* of Toulouse but was confirmed in July. Jouve's case prompted a renewal of the decree against illegal practitioners in the same year.[68] In 1581, Besionne, from Castres, was brought before the Faculty of Medicine at Montpellier for illegal practice of medicine, surgery and pharmacy. She was threatened with whipping and banishment should she re-offend.[69]

It is difficult to draw conclusions from such scanty evidence, although it seems that, in Montpellier too, female practitioners were not a disproportionate concern to the faculty. None was involved in child care or midwifery, but rather one was accused of witchcraft (probably as a result of sicknursing) and the others of the competitive practices of surgery and medicine. Of the ten cases, the origins of six practitioners are unknown, although the four who are known were all strangers to Montpellier (Spain, Lyon, Paris and Castres) so we might tentatively conclude that there, too, non-local providers were a concern to the faculty. In Montpellier too, the personality of individuals on the faculty staff was instrumental in pursuing practitioners. Klairmont Lingo suggests that the influence of Laurent Joubert who became chancellor in 1573 is evident in the fact that half of the ten cases were brought after that year. As in Paris, the ability of healers was not central to the prosecutions (the woodworker's wife may be an exception here) but rather, their licensing. In the case of Simon de Challieu, brought before the royal court of Montpellier in 1584, Klairmont Lingo argued that physicians showed no interest in the efficacy of his healing talents but focused on whether he was licensed to practise within the jurisdiction of the Montpellier physicians.[70] Moreover, as in Paris, the Montpellier faculty had support for its prosecution of cases from other local authoritative bodies: the bishop, the governor, the local municipal court as well as the regional *Parlement*, who recognised the public utility of the physicians' surveillance.[71]

Although Avignon was papal, not French, territory during the sixteenth century, it drew French physicians both to practise and teach in the town. The medical faculty there formed part of the papal-established university, but its preoccupations with status over guild-regulated medical work and its policies on other medical practitioners show little difference from those of contemporary French faculties. Statutes drawn up for the town in 1558, with the participation of the medical faculty, appealed to the logic of acting in the public good as a means of establishing superiority over medical competitors. For example, master surgeons, when faced with serious operations such as amputations or incisions, 'in anything that requires the simultaneous use of a regime, bleeding, and purgatives, are to call one or several physicians to prescribe such remedies that are not of the knowledge of surgeons. In this way, individuals suffering such afflictions both dangerous and difficult to treat will be better cared for and more certainly healed.'[72] The same regulations are of particular interest to us here because they set out clearly how the faculty's preoccupation with other practitioners did not by any means encompass the range of medical service providers. The statutes permitted 'all operators without licences in surgery nor the approbation of some master, to operate with their hands, such as drawing the stone, removing cataracts from the eyes, healing hernias or ruptures, with manual operations, pulling teeth and doing other works that they have learnt by the sole means of long experience'.[73] As far as the faculty was concerned, manual operators who claimed no theoretical underpinning to their practice could perform a range of medical procedures without fear of prosecution from the university, or apparently representing any danger to public welfare.

So far our examination of the university's relationship with women as medical practitioners suggests that they were largely concerned to eradicate only those women whose medical services crossed paths with their own. The physicians argued that providers who had not drawn their training from textual knowledge could not 'know' the true science of medicine as they did and might therefore harm rather than heal their patients. However, we have also seen that as well as this argument, a key concern of the physicians was the very real competition that such providers constituted both to their clientele and, by the efficacy of their services, to their claims to provide the correct knowledge of medicine. Despite their public arguments dismissing the value of services provided by 'other' providers, physicians' efforts to bar competing practitioners demonstrates how seriously they respected their challenge.

Moreover, we have seen that the authority of the faculty was by no means perceived by other medical providers as superior to their own. Women whose medical practice competed with that of the faculty refused to accept their injunctions to stop work. Women, like the old woman of Champgaillard, refused to appear before the faculty to discuss their medical work. Others, like Peretta Peronne, expected the faculty to treat them with respect and to honour their medical duty to their patients. We know too from the arguments of both male and female practitioners that many more women practised with no interference from physicians, either because they worked in areas that the faculty did not, or because the faculty could not gather sufficient evidence to pursue a case.

Women and university medicine

The university pursued female practitioners in their own domains of medical competence but who practised with diverse sources of medical knowledge. But what opportunities did the medical faculties provide for women to gain their version of correct medical knowledge and practices? In this section of the chapter, I want to explore how the university interacted with women as students of their forms of medicine. To do so, I will examine what opportunities women had to access university medical learning, read their texts and observe their practices at work. Obviously some (usually elite) women observed physicians at work and developed relationships to doctors and university medicine through their interactions as patients.

Most commentators observe women's lack of access to university education generally throughout the medieval and early modern period. Only Catholic men could attend the Faculty of Medicine in Paris, and although historians have commented on the range of men who did attend its courses, including both poor men on scholarships and some nobles, the majority constituted nonetheless a small cross section of society. If the faculty at Montpellier allowed Protestants to its courses, it too catered to a small number of individuals in the population. Neither of these institutions, nor indeed any of the university medical faculties in France, permitted women as formal students.

Yet we know that a select group of women did have access to observe some aspects of university medicine. Attending the faculty anatomy classes in Montpellier in 1595, Thomas Platter reported on two occasions in his journal seeing women in the audience. 'Sometimes, as I have seen, there are women among the spectators, and they hide their faces behind their masks, especially when the subject is a woman.'[74] 'On the 2nd of December we dissected the body of a woman who had died in the hospital. In her womb she had a tumour as hard as a stone. The autopsy was completed on the 5th, in the presence of some elegant ladies'.[75] The very fact that Platter noted the female presence at dissections suggests that women were not usually present in other medical classes. Platter's description of elegant ladies suggests these women were curious onlookers, rather than practitioners seeking anatomical expertise. Dissections were open to a wider public than other university courses. Dissections could be, in some measure, a public, revenue-raising event for medical faculties: a kind of refined public spectacle in the same vein as public executions. Indeed, the bodies involved in such displays were often those of executed criminals. Medical faculties could allow a certain clientele to witness these classes, charging their guild counterparts a small fee to attend, and permitting the attendance of elite women and some midwives. Medical faculties probably allowed elite women to attend dissections not because of any perception that anatomical knowledge could or should be provided to women, but because they were a curious and paying audience.

However, Laurent Joubert's description of Montpellier's late sixteenth-century dissections suggests that the faculty did see anatomical dissections as an opportunity for female practitioners to learn medical skills. He praised a local matron Gervaise, as 'truly a wise woman and well advised', not by mentioning her practical experience, but commenting that she did 'not fail to attend public anatomies when we have a female to hand'.[76] If dissection afforded a few women the chance to see (but by no means conduct) some university practices, was it possible that other means for accessing university medicine were available to women in physicians' families? Did they, like women in guild-regulated practitioners' families, have opportunities to learn about their male family members' medical work? In particular, did women in physicians' families have access, not available to other women, to university medical texts: the very basis for its alleged superiority over other forms of medical practice? While Chapter 5 will focus on women's reading of medical texts more generally, here I will analyse whether women in physicians' families had increased opportunities to understand university medicine.

Of the 66 Parisian physicians in the sixteenth and seventeenth centuries analysed by Françoise Lehoux, she found 50 had inventoried libraries for which records still remain.[77] Many physicians kept their texts in studies or library rooms. Designating a space particularly for holding texts, including medical literature, may have lessened women's chances to read the material held within it. As Roger Chartier has argued, libraries often had the function of withdrawing its owner from activities and people inside the household.[78] The late sixteenth-century essayist Michel de Montaigne enjoyed an isolated library, in a tower separated from the goings-on of family and domestics: 'I try...to withdraw this one corner from all society, conjugal, filial and civil'.[79] Physicians such as Philibert Guibert even refused to open his medical cabinet for the notaries to inventory, because it contained drugs and compositions he did not want to divulge. Two physicians from the Paris faculty were called upon to make an assessment of its value, but even they did not disclose what was held in the two rooms.[80] Such secrecy surrounding the private household space of a physician might mean that not only the herbs, drugs and instruments but also the books contained within it, might be off limits to others in the family. Lehoux also notes, however, that some physicians held books but no study to contain them, and perhaps here, if the books were readily accessible, other family members could read them.[81] Whether women could peruse the texts held in physicians' homes probably depended on individual relationships in physicians' families, but it seems likely that where medical texts were held within a specific library setting, this was a space set apart from other household members.

When physicians died, however, widows could inherit their medical texts and therefore gain access to university knowledge. Yet Lehoux's survey of the libraries of Parisian physicians' widows suggests that they did not especially retain their husband's medical texts. Only two widows had retained some of the books belonging to their husbands; most held libraries of devotional books or others that the notaries did not bother to describe at all. Since notaries recorded valuable items for inventories it is possible that some widows did retain scrapbooks of medical knowledge, but little of much economic value. Lehoux concludes that widows disposed of texts which they did not think they would read themselves.[82]

Why did widows not retain and want to read medical texts then? We might need to ask whether physicians' wives were in fact capable of reading their texts. University education was transmitted both orally and in written documents, through Latin. This was a language that few women learnt. Although some elite women could have extensive knowledge of Latin and some Greek, the wives of physicians were more commonly of middling, mercantile origins. If they had some learning and literacy, it was unlikely to include Latin sufficient to understand medical texts. Indeed, it was by no means certain that all physicians' wives were literate in the vernacular: as late as 1584–85, the wives of Pierre Ravyn and Pierre Thouzet were both recorded as illiterate in legal documents.[83]

Unlike most university education, medicine had an element that was practical and observable. The work of physicians, their methods of diagnosis, their discussion with patients, made elements of their knowledge observable in ways other university disciplines such as theology or law did not. Did women in physicians' families have exposure to medical work in such ways?

Physicians worked most commonly by attending patients in housecalls. In this way, they differed from guild-regulated medical practitioners such as barbers and apothecaries whom patients consulted in their workshops, which were often located near or in the practitioners' homes. As a consequence, women in barbers' or apothecaries' families might see and hear consultations with patients regularly, but a physicians' wife or daughter was unlikely to do so. The divide in physicians' households between the domestic, female sphere and the public work place of the physician was distinct. Lehoux comments in her chapter concerning the daily life of Parisian physicians' families how different husband and wives' days probably were since his was external or segregated in the library, while her day was almost wholly domestic.[84]

It is interesting and significant to note that marriage patterns among physicians differed from those of guild-regulated medical practitioners. Klairmont Lingo's study of Lyon and Montpellier physicians suggests that they married among their social equals or sought upward social mobility through their marriage to better-placed female partners.[85] In contrast, apothecaries tended to marry among other apothecaries or other medical service providers. For the apothecaries, then, the 'family was the basic unit for professional and social advance.'[86] Lehoux's evidence for Paris bears out a similar pattern. While a large number of physicians do marry daughters of men in medical fields (10 from 29 marriages where the professions of fathers-in-law are known), more married daughters of similar or better social origins in unrelated areas, such as merchants and royal officers.[87] This suggests that, in guild-regulated professions, the connections, utensils and knowledge of a female partner could be essential for establishment in the medical area. For physicians, however, women were not seen to have useful medical knowledge to contribute, nor were they likely to bring to the marriage utensils useful to husbands' work. Physicians' partners were also frequently in their teens at marriage.[88] Some women from medical families might provide connections to clientele and patronage, but physicians backed their own ability to establish such links through their knowledge and practice in marrying women from families in other fields who might bring large dowries or social mobility instead.[89]

Even where physicians did marry into families of other physicians or medical practitioners, it did not appear that the knowledge a woman might bring to the relationship was key. Rather it seems likely that the woman's networks were more important in establishing a young physician's clientele, patronage and networks to apothecaries and other providers. In contrast to guild medical occupations, women in physicians' families had fewer opportunities to observe or understand the work of their husbands, fathers or brothers. Louise Guichard, the wife of the Montpellier medical faculty chancellor, Laurent Joubert, came from a medical family herself. Her brother Jean was a doctor at the University of Montpellier and the *médecin ordinaire* of the king of Navarre.[90] Yet Joubert never made reference to her particular medical knowledge. He did, however, praise the botanical practices of his mother in one of his medical texts. Joubert cited several of her distilled waters, fortified wines and jams as famous across the region.⁹¹ Although he cited his mother as having exceptional herbal expertise, it is not an expertise that he defines as based on university medical knowledge, or indeed through any interaction with learned medicine in her family.

The Du Laurens family shows a similar example. Jeanne du Laurens' father was a doctor at Tarascon, then at Arles; her brother André du Laurens was the premier physician to Henri IV, and a professor of the medical faculty at Montpellier; her brother Charles was a physician at Arles; and her brother Richard practised medicine at Lyon and then Arles. Her mother was the sister of Honoré de Castellan, a professor at the Montpellier medical faculty. Jeanne's memoirs of family life, *Généalogie de Messieurs du Laurens, descrite par moy Jeanne du laurens*, one of the few documents composed by a woman from a medical family, gives no real hint of the existence or extent of medical knowledge that she might have picked up in the household, though this was clearly not the object of the work.⁹² Describing her father's practice she says:

> he had a good method and great care of his patients whom he attended as a rule when they took medicine, rising every morning very early for this reason. And being asked why he took this trouble, he responded that it was to see in what state was the patient and to interrogate him as to how he slept the previous night, for fear that should some accident arise, he had not taken his medicine, saying often that one must be concerned with this on all occasions, if one wanted to acquit oneself well, when it concerned many times the life of a man.⁹³

Du Laurens' memories of her father's housecalls to patients seems to confirm that women in medical household may not have had opportunities to observe the daily practices of the physician who visited patients in their own homes.

If the university appears to have provided few opportunities for women to explore its knowledge of medicine, there is some evidence that women as members of physicians' families could be involved in some of the ritual activities associated with the corporate medical body. In the Parisian medical faculty, when a physician died, twelve other physicians attended the funeral to represent the faculty. Physicians trained at the faculty were also entitled to a mass held in the faculty chapel, where staff and students were in attendance.⁹⁴ In such ways, the corporate body of physicians in Paris, the faculty, stood by the widow of one of its own.

In towns without university faculties, physicians often formed a college or corporate body, which acted as a regulatory power authorising the practice of university medicine in that town, and was often called upon to oversee the work of guild-regulated medicine. In Amiens, the physicians had a responsibility to inspect the offices of apothecaries each year and to oversee examination and induction of new apothecaries: roles that accredited them with authority over a hierarchy of medical providers. The 1576 statutes of the apothecaries stated for the feast of St Luke the compulsory attendance of 'all the physicians and apothecaries with their wives and widows of physicians and apothecaries'.[95] Women in medical providers' families could partake in, indeed were required to attend, the ritual ceremonies of the medical corporate body. Such ceremonies were important, not only in the formation of a collective consciousness among the practitioners but also as a public display of their status in the community: a status from which women as well as men in medical families could benefit. The statutes also demanded as a corollary to this that 'the costs of the church, as much on that day as during the year, each will contribute to it, and widows in equal portion'.[96] Although this probably disadvantaged widows financially compared to their male confraternity members with higher incomes, it also gave women a sense of contributing on an equal basis to them. As we have seen, women in guilds fought for the right to contribute fees to the corporation, most likely because of the attendant status which accompanied the act.

Moreover, the 1576 statutes clearly allowed for wives as well as widows of physicians and apothecaries who practised at Amiens to attend the banquets associated with induction ceremonies. As part of the proceedings of the induction, the candidate owed a general banquet or dinner for all the physicians, apothecaries, their wives and widows. What is fascinating about this document is the explicit manner in which university (and university-approved) medicine was gender segregated. While women as wives and widows could share in the banquet and listen to the speech of the most senior physician, they were not invited when the new inductee was required to demonstrate his medical knowledge.[97] Thus while corporate bodies in towns without medical faculties might provide women more means to partake in the company's celebrations, identity and status, its medical knowledge was still guarded from them.

In conclusion, it is evident that 'the university' as an institution certainly restricted women both consciously and unconsciously, as students, daughters, wives and widows, from most of the means by which they might gain some understanding of university medicine. My focus in this study is on the experiences of women but it is also important to note that there were similarly many men too who were restricted from such knowledge, though for different reasons. I do not think that the evidence presented here demonstrates that the Faculty of Medicine, at least in Paris, had any particular motivation to exclude female practitioners *per se*, and most women continued to practise medical services unhindered. It seems that the activities of the faculty, in the restricted access to its learning and practices as well as its limited prosecutions, had little impact or significance on the medical work with which many female practitioners were involved. The next chapter will investigate an area of women's medical work which barely impinged on that of the faculty, that of hospital nursing.

Notes

1 The details of her case can be found in *Chartularium Universitatis Parisiensis*, ed. Henri Denifle, vol. 2 (1891) (Brussels: Culture et Civilisation, 1964), no. 811–16 and are summarised by Pearl Kibre, 'The Faculty of Medicine at Paris, charlatanism, and unlicensed medical practices in the later middle ages', *Bulletin of the History of Medicine*, 27:1 (1953), pp. 8–11.

2 Iain M. Lonie, 'The 'Paris Hippocratics': teaching and research in Paris in the second half of the sixteenth century', in A. Wear, R. K. French and I. M. Lonie (eds), *The Medical Renaissance of the Sixteenth Century* (Cambridge: Cambridge University Press, 1985), pp. 155–74, p. 157.

3 *Commentaires de la Faculté de Médecine de l'Université de Paris*, vol. 1 *(1395–1516)* ed. C. A. E. Wickersheimer (Paris: Imprimerie Nationale, 1915); vol. 2 *(1516–1560)* ed. Marie Concasty (Paris: Imprimerie Nationale, 1964).

4 H. Denifle (ed.), *Chartularium Universitatis Parisiensis*, 4 vols (1891–99) (Brussels: Culture et Civilisation, 1964), and *Index Chronologicus Chartarum pertinentium ad historiam Universitatis Parisiensis ad ejus originibus ad finem decimi sexti sæculi*, ed. C. Jourdain (Paris, 1862) (Brussels: Culture et Civilisation, 1966).

5 There are a number of excellent works devoted to the Parisian medical faculty: see particularly the introductions by Wickersheimer and Concasty to the *Commentaires* and Cornelius O'Boyle, *The Art of Medicine: Medical Teaching at the University of Paris, 1250–1400* (Leiden: Brill, 1998).

6 Françoise Lehoux, *Le Cadre de vie des médecins parisiens aux XVIe et XVIIe siècles* (Paris: A. and J. Picard, 1976).

7 O'Boyle, *The Art of Medicine*, p. 266.

8 *Ibid.*, p. 269.

9 Vern L. Bullough, *The Development of Medicine as a Profession: The Contribution of the Medieval University to Modern Medicine* (Basel: S. Karger, 1966).

10 Alison Klairmont Lingo, *The Rise of Medical Practitioners in Sixteenth-Century France: The Case of Lyon and Montpellier* (PhD, University of California-Berkeley, 1980), p. 22.

11 *Ibid.*, pp. 27-8.
12 Wear, French and Lonie (eds), *The Medical Renaissance of the Sixteenth Century* (Cambridge: Cambridge University Press, 1985), p. xi.
13 See especially the *Chart. univ. Paris.* vols 1-4, Pearl Kibre, *Scholarly Privileges in the Middle Ages: The Rights, Privileges and Immunities of Scholars and Universities at Bologna, Padua, Paris and Oxford* (Cambridge, Mass.: Medieval Academy of America, 1962); as well as Kibre, 'The Faculty of Medicine at Paris'.
14 Chart, I, 488-90, in L. Thorndike, *University Records and Life in the Middle Ages* (New York: Octagon Books, 1971), p. 83.
15 *Ibid.*, p. 84.
16 *Ibid.*, p. 84.
17 O'Boyle, 'Surgical texts and social contexts: physicians and surgeons in Paris, c. 1270 to 1430', in Luis Garcia-Ballester, Roger French, Jon Arrizabalaga and Andrew Cunningham (eds), *Practical Medicine from Salerno to the Black Death* (Cambridge: Cambridge University Press, 1994), p. 173.
18 MMCLXXIII, *Index Chronologicus Chartarum*, p. 410.
19 MMLXXXVI, *Ibid.*, p. 398.
20 Alison Klairmont Lingo, 'Empirics and charlatans in early modern France: the genesis of the classification of the 'Other' in medical practice', *Journal of Social History*, 19 (1985-86), pp. 583-603.
21 MDCCIV, *Index Chronologicus Chartarum*, pp. 339-40.
22 MMLXXXIII, *Ibid.*, p. 396.
23 See Danielle Jacquart, *Le Milieu médical en France du XIIe au XVe siècle* (Geneva: Droz, 1981), pp. 246-7 and her 'Medical practice in Paris in the first half of the fourteenth century', in Garcia-Ballester *et al.*, *Practical Medicine from Salerno to the Black Death*.
24 Allen G. Debus, *The French Paracelsians: The Chemical Challenge to Medical and Scientific Tradition in Early Modern France* (Cambridge: Cambridge University Press, 1991), pp. 49-50.
25 *Commentaires (1516-1560)*, p. 2.
26 *Ibid.*, p. 35.
27 *Ibid.*, p. 180.
28 *Ibid.*, p. 35.
29 *Ibid.*, p. 194.
30 *Ibid.*, p. 479.
31 *Ibid.*, p. lxix.
32 *Ibid.*, pp. 351-2.
33 See *Chart. Univ. Paris.*, vol. 2.
34 Chart, III, 16-17 in Thorndike, *University Records*, p. 235.
35 *Ibid.*, p. 236.
36 André du Breil, *La Police de l'art et science de medecine, contenant la refutation des erreurs, & insignes abus, qui s'y commettent pour le iourd'huy* (Paris: Leon Cavellat, 1580). See also Klairmont Lingo, 'Empirics and charlatans in early modern France', pp. 583-603.
37 Klairmont Lingo, 'Empirics and charlatans in early modern France', p. 596.
38 Du Breil, *La Police de l'art et science de medecine*, p. 89.

39 *Ibid.*, p. 90.
40 *Commentaires (1395–1516)*, p. 490.
41 *Ibid.*, p. 529.
42 *Commentaires (1516–1560)*, p. 479.
43 *Chart. univ. Paris*, t.2, nos. 811–16, pp. 255–67.
44 Monica H. Green, 'Women's medical practice and health care in medieval Europe', in Judith M. Bennett *et al.* (eds), *Sisters and Workers in the Middle Ages* (Chicago: Chicago University Press, 1989), pp. 61–2.
45 *Commentaires (1516–1560)*, p. lxxi.
46 *Ibid.*, p. lxxii.
47 MDXLV, *Index Chronologicus Chartarum*, p. 319.
48 MDXLVII, *Ibid.*, p. 319.
49 Monica H. Green, 'Documenting medieval women's medical practice', in Garcia-Ballester, French, Arrizabalaga and Cunningham (eds), *Practical Medicine from Salerno to the Black Death*, pp. 340–1, n. 72.
50 *Chart. univ. Paris*, vol. 4, p. 426.
51 *Ibid.*, p. 425.
52 *Ibid.*, p. 426.
53 *Ibid.*, p. 427.
54 *Ibid.*, p. 427.
55 Richard L. Petrelli, 'The regulation of French midwifery during the Ancien Régime', *Journal of the History of Medicine* (1971), pp. 276–92, pp. 277–8.
56 *Chart. univ. Paris*, vol. 2, p. 267.
57 O'Boyle, 'Surgical texts and social contexts', p. 182, n. 79.
58 Further details of this case can be found in Geneviève Dumas, 'Les femmes et les pratiques de la santé dans le "Registre des plaidoiries du Parlement de Paris, 1364–1427"', *Canadian Bulletin of Medicine*, 13 (1996), pp. 13–27.
59 Chart IV, 198–99, in Thorndike, *University Records*, p. 290.
60 *Ibid.*, p. 290.
61 For details on Paracelsianism in France, see Debus, *The French Paracelsians*.
62 Klairmont Lingo, *The Rise of Medical Practitioners*, p. 119.
63 Laurent Joubert, *La Médecine et le régime de santé, des erreurs populaires et propos vulgaires* (Bordeaux: Simon Millanges, 1578) ed. Madeleine Tiollais, vol. 1 (Paris: L'Harmattan, 1997), pp. 163–4.
64 *Ibid.*, p. 152.
65 Klairmont Lingo, *The Rise of Medical Practitioners*, pp. 254–5.
66 Louis Dulieu, *La Médecine à Montpellier: la Renaissance*, vol. 2 (Avignon: Les Presses universelles, 1979), p. 268 and Klairmont Lingo, *The Rise of Medical Practitioners*, pp. 224–5.
67 J. Barbot, *Les Chroniques de la Faculté de Médecine de Toulouse du treizième au vingtième siècle*, vol. 1: *1229–1793* (Toulouse: Charles Dirion, 1905), p. 74.
68 Klairmont Lingo, *The Rise of Medical Practitioners*, p. 222.
69 Dulieu, *La Médecine à Montpellier: la Renaissance*, vol. 2, p. 268.
70 Klairmont Lingo, 'Empirics and charlatans in early modern France', p. 592.
71 For an interesting argument about the faculty's lobbying to the king to avoid the *taille* on the basis of public utility, see James Eastgate Brink, 'A tax loop-hole in the sixteenth century: the battle over the claim of the medical school of Montpellier to

exemptions from the taille', *Proceedings of the Annual Meeting of the Western Society for French History*, 3 (1975), pp. 2–12.

72 Victorin Laval, *Histoire de la Faculté de Médecine d'Avignon: ses origines, son organisation et son enseignement (1303–1791)*, vol. 1 (Paris: E. Lechevalier, 1889), p. 78.

73 *Ibid.*, vol. 1, p. 78.

74 *Journal of a Younger Brother: The Life of Thomas Platter as a Medical Student in Montpellier at the Close of the Sixteenth Century*, ed. Sean Jennett (London: Frederick Muller, 1963), pp. 36–7.

75 *Ibid.*, p. 54.

76 Laurent Joubert, *La Médecine et le régime de santé*, vol. 2, p. 234.

77 Lehoux, *Le Cadre de vie des médecins parisiens*, p. 205.

78 Roger Chartier, 'The practical impact of writing', in Roger Chartier (ed.), *A History of Private Life* vol. 3, *Passions of the Renaissance*, trans. A. Goldhammer (Cambridge, Mass.: The Belknap Press of the Harvard University Press, 1989), p. 136.

79 *Ibid.*, pp. 135–6.

80 Lehoux, *Le Cadre de vie des médecins parisiens*, p. 443.

81 *Ibid.*, p. 205.

82 *Ibid.*, p. 462.

83 *Ibid.*, p. 97.

84 See *Ibid.*, pp. 515–23.

85 Klairmont Lingo, *The Rise of Medical Practitioners*, p. 53.

86 *Ibid.*, p. 60.

87 Lehoux, *Le Cadre de vie des médecins parisiens*, p. 24.

88 *Ibid.*, p. 30.

89 Margaret Pelling offers an interesting contrast to this data for her study of English doctors at this period. She argues that at a time when university medicine was based around the domestic setting, moving into homes through physicians' housecalls, and compromised by congruences with stereotypes of women's work, physicians responded to the feminisation of their profession by a rejection of marriage, a pattern of anti-natalism and increased celibacy. Although university medicine in France had developed from a clerical base, indeed students of the Parisian medical faculty were only permitted to be married after 1542, the available evidence suggests celibacy was not a dominant pattern. Only 8 of the 66 physicians surveyed by Lehoux were single in the period 1522–1660. See Pelling's 'The women of the family? Speculations around early modern British physicians', *Social History of Medicine*, 8:3 (1995), pp. 383–401 and 'Compromised by gender: the role of the male medical practitioner in early modern England', in Hilary Marland and Margaret Pelling (eds), *The Task of Healing: Medicine, Religion and Gender in England and the Netherlands, 1450–1800* (Rotterdam: Erasmus Publishing, 1996), pp. 101–33.

90 Evelyne Berriot-Salvadore, *Les Femmes dans la société française de la Renaissance* (Geneva: Droz, 1990), p. 175.

91 Laurent Joubert, *La Grande Chirurgie de M. Gui Chauliac* (Lyon: Estienne Michel, 1580), p. 28.

92 *Généalogie de Messieurs du Laurens, descrite par moy Jeanne du Laurens, veufve à M. Gleyse, & couchée nayvement en ces termes*, ed. Charles de Ribbe, *Une famille au XVIe siècle* (Paris: Joseph Albanel, 1868).

93 *Ibid.*, pp. 47–8.

94 Lehoux, *Le Cadre de vie des médecins parisiens*, p. 435.
95 *Recueil des monuments inédits de l'histoire du tiers état: première série, chartes, coutumes, actes municipaux, statuts des corporations d'arts et metiers des villes et communes de France, region du nord*, ed. Augustin Thierry, vol. 2 (Paris: Firmin-Didot, 1853), p. 849.
96 Ibid., p. 850.
97 Ibid., p. 847.

3

Hospital nursing by women religious: the Hôtel-Dieu in Paris

THIS CHAPTER will focus on the nursing work of women in late fifteenth- and early sixteenth-century hospitals. The sixteenth century was a period of great change where the organisation of hospitals shifted from ecclesiastical control to one of the many poor relief services managed by municipal councils. Most of the work on early modern hospitals examines the changes in administration, from ecclesiastical to municipal,[1] and the resistance to these moves at the local level.[2] But how much did this shift affect medical provision in hospitals? In particular what effects did it have on the medical services provided by women? Marie-Claude Dinet-Lecomte has critiqued the work of perhaps the best known historian of French hospitals, Jean Imbert, for his almost exclusive focus on the perspectives of administrators in the history of the early modern hospitals. She argues that the sisters too need to be studied as an indispensable part of the hospital equation.[3] As studies of women's nursing in early modern France increase, almost all of these focus on the new nursing orders founded in the seventeenth century, such as the Daughters of Charity created by St Vincent de Paul in 1633.[4] In this chapter, I want to examine religious women's work as nursing staff in the Hôtel-Dieu in Paris during the early sixteenth century, a period that allows us to understand how the change from ecclesiastical to lay governors affected provision of their medical services.

There were complex issues surrounding women's participation in the medical realm as nursing staff. The nuns of the Hôtel-Dieu of Paris were involved in a range of medical practices that required them to have knowledge of both diagnosis and treatment of illness, to care for patients and to administer treatment prescribed by the hospital's physician. Yet they had great difficulties in having their work recognised as medical, in a period when women's nursing role was so naturalised as a part of feminine nature and as part of their sworn religious duties that it often went unrecognised as a vocation or occupation. Although even the nuns themselves did not clearly articulate their work as a vocation to nurse, they expressed a perception that their type of care-giving work was unique, specialist and different to that performed by other women. However, even in recent histories, the work of the nursing staff is still segregated from that of other medical staff such as doctors and surgeons. Jean Imbert, in his recent 1993 work *Le Droit hospitalier de l'Ancien Régime*, distinguishes between the hospital personnel, which includes the nursing staff, and the medical personnel. Was this a universal perception of contemporaries: administrators, patients and women religious alike?

The documents with which this chapter is concerned encompass a time period from 1480 until 1539. I have deliberately selected such a period, in order to demonstrate that the difficulties and conflicts that women faced in pursuing their nursing work were not issues related to a single 'regime' or a particular prioress. Furthermore, the period from 1480 to 1539 marks a significant phase in the history of the Hôtel-Dieu. In 1505 by *arrêt* of the *Parlement* of Paris, the temporal administration of the Hôtel-Dieu ceased to be governed by the chapter of Nôtre-Dame, at their request, and was placed under the control of a bureau composed of eight bourgeois of Paris.[5] The documents studied here, therefore, involved the management of the work of nuns by both religious and lay authorities.

Religious women's work in the Hôtel-Dieu

The Hôtel-Dieu in Paris, like most in early modern France, was a medical sphere administered and governed on a daily basis by women. Although most hospitals of this kind had a male supervisor, and brothers who confessed the poor and sick as they arrived at the Hôtel-Dieu, as well as a male governing body in either lay administrators or a chapter head, the vast majority of the health-care work in these institutions was performed by women. In the Hôtel-Dieu in Paris, nuns greatly outnumbered the male staff, as one 1481 document indicates: 'they have twenty religious brothers, forty veiled nuns and thirty novices serving the patients'[6] as well as a number of domestic staff. Most large hospitals in France were run by religious orders who followed some form of the Augustinian rule. Many had adapted and developed the rule with their own specific statutes.[7] The accounts of the Hôtel-Dieu in Paris indicate that, upon profession, nuns swore to the particular statutes of the

Hôtel-Dieu, not to the Augustinian rule generally. Not all hospitals were run directly by religious orders. Often in the countryside, the staff of small Maisons-Dieu took no vows, and could be married.[8] At the Hôtel-Dieu in Chinon, a single maid was responsible for the everyday care of the patients until the early seventeenth century.[9] Similarly, in the Maison-Dieu at Châteaudun, nursing the patients and administration of the hospital were just a few of the duties of the maid.[10]

The prioress occupied a powerful and controlling position at the head of the daily organisation of the Hôtel-Dieu in Paris.[11] The seventy or so nuns and novices who lived there were answerable only to the prioress within the hospital, and to the governing body outside of it. The positions of prioress and master were independent of each other, as more than one record in the Hôtel-Dieu made clear.[12] As Ernest Coyecque has demonstrated, the prioress dealt directly with the chapter, presented her own accounts (with an impressive budget encompassing the massive task of constant replacement of the linen), had her own seal and managed her rural and Parisian domains herself.[13] The prioress' authority was not unique to the Hôtel-Dieu in Paris, as a survey of other hospitals' statutes demonstrates.[14] As Jean Imbert has argued, the prioress of some regional hospitals held so much power that the position of master seems redundant.[15]

It was the prioress, sisters and novices who were primarily responsible for the care and well-being of the Hôtel-Dieu's patients, be they poor or ill. In the 1482 statutes and declarations, 'to administer necessities to the poor patients, and nurse and visit them in their illnesses and bury them . . . there are at present fifty five patients, men and women: forty professed nuns and twenty two novices are appointed to them'.[16] The nuns' nursing work was divided into specialised areas. In the linen room were four sisters and the prioress. In the convalescents' room, Saint-Thomas, there were three sisters and a novice; in Saint-Denis where those with light illnesses or injuries were received, the staff consisted of two sisters and a novice. In the infirmary, for those seriously ill, were four sisters and three novices; in the *Salle Neuve*, or New Room, set aside for female patients, worked three sisters and three novices. The great laundry was run by six sisters and three novices, and in the smaller laundry, there were three sisters and three novices. Three sisters and three novices were appointed to night rounds, replaced at 6 a.m. by the daytime sisters; in the room for pregnant and newly delivered mothers was one sister; in the accounts room two sisters; two further sisters managed the alms boxes, two sisters minded the house in the daytime, and one further sister worked at the press-house.[17]

The nuns progressed through these specialisations until they had expertise in a range of care-giving and administrative domains. One aged sister demonstrates well the model of cumulative experience women gained in doing so:

> during her time she has had charge of all the offices of the said house and hospital ordained to the nuns from ancient times, from the smaller laundry to the great laundry, as *poulliere* which is she who presses the robes, apothicaress, *chevetayne*, which is the office in charge of the services and treatment of the poor, as well as other charges and offices of the said place... [including] the infirmary... where she has been for twenty-five years.[18]

Such experience was recognised in one position requiring some expertise in a range of illnesses: that of the *sœur portière*. Ordinarily this position was filled by an older sister who 'sends the patients that she received into the various rooms and to various *chevetaines* to be treated according to their illness'.[19] It was the *sœur portière*'s duty to assess the gravity of the patient's illness or situation, and to determine to which room the patient should be admitted, skills that required considerable training and knowledge.

Much of the nuns' daily work consisted of hard and demanding labour. Such was the view Jehan Henry portrayed in his stylised account of the life of those who worked at the Hôtel-Dieu, in the *Livre de vie active de l'Hôtel-Dieu de Paris*. Henry was in a position to know firsthand the challenges of managing the Hôtel-Dieu: he was twice one of its governors, from 1471–79 and in 1482. Dedicated to Perrenelle Hélène, a nun in the Hôtel-Dieu, the text was composed at the beginning of the period under consideration in this chapter, around 1480.

> The work in this house is extremely taxing, as quite often here day must become night, and night day, so the sick poor can be tended ... cleaned up, washed, put to bed, bathed, dried, fed, given drinks, carried from one bed to another and lifted; so beds can be made and remade, personal linen washed out every day in clean water and cloths warmed to wrap around the patients' feet; so every week between eight and nine hundred sheets can be laundered, rinsed out in clean water and put in the wash tub; so ashes can be kindled and wood thrown into the furnace; so the sheets can be washed in the River Seine, whether it is freezing, windy or raining, then hung out on walk-ways in summer or dried by a great fire in winter and then folded up; so the dead can be buried, and other innumerable, laborious and exhausting services can be performed ... Some patients, hard to look after and impossible to please, abuse [the nurse] with hostile

and defamatory language, while others, in a frenzy brought on by sickness, strike and wound her, and others pull at her clothing.[20]

Although the account was designed to reinforce the notion that the active life of a nun was one of hardship and suffering in imitation of Christ, it demonstrates well the range of tasks performed by the nuns in their daily work.

Such was the work of the Hôtel-Dieu female staff. However, there were also other medical staff adjunct to the Hôtel-Dieu, including 'several surgeons, barbers, physicians, all salaried by the Hôtel-Dieu to visit and heal each day the patients in need of a surgeon'.[21] That surgeons and other medical practitioners were actually visiting on a daily basis seems doubtful, since in 1536, in attempts to improve medical provision at the hospital, *Parlement* demanded that the governors elect both a doctor and apothecary to visit the patients once a week to prescribe treatments and medication.[22] Occupying a position of apparently lesser importance was the midwife: she was named among the servants of the Hôtel-Dieu staff. The room for newly delivered mothers was beneath the *Salle Neuve*, 'for it is reasonable and a most suitable thing that pregnant women are in an enclosed, secret and out of the way place and not visible like the other patients'.[23] The midwife was paid per delivery, and assisted by a female servant,[24] possibly an apprentice. It was she who, in conjunction with the *dame des accouchées*, the nun in charge of this room, determined whether a pregnant woman had reached the eighth month, from which time she could be admitted. From then on, she could not leave or receive visitors. The room was one of the few places where even the nuns had limited access, forbidden to enter the room unless accompanied by 'an honest matron' for their moral wellbeing.[25]

Given that physicians and apothecaries only visited the hospital once a week after 1536, and probably somewhat less frequently before, a great deal of the administration of these medical practitioners' orders lay in the hands of female medical personnel who cared for the patients around the clock. This did not mean that nuns and novices carried out the same functions as physicians: nuns' training was practical and lacked the theoretical underpinnings of the university-trained physicians. For example, the *sœur portière's* duty was not to determine the nature of the patient's illness, though she may well have recognised it from her experience, but only to assess its gravity. Equally, when a pharmacy was installed in 1495 and staffed by two sisters, their role was not to prescribe medication but to prepare their prescriptions according to the physician or apothecary's orders, although this too required specific pharmaceutical knowledge and experience. Clearly the religious women gained medical knowledge and practices from their experiences, but contemporaries perceived these to be different from the textual knowledge of physicians and apothecaries.

Women's work as nurses in early sixteenth-century hospitals displayed aspects of curing, caring and hygiene that today might be separated as the work of physicians, nursing personnel and cleaning staff. They diagnosed and treated (sometimes without intervention by surgeons, apothecaries or physicians), nursed and attended the needs of the patients, as well as cleaned and laundered. All of these functions brought them into direct and everyday contact with the patients.

The problems

Despite the picture of harmonious co-operation that Jehan Henry's description sought to present, all was not satisfactory between 1480 and 1539 at the Hôtel-Dieu. The second half of the fifteenth century had been marked by an active policy of hospital reform across France which regrouped and consolidated small hospitals, and created large specialised establishments. At Montpellier, the small inner-city hospitals were closed and a new larger one opened in the outskirts of the town.[26] In 1478, when the Hôtel-Dieu in Lyon had shown itself incapable of handling the crisis during the plague, it was officially taken over by the town council. All ecclesiastical links were severed in the bull of 1480, and the city council passed over its management to four bourgeois of the town.[27]

The sixteenth century was to see a royal push towards lay administration, principally, it claimed, in response to corruption of hospital management and defraud of resources destined for the poor. In 1545 the edict of St Germain-en-Laye complained of the abuses of hospital revenues and ordered judges to have hospital governors show them the accounts.[28] In 1547, commissioners were created whose role was to oversee hospital management and accounts.[29] In 1561, the crown decreed that governance of all hospitals, not just those with known problems, would be confined to two lay administrators, to be elected every three years. Thus, in the sixteenth century, the crown continued a policy of renovation of the hospital order in France. Increasingly, government officials sought to close smaller hospitals in order to make way for larger, centralised institutions offering specialised treatment and care. 'To justify their closure, charges of corruption and inefficiency were regularly levelled at small, local hospitals by crown officials.'[30] However, the efficacy of this royal policy was far from evident. Change was hampered by the non-implementation of edicts, as well as contradictory edicts from the crown. There were also conflicting ecclesiastical prescriptions complicated by the debate over implementation of the decrees of the Council of Trent.[31] Local and rural areas objected to what were seen as urban policies. As Daniel Hickey has argued, many of these older, local arenas of care demonstrated a 'long term grass roots effort to resist the forces of centralization and rationalization'.[32]

As early as the 1490s there were clear conflicts in the Hôtel-Dieu in Paris between the administration and resources provided by the governors, and the day-to-day management provided by its staff. In a complaint made to *Parlement* in 1498, the personnel protested that they could no longer care for the poor as they saw fit since the chapter heads had altered the arrangements for the services of the kitchens: 'for lack of bakers, cooks and others that have been put out, the poor wait for treatment and are in great poverty and misery'.[33] Furthermore, they complained that it was not the role of the governors to punish the staff of the Hôtel-Dieu themselves: 'the punishment of monks and nuns belongs to the master *primo loco*, as it is for the monks, and the prioress for the nuns, without the chapter having the practice to give correction to the nuns or novices'.[34] Having heard complaints from both sides, in April 1498 *Parlement* produced an *arrêt* in which it demanded that the master and prioress 'look carefully into faults . . . and that they punish without any concealment' and that 'all the brothers, sisters and novices of the hospital obey from now on . . . according to the regulations of the house.' The *arrêt* equally enjoined the chapter to provide such good order and provision to the Hôtel-Dieu that hereafter 'no complaints or grievances come to the Court.'[35] In 1505 the chapter of Nôtre-Dame had encountered so many difficulties in controlling the personnel of the Hôtel-Dieu that it requested the municipality of Paris assume its control.

Problems continued, however, under the new management. In 1525, Jean Briçonnet approached *Parlement* about creating distinct hospitals in Paris catering to particular illnesses. To support his case, he described a vision of disorganisation at the Hôtel-Dieu where 'the disorder is so great that they put twelve and fifteen to a bed'.[36] In 1528, the difficulties of swelling numbers with 'the poor in a pitiful state' in the Hôtel-Dieu forced the personnel themselves once again to go to court 'to remonstrate the many problems that arise each day at the Hôtel-Dieu because of the great multitude of poor who flocked there, even little children;

who because of the small space in which they are constrained to stay and for lack of air, die each day like animals'.[37] The staff proposed that the *Parlement* speed up a trial between the Hôtel-Dieu and the chapter of Nôtre-Dame concerning a house that could be used for their expansion.

When, in 1534, the governors attempted to outsource the services of the cellar and kitchens, and the accounting, the staff went to *Parlement* in defence of their abilities to manage these functions.[38] They argued that to guarantee the smooth operation of the Hôtel-Dieu they needed to retain these services, 'for the good and utility of the Hôtel-Dieu'.[39] These were core offices of the Hôtel-Dieu, which according to its statutes, 'secular people are not capable of holding'.[40] In particular, they argued that the governors had vested interests in the privatisation of these services: 'it is rather to deprive [the staff] of the knowledge of the assets of the Hôtel-Dieu than for the charity that they claim to have'.[41] As Chapter 5 examines, food was judged a primary component in medical and health care by both the medical and non-medical community. To understand the emphasis placed upon the supply and preparation of the patients' portions, one must remember that food was the primary medication given to the patients of the Hôtel-Dieu. Since many of the Hôtel-Dieu's patients were not sick but primarily poor, this was probably the most important care and treatment that the Hôtel-Dieu could provide for them. Therefore, to have this service removed from their control, was a major diminution of the staff's ability to give care to the patients.

By May 1535, the canons delegated by the chapter recommended that in order to carry out reform in the convent, Hélène la Petite, the prioress, would have to be removed along with the sub-prioress and the master. She was to be replaced by Perrenelle la Tache, with Johanna de Costes as sub-prioress. However, the situation only worsened, suggesting the problems were not related to the particular management of a few personalities, but were, rather, inherent. By September, the Court ordered the chapter to investigate and produce new regulations for the hospital within a month.[42] In the enquiries that followed over a two-week period in the Hôtel-Dieu, the new prioress and sub-prioress did not hesitate to raise an important number of issues in their complaints about the governors.

La Tache who had been at the Hôtel-Dieu thirty years by 1535 when interviewed about the treatment of the poor, complained primarily about the insufficiency of the portions. She remonstrated that 'since Easter, the poor had only had mutton and beef and no veal nor chicken, as the governors had ordered, and they could not administer sufficient wine, and it was often full of water'.[43] Marie Gilles, a sister with seventeen years of experience, remarked upon the present portions, saying 'often the portions for the poor are so small that she dares not present them to the patients'.[44] Jacqueline la Vielzville noticed that 'the baker often provides such hard bread that the patients cannot eat it'.[45]

In their complaints, the sisters were supported by the Hôtel-Dieu's male staff. One of the priests, Claudius Parius, confirmed that 'the portions are so small and not sufficient for the number of poor, and the nuns had complained to the governors of it, when they came into the house and saw for themselves the portions'.[46] The sub-prioress Johanna de Costes had already received a dismissive response from one of the governors, Jean Briçonnet, whose criticisms of the Hôtel-Dieu's effectiveness had already been apparent in 1525, when she had raised problems about the patients' meal sizes.

> She says also that seeing the pity and necessity of the poor patients, she was constrained sometimes to buy marlings, fishing nets to do it, to sustain the poor, and asked for money from her relatives and others ... and said that one day the president Brissonnet arrived at the office of the room Saint-Denis, where she was complaining that the poor had only a little herring for the day, and he said to her these words: "When I'm at the table of herrings, I take the smallest ones".[47]

When Marie Gilles complained to the cellarer that she did not have enough wine for the patients, he 'locked her in the store-cupboard with one of the servants of the house, where she remained for about half an hour'.[48] Gilles was furious, not least for the damage it could do to her reputation of chastity and of all the sisters at the Hôtel-Dieu.

Another complaint was the lack of heating provided by the governors in the Hôtel-Dieu. Johanna de Costes remembered 'that the two last winters ... there were in her care more than forty poor who died of cold; for the poor cried out that they would rather be provided means to heat them rather than to care and feed them'.[49] As to other medical attention, the Hôtel-Dieu saw little of it, either for its staff or patients. 'Asked if there was a physician to treat the sick sisters and novices,' the prioress, Perrenelle la Tache, responded 'that no, and it was more than six years since they had had one'.[50] Jehanne Vauverde attested that 'when the sisters are sick, their relatives sent them physicians and medicines, for none is provided in the house, and the pharmacy room has great trouble providing for the poor.'[51]

Even the patients protested about the lack of facilities provided for their care in the Hôtel-Dieu. One patient, Michelle Derrée, remarked 'that the nuns treated them well, but the wine and the portions was not sufficient', and that she had not seen a fire since she'd been in the hospital.[52] Significantly, several made clear that the sisters were not at fault in their duties, as did Martin Cheval and Pierre Marchal, who 'say that the nuns do their duty well in serving them'.[53] Importantly, they distinguished between the nuns' interest in their patients' welfare and the services they were actually able to provide them. Their perception of the Hôtel-Dieu is all the more vital, because when asked about their treatment in the hospital, it was about the nuns and the daily service in the hospital that the patients commented. The patients themselves did not immediately think to comment on the quality of the health-care services provided by either the doctor or surgeon, it was the nursing staff with whom they had most contact and whom they saw as the providers of their medical assistance and treatment.

The sort of problems experienced by personnel at the Hôtel-Dieu in Paris were certainly not specific to them. Elsewhere too, Hôtels-Dieu were experiencing increasing financial difficulties. In Orléans, successive requests and criticisms in 1524, 1529 and 1555 which complained about the insufficiency of the buildings, the food and the staff preceded reforms to the administration in 1558.[54] The enquiry into the Hôtel-Dieu in Meaux in 1518 demonstrates that similar experiences were faced by its staff. The nuns complained that 'there was no surgeon, physician nor apothecary to send them drugs and medicines... to help the poor and that when they have seriously ill patients, they help them with the alms and assets of the hospitals as best they can'.[55] There too, when the prioress and sisters had raised these inadequacies with the chapter, they had met with little success and a clear disregard for the requirements of the sisters to perform their work.

> the prioress one time went to see the minister to remonstrate to him about the poor of the hospital; to which he responded that "she was always talking to him about her poor"; and sisters Guillemette, Nicolle, Jehanne Converse and Jehanne Morisette affirmed that when they went to the minister for wood and other things, he did not want to hear of it and told them that they were destroying the house and that there were too many poor there, holding them in fear and threatening them in various ways, and even further, he himself put Jehanne Converse in prison at the prisons of the Hôtel-Dieu.[56]

The poverty of the Hôtel-Dieu de Meaux was such that the patients themselves were forced to gather alms in the churches of the town to buy something to eat.[57]

The attitude of the governors

We have seen the nature of difficulties which the nuns faced in participating in the hospital's management as nursing staff. What then were the underlying causes and tacit assumptions that underpinned these problems? Primarily, it seems that those who possessed the funds to improve the quality of services offered to the ill did not recognise the importance of the nuns' nursing work. These men did not belong to either the university or guild medical community but were members of the religious or municipal governing bodies.

The problem was twofold. Firstly, as professed nuns, or novices, the duty of *caritas*, as well as hardship and suffering, was part of their religious observance within the active life. Although it was given a very minor consideration in the regulations, statutes for hospitals do nonetheless give some indication of what religious women were expected to do in regards to their patients. The statutes for the hospital at Pontoise, from 1265, indicate that at their profession, nuns accepted

> to serve and administer the poor patients what they need, help them in their indigence according to the faculty of the place, feed them and assist them, as they are held to do, supporting their imperfections and making charitable remonstrances, teaching and admonishing their salvation in the great necessity that is death, and by you they cannot lose the sacraments of the Church, also consoling them and encouraging them always to have patience.[58]

Most of the rules made even less mention of the actual nature of the work expected of the staff in their rules or profession statements. Where it was mentioned, the emphasis was for the salvation of the patient, not necessarily for a medical cure.

Moreover, regulations often emphasised the hardship of the care-giving labour for the nun, as imitation of the sufferings of Christ, as did Jehan Henry's manuscript for the Hôtel-Dieu in Paris. Reforms to the statutes of the Hôtel-Dieu in Reims in 1643, highlighted 'the continuity of the work, tiresome humours of the patients, the bad air in the place and the other inconveniences rendering this way of life quite difficult'.[59] Treating the ill, a humbling and monotonous chore, was beneficial to the salvation of the nun herself. Thus curing the patient, and specification of medical skills to do so, was an entirely secondary concern in this religious framework of salvation of both patient and nun.

Secondly, in the wider community, the discourse surrounding women and their nursing role so naturalised women as carers, that there was no *vocation* of nursing. Care-giving was a role all women performed in their families and household. As Yvonne Knibiehler and Catherine Fouquet have argued, the very definition of 'feminine nature' – sensitive, patient, devoted – designated women especially apt to give care.[60] Humanist authors in particular, such as Jean-Louis Vives, encouraged women to be occupied with the care of their husbands and family.[61] These views were certainly not new to the early modern period. Many a medieval handbook for women reminded her of her duties to nurse. The *Mesnagier de Paris* even provided curative recipes to his young wife to help her nurse those in her household, in a tradition which continued well into the sixteenth century as Chapter 5 explores.[62]

There were women paid to nurse in the sixteenth century, but they were rarely perceived by contemporaries as members of a medical community.[63] One reason was that women who worked as sick nurses tended to come from modest social origins, like Jeanne Marguerite, widow of the manual worker Jean Françoys, in Paris.[64] Working as a sicknurse may have provided women with a supplementary income, and many women may have taken on the work since it required no recognised training. Furthermore, many women who nursed frequently did so part time, like Marion Le Febvre in 1543, who identified herself in notarial documents as a launderer and sicknurse[65] and the fifty-year-old Catherine Oquefre, sicknurse and launderer at Saint Marcel in 1540.[66] Thus they did not privilege their nursing work over other forms of work nor commit themselves full time to nursing as a vocation within a medical community, as did physicians and surgeons.

Unsurprisingly, the work of sicknurses was poorly paid since it was not perceived to require special skills, practices or knowledge. Marion Guillotine was paid 11 livres, 4 sols tournois for having nursed Jean Baudet, a student at the university of Paris, back to health from a knee injury, at a rate of 3 sol tournois a day. Baudet's physician was paid 4 livres tournois for his expertise.[67] Some sicknurses might be lucky to benefit from donations in the will of a dying patient as did Geneviève Bourgenymée, sicknurse and servant, who in 1539 nursed Nicole Rabeau in her last illness and received 60 sol tournois and two shirts.[68] Sicknurses were not especially likely to be exposed to learned knowledge of the diseases they treated. In 1522, Marguerite Deshayes, widow of Guillaume Deshayes, testified about the death of Jean Denison, a priest and chaplain at Nôtre-Dame, whom she had nursed and been chambermaid for, that he had died only of 'a very dangerous illness'.[69] The sisters of the Hôtel-Dieu in Paris were likely to have more knowledge of elite medical theory than this, since they mixed with physicians, surgeons and prepared the remedies advised by their learned counterparts.

Since there was no clear recognition of a nursing *vocation* contributing to the early sixteenth-century health-care realm, the work of the women of the Hôtel-Dieu was not viewed by the religious or lay community that administered it as either medical, or as a profession requiring specific resources. Even if the nuns themselves did not clearly articulate their work as a vocation to nurse, they did express a perception of their work as unique, and in need of special assistance – even if that assistance was simply sufficient heating, food and the ability to control its administration to the patients.

If all women were supposed to care for those around them, what was different about the nuns of the Hôtel-Dieu? Why did they need special assistance to do what all women should be doing anyway? Moreover, these women had made a conscious commitment to an active religious life in which their primary duty was to care for the needy. By claiming that they did not have sufficient means to carry out their work, were they not highlighting their own inefficiency and lack of success? Surely they must be bad women if they could not achieve what was the natural duty of all 'good women' and the sworn role of an active nun. In complaining, the nuns demonstrated, in the eyes of the administrators, that they had failed as good women and good nuns.

The governing bodies, both religious and lay, demonstrated a concern about 'bad women' in their enquiries into the management of the Hôtel-Dieu. In the mixed-sex environment that the Hôtel-Dieu constituted, both religious and lay governors seemed especially concerned with sexually uncontrolled women. In 1498, the governors had recognised this problem of chastity, 'they would like to keep it, but to see their lifestyle, liberty and communication, they do not keep their rule'.[70] However, as the staff claimed in response, the very nature of the Hôtel-Dieu meant that 'the monks and nuns must be together; but each to their own head, that is the master and prioress, and if they are well governed by them there will be no scandal nor rumour of it'.[71] Yet it seems the very fact that the sisters were controlled only by another female, the prioress, concerned the chapter council. Although there were equally complaints from patients about the lack of care taken by certain nuns, and others who claimed sisters pushed dying patients to leave their goods to the Hôtel-Dieu in their wills, the governors showed a particular interest in the sexual behaviour of the nuns. In 1498, the staff had to complain to *Parlement* about one master installed by the chapter head who was 'so indiscreet, so ignorant that he demanded of one poor girl if she had ever had carnal company with her father and how many children they had had'.[72] They furthermore objected to his previous experience since he 'had at other times governed repentant girls, who, for lack of good government, returned *ad vomitum*'.[73]

In 1533, the governors investigated whether the sisters had invited several dyers to sleep the night in the *salle des accouchés*. In the enquiry made in October 1535, the chapter vicars were keen to examine the conduct of the sisters and novices. The priest Claudius Parius was 'asked if he knew that several young men and boys frequented the house to be with the nuns every day'.[74] Certainly some of the staff did testify to such behaviour and a few made reference to pregnant sisters in the Hôtel-Dieu in years gone by. Equally, however, nuns complained about their treatment by the domestics in the Hôtel-Dieu, 'who often say insults to the nuns . . . calling them wanton and ribald and other insults'.[75] Such insults of a sexual nature made in public, in the hearing of the patients, could be very dangerous to women and to the way the Hôtel-Dieu was perceived by the community outside.

One concern that warranted much discussion was the practice of nuns visiting patients in their homes outside the Hôtel-Dieu. An anonymous letter received by the chapter of Nôtre-Dame claimed that Jehanne la Chacheleuse came and went as she pleased from the Hôtel-Dieu in the company of men, with the full knowledge of the prioress and sub-prioress.[76] When the governors and Hôtel-Dieu staff were brought to court, one of the major complaints of the governors was the nuns' freedom in leaving the Hôtel-Dieu. They 'do nothing but go about the town', they complained,[77] 'the older nuns want to go and scamper around town, and do not listen to the patients, as they should'.[78] Nuns' freedom and lax sexual behaviour were the reasons that patients were uncared for, they argued.

The governors continually confounded sexual licentiousness with the nuns' freedom to leave the convent to nurse patients. The nuns argued that theirs was an active apostolate which, to undertake properly, required them to leave the Hôtel-Dieu, and one which also enriched the Hôtel-Dieu's coffers: 'As to that the poor are badly cared for and the nuns do not want to serve them, the nuns say that theirs is not the contemplative life, but the active, like Martha, for they are commanded to serve the poor and the bourgeois and those of the town, from which come the acquisitions and assets of the house'.[79] This duty could also be dangerous. In times of plague, it was these same sisters who visited patients who were quarantined inside their houses, as did sisters of the Hôtel-Dieu de Tours, who were paid 7 sous, 6 deniers per week during the contagion to carry food and drink to the pestiferous.

In the epidemic of 1531, Jehanne Janotine, dame de l'Hôtel-Dieu, and Jehanne Poztier cared for the victims for over five months.[80] Such accusations were not only encountered at the Hôtel-Dieu in Paris. Across the country, similar claims of licentiousness and inobservance of their rules were cast upon the sisters of Hôtels-Dieu in ways which suggest that the active apostolate of women religious caused concern to both lay and religious male authorities. Many Hôtels-Dieu offered a rare location in which women could be both unmarried and reasonably independent. At the Hôtel-Dieu in Lyon and at Beaune, the sisters did not take strict vows as did the nuns in the Hôtel-Dieu in Paris.[81] As Natalie Zemon Davis has shown, sexual connotations were linked to the Hôtel-Dieu in Lyon where many of the nursing staff were ex-prostitutes. These women, of modest social origins, wore habits like nuns and received no salary for their work, but were free to leave when they wished.[82] When the question was raised about forming a religious order for the women, in 1589, the lay governors rejected it on the basis that the hospital was created for the poor, not for nuns, that the poor needed corporal not spiritual aid in their treatment, and that it was more expedient to have active women free of any monastic rule rather than nuns continually at prayer.[83] What is all the more remarkable is that the staff at the Hôtel-Dieu in Lyon provide a rare example of female administration from among the lower orders.[84] As Davis argues, they were the only women in Lyon who held offices of municipal administration, with the exception of the mistress of the orphanage Sainte Catherine, and their authority was exercised over a large number of people of both sexes.[85]

The threat that contemporaries felt in such a dangerous cocktail of female power and independence was clear in their satires portraying the sexual licentiousness of the Hôtel-Dieu in Lyon. The 1502 *Sensuit le droit chemin de lhopital et les gens qui le trouvent par leurs œuvres et manière de vivre*, published by the physician Symphorien Champier (probably written by Robert de Balzac) emphasised the poor governance of the hospital indicating that the elite medical community in Lyon was uncomfortable with the idea of female medical administration.[86] The nursing sisters' independence was all the more apparent because until 1526 they had no common uniform to signify their professional activities, but dressed as they wished according to their resources.[87] In comparison to the professed nuns to be found in other contemporary hospitals, the nursing staff of the Hôtel-Dieu in Lyon, ex-prostitutes wearing their own clothes and commanding the most important welfare establishment in the city, must have appeared extraordinary indeed.

However, no perception was universal. Marguerite de Navarre provides an alternative female view in her tale of a foolish but unfortunate young sister seduced by one of the brothers in a wealthy hospital among those of the *Heptaméron*. She too is aware of the sexual innuendo of the mixed sex environment but it is significant that, although Marguerite depicts the nun as foolish, it is the brother who is depicted as licentious.[88] Undoubtedly not all women religious were good and pious, but it seems likely that the charge of sexual licentiousness often functioned as an successful means to affect change in hospitals.

The response of the Hôtel-Dieu staff to the administrators' criticisms claimed the scandals that the governing bodies feared so much were in part created by their own mistrust of the sisters which led to rumours around Paris. As they argued, 'the governors had spread around the town that . . . it is the biggest brothel in Paris'.[89] Furthermore, they claimed 'that in the house, one hundred years ago, there was no scandal or disorder as at present, and there was no Hôtel-Dieu more beautiful nor where the poor were better treated that they were here'. They even provided the Court with a list of names of cured patients who had left the house in the last forty years treated by the 'good diligence of the nuns'.[90]

In the April 1536 parliamentary *arrêt* that followed the enquiry of 1535, one of the few immediate recommendations, beyond general 'reform in the Hôtel-Dieu', was the enclosure and separation of the nuns of the Hôtel-Dieu, from the monks brought in to conduct reform.[91] This tacitly suggested the greatest obstacle to reform in the convent was the sexual licentiousness of the Hôtel-Dieu's female staff who might tempt the incoming brothers appointed for its reform. The more specific recommendations that followed in the *arrêt* of September 1536 went further, appointing 'visiting fathers . . . to visit the nuns and make the usual enquiries, if they observe the rule' as well as that of the male staff.[92] An administrator was also appointed to visit the kitchens twice a week to oversee the preparation and distribution of the food portions and 'take care that the nuns are appointed to the treatment of the poor patients, and do their duties to treat and care for them'.[93]

The authority to care for the sick

The means by which women argued their rights, and those of their patients, were not always rational, though they were certainly passionate. They tended to resist and fight against changes of any nature within the Hôtel-Dieu, particularly the imposition of personnel from outside. The sisters acted aggressively towards changes within the hospital management and were defensive about the care they took with patients. In 1497, when rumours spread within the Hôtel-Dieu that the dean was coming to instruct the sisters to take better care of the patients, the sisters gathered a collection of the staff and patients to meet the dean and his colleagues as they arrived at the Hôtel-Dieu. The twenty or thirty chased them away from the Hôtel-Dieu shouting 'Stop thieves! Stop ribalds! Stop Jews! they are only coming here to fleece the poor, we must bash them!' creating public scandal and infuriating the chapter head in the process.[94]

Further problems occurred with the installation of the new master, Martin Grevin, appointed by the chapter head to proceed with reform in the Hôtel-Dieu. By November 1497 an enquiry was called into the behaviour of the prioress, Jeanne Asseline, and sisters who refused to obey Grevin. The staff complained that Grevin had not been chosen according to the statutes of the Hôtel-Dieu, from one of the staff themselves. As an outsider, he did not understand the management of the Hôtel-Dieu. The sisters and prioress consequently refused to work in co-operation with him, creating difficulties and disturbances. As he complained to the commission,

> some of the monks and nuns, in contempt of our ordinances and appointment and the injunctions that have been made by the chapter and governors, make derision and mockeries in the Hôtel-Dieu, and do not want to obey master Martin nor confess to him, as the statutes say, and scoff him and the novices who go to confess to him, showing them the finger and calling them bigots, in order to induce them not to go.[95]

The sisters adopted simple but effective methods of resistance that they could enact in their everyday lives.

Before 1505, concerned with the shortage of sisters to carry out the daily tasks of the Hôtel-Dieu and to assist with the reforms to its management, the chapter of Nôtre-Dame introduced grey hospitalier sisters in the hospital to live there and administer its patients, in the hopes of allowing the reforms to proceed.[96] Within the Hôtel-Dieu, this decision met with widespread disapproval and the grey sisters were subject to insults and appalling behaviour from the other nuns. The original nuns greeted the 'intruders' with insults and blows, and refused to assist them in treating the patients or in carrying out their tasks.[97] Although both groups were sworn to a vocation which encompassed care for the poor and ill, the sisters of the Hôtel-Dieu seem to have seen the grey sisters as a threat to their control of the institution, imposed upon them by the administration outside the Hôtel-Dieu. Again, another measure of reform had been rejected by the Hôtel-Dieu staff because it conflicted with their authority, and was enacted without their consultation. By 1505, two of the grey sisters had died, three had received extreme unction, twenty were ill and the rest asked to be returned to their convent.[98] The unruly behaviour of the sisters probably only enhanced the view among the governors that further and stricter controls were needed. In the deliberations in May 1505 the chapter governors despaired of the staff's behaviour:

> for more than twenty five years, the governors have continually supported numerous complaints about the lack of piety, harshness and insolence of the monks and nuns of the Hôtel-Dieu; that they applied all their care to correct and eradicate these bad habits against the obstinate resistance and inveterate malice of the monks and nuns, who were supported by various influential people in the Parisian city, they can do no more.[99]

The nuns and monks of the Hôtel-Dieu had difficulty articulating, in a way that would convince the male authorities, their demands for better facilities, and for consultation, in the Hôtel-Dieu. In March 1537 a parliamentary *arrêt* gave extensive punitive powers to the canons Merlin and Berthoul, the abbot of Saint-Victor and the prior of Saint-Ladre, to enact reforms within the Hôtel-Dieu, and another in June, to verify that the new rule was being followed. In July 1537, the sisters showed their defiance of the new regime in the Hôtel-Dieu once more, publicly announcing their opposition in a notarial act. Claude Gruot, the prioress, Cecille Mareschal, the sub-prioress, and eight of the sisters (including the former prioress, Perrenelle la Tache) proclaimed 'that they were ready to obey God, the King, the Court, monseigneur de Lizeulx and the chapter governors, but it was impossible for them to keep the statutes entirely with their labour for the poor, or the poor would be uncared for'.[100] They had evidently first voiced their concerns privately, in correspondence 'already they had sent in writing to La Fontaine the articles and things which they could not hold to and he had sent them no response'.[101] The governors' dismissal of the sisters' objections was undoubtedly one of the reasons for their disruptive behaviour in the Hôtel-Dieu. In refusing to take seriously their arguments and to discuss the problems, the administrators left the nuns no other way but physically to demonstrate their discontent.

By November of the same year, fresh troubles had arisen in the Hôtel-Dieu. On the sixth, there had been near riots between pro- and anti-reform staff within the Hôtel-Dieu, among which a number of the 'nuns and novices were the most vehement and riotous'.[102] One Françoise Cullotte, 'in the middle of the house, among the patients, made a great uproar and injurious noise',[103] another, a novice named Catherine Patine, 'crying to people outside "Break down the door!" in order to excite the townspeople to come to their aid'.[104] Another 'heard Perpette and other nuns and novices saying the words: What are these traitors coming to do here?'[105] Another witness testified to seeing Catherine Chambaulde call Jehan Bernard, a brother, a traitor and wicked man among other insults.[106] Their words show clearly that they were angry with the 'traitors' who supported the reforms because these would alter the management of the Hôtel-Dieu which had always existed. The very uniqueness of the Hôtel-Dieu's organisation was being betrayed by its own members, they felt. But such behaviour was unlikely to convince the governors of the nuns' seriousness to be counted in the decisions about the provision of health-care services at the Hôtel-Dieu. By 1540, a new constitution agreed upon by the male supervisory bodies was ratified by *Parlement*. Despite the protests of the sisters of the Hôtel-Dieu and without their participation, the reforms so desired by the governors would eventually take place.

It is significant to note that throughout this period of conflict and transformation at the Hôtel-Dieu, that elsewhere in France the Hôtel-Dieu in Paris was seen as the model of hospital administration and nursing expertise in the kingdom. In 1526 sister Marie de Pardieu from the Hôtel-Dieu de Pontoise was sent to Paris for three months to learn to the skills of hospital nursing.[107] There was no question that governors of other Hôtels-Dieu looked upon the women of the Hôtel-Dieu in Paris as having expertise in nursing care. The governors of the Hôtel-Dieu d'Orléans wrote to the Hôtel-Dieu in Paris in 1531 to ask if they could exchange some of their staff in order to gain medical and administrative experience from Paris.[108]

In conclusion, the health-care work of women religious continued to be a vital contribution to hospitals under both ecclesiastical and lay administration.[109] As the work of Colin Jones has demonstrated, new female religious nursing orders such as that founded by St Vincent de Paul and Louise de Marillac sprang up in the seventeenth century and they continued to underpin the functionality of most hospitals until the Revolution.[110] This chapter has shown how complex were the ongoing negotiations of the basis and nature of women's medical expertise and authority as nurses in early modern hospitals, as both carers and administrators. Women involved in heath-care provision within the Hôtel-Dieu were unable to have their work recognised, valued and provided for in an appropriate manner under both ecclesiastical and lay administration. It becomes clear in these documents that successive generations of nuns, under different governing bodies, encountered similar challenges in having their role as nursing staff recognised. The governors viewed the hospital staff as passive employees, rather than as active contributors to the Hôtel-Dieu's management plans, and denied their participation in important decisions to change the administration. They did not perceive the women who provided for the patients on a daily basis as authoritative participants in health-care management whose knowledge and opinions were to be respected. The administrators left them no means to debate decisions taken in the Hôtel-Dieu in a rational way. The nuns' resort to generally public displays of violent, angry and disruptive behaviour may have been the only means by which the women were able to enter into discussion with the governors about the changing administration of the Hôtel-Dieu.[111] These conflicts over the meaning and authority of their nursing role were not the first that religious women faced, nor would they be the last.[112] Unfortunately for them, the governors became convinced that this irrational behaviour and conduct required even stricter control. In the long term it resulted in reducing the nuns' authority to participate in the decisions concerning caregiving in the Hôtel-Dieu.

Notes

1 See particularly the works of Jean Imbert, 'L'église et l'état face au problème hospitalier au XVIe siècle', *Etudes d'histoire du Droit Canonique dédiées à Gabriel Le Bras*, vol. 1 (Paris: Sirey, 1965), pp. 577–92; 'Les prescriptions hospitalières du Concile de Trente et leur diffusion en France', *Revue d'histoire de l'Eglise de France*, 42 (1965), pp. 5–28; *Le Droit hospitalier de l'ancien régime* (Paris: Presses universitaires de France, 1993).
2 Daniel Hickey, *Local Hospitals in Ancien Régime France: Rationalization, Resistance, Renewal, 1530–1789* (Montreal and Kingston: McGill-Queens University Press, 1997).
3 Marie-Claude Dinet-Lecomte, 'Les Sœurs hospitalières au service des pauvres malades aux XVIIe et XVIIIe siècles', *Annales de démographie historique* (1994), pp. 277–92, p. 277.
4 See recent studies by Colin Jones, *The Charitable Imperative: Hospitals and Nursing in Ancien Régime and Revolutionary France* (London: Routledge, 1989) and M.-C. Dinet-Lecomte, 'Les religieuses hospitalières à Blois aux XVIIe et XVIIIe siècles', *Annales de Bretagne et des Pays de l'Ouest*, 96:1 (1989), pp. 15–40; 'Les hôpitaux sous l'Ancien Régime: des entreprises difficiles à gérer?', *Histoire, économie et société*, 18:3 (1999), pp. 527–45.

5 E. Coyecque, *L'Hôtel-Dieu de Paris au moyen âge: histoire et documents*, vol. 1: *Documents (1316–1552)* (Paris: H. Champion, 1891), p. 181.
6 Mémoires du Parlement, vol. 3, fol. 172, Arsenal, ms. 2392, in *Ibid.*, p. 27.
7 Léon Le Grand, *Statuts d'Hôtels-Dieu et de léproseries: recueil de textes du XIIe au XIVe siècles* (Paris: A. Picard, 1901), pp. v–vii.
8 J. Imbert, *Les Hôpitaux en droit canonique* (Paris: J. Vrin, 1947), p. 262.
9 A. Boucher, 'L'ancien Hôtel-Dieu de Chinon', *Bulletin de la Société des Amis de Vieux Chinon*, 7 (1975), p. 848.
10 A. de Belfort, *Archives de la Maison-Dieu de Châteaudun* (Paris/Châteaudun: Pouiller-Vandegraine, 1888), p. xxiv.
11 Jean Imbert (ed.), *Histoire des hôpitaux en France* (Toulouse: Privat, 1982) provides an excellent general introduction to the daily work of an early modern hospital.
12 Comptes, XV, 231, in Coyecque, *L'Hôtel-Dieu de Paris au moyen âge*, vol. 1, p. 47.
13 Coyecque, *L'Hôtel-Dieu de Paris au moyen âge*, vol. 1, p. 46.
14 See Le Grand, *Statuts d'Hôtels-Dieu et de léproseries*.
15 Imbert, *Les Hôpitaux en droit canonique*, p. 261.
16 E. Coyecque (ed.), *L'Hôtel-Dieu de Paris au moyen âge: Histoire et Documents*, vol. 2: *Déliberations du Chapitre de Nôtre-Dame de Paris relatives à l'Hôtel-Dieu (1326–1539)* (Paris: H. Champion, 1889), pp. 193–4.
17 Coyecque, *L'Hôtel-Dieu de Paris au moyen âge*, vol. 2, p. 195.
18 *Ibid.*, vol. 1, p. 35.
19 Livre de vie active, 95, in *Ibid.*, p. 64, n 1.
20 (Rawcliffe's translation) Carol Rawcliffe, *Medicine and Society in Later Medieval England* (Stroud: Sutton, 1997), p. 207 and Comptes XV, 113–15, Livre de vie active, in Coyecque, *L'Hôtel-Dieu de Paris au moyen âge*, vol. 1, pp. 34–5.
21 Charte de XVe siècle, in Henriette Carrier, *Origines de la Maternité de Paris: les maitresses sages-femmes et l'office des accouchées de l'ancien Hôtel-Dieu (1378–1796)* (Paris: Georges Steinhal, 1888), p. 5.
22 30 September 1536, Arrêt du Parlement (Arch. Nat. L 53321, expédition, 4 feuillets, paper) in Coyecque, *L'Hôtel-Dieu de Paris au moyen âge*, vol. 1, p. 374.
23 Charte de XVe siècle, in Carrier, *Origines de la maternité de Paris*, p. 4.
24 Coyecque, *L'Hôtel-Dieu de Paris au moyen âge*, vol. 2, p. 195.
25 Extrait des registres du Parlement, 10 septembre 1535, in Carrier, *Origines de la Maternité de Paris*, p. 156, fn 1.
26 Pierre de Spiegeler, *Les Hôpitaux et l'assistance à Liège (X–XVe siècles): aspects institutionnels et sociaux*, Bibliothèque de la Faculté de Philosophie et Lettres de l'Université de Liège, Fascicule CCXLIX (Paris: Société d'Edition 'Les Belles Lettres', 1987), p. 128.
27 Imbert, *Le Droit hospitalier de l'ancien régime*, p. 12. For the history of hospitals in Lyons, see Jean Artaud, *Le Grand Hôtel-Dieu de Lyon* (n.p. 1898); J. Drivon, *Les Anciens Hôpitaux de Lyon: hôpital des passants* (Lyon: Association Typographique, 1905); Drivon, *Miscellanées médicales et historiques: notes pour servir à l'histoire de la médecine à Lyon* (Lyon: Association Typographique, 1908, 1910 and 1913); A. Croze, 'Etudes et documents pour servir à l'histoire hospitalière lyonnaise', *Revue d'histoire de Lyon* (1912 and 1915); Jean-Pierre Gutton, *La Société et les pauvres, l'exemple de la généralité de Lyon. 1534–1789* (Paris: Les Belles Lettres, 1971); Nicole Gonthier, 'Les

hôpitaux et les pauvres à la fin du moyen âge: l'exemple de Lyon', *Le Moyen Age* (1978), pp. 279–308.
28 Imbert, *Le Droit hospitalier de l'ancien régime*, p. 18.
29 *Ibid.*, p. 19.
30 Hickey, *Local Hospitals in Ancien Régime France*, pp. 3–4.
31 For elaboration of royal and ecclesiastical hospital politics, see Imbert, 'L'église et l'état face au problème hospitalier au XVIe siècle'; 'Les prescriptions hospitalières du Concile de Trente et leur diffusion en France'; *Le Droit hospitalier de l'ancien régime*.
32 Hickey, *Local Hospitals in Ancien Régime France*, p. 198.
33 Arch. Nat., Parlement, Après-dînées, X 1a 8325, fol. 125 in Coyecque, *L'Hôtel-Dieu de Paris au moyen âge*, vol. 1, p. 312.
34 Coyecque, *L'Hôtel-Dieu de Paris au moyen âge*, vol. 1, p. 311.
35 Arrêt du Parlement, 4/4/1498, Arch. Nat. Parlement, Conseil, X1a 1504 in *Ibid.*, p. 323.
36 Arch. Nat. Parlement, Conseil, X1a 1528, fol. 583v in *Ibid.*, p. 334.
37 11 dec 1528 Arch. Nat. Parlement, Conseil, X1a 1532, fol. 22v in *Ibid.*, p. 337.
38 16/10/1534 to 27/3/1535 'Inventaire des pièces produites en Parlement par les religieux de l'Hôtel-Dieu contre l'entérinement des requêtes des gouverneurs tendant à la laïcisation de certaines services' (Archives de l'Assistance publique, liasse 869, côte 1, numéro 4714 de l'*Inventaire-Sommaire*, 10 feuillets), in *Ibid.*, p. 194.
39 Coyecque, *L'Hôtel-Dieu de Paris au moyen âge*, vol. 1, p. 347.
40 *Ibid.*, p. 347.
41 *Ibid.*, p. 351.
42 *Ibid.*, p. 195.
43 'Enquête des vicaires capitulaires sur l'état de l'hôpital; interrogatoire du personnel et des malades; visite de la maison: extract' (A.N. L5364, orig. 32 ff., papier) in *Ibid.*, p. 356.
44 *Ibid.*, pp. 357–8.
45 *Ibid.*, p. 359.
46 *Ibid.*, p. 354.
47 *Ibid.*, p. 357.
48 *Ibid.*, p. 358.
49 *Ibid.*, p. 357.
50 *Ibid.*, p. 356.
51 *Ibid.*, p. 359.
52 *Ibid.*, p. 360.
53 *Ibid.*, p. 360.
54 Pierre Bouvier, *Etude sur l'Hôtel-Dieu d'Orléans au moyen-âge et au XVIe siècle* (Orléans: Paul Pigelet, 1914), p. 73.
55 Coyecque, *L'Hôtel-Dieu de Paris au moyen âge*, vol. 1, p. 328.
56 *Ibid.*, pp. 328–9.
57 *Ibid.*, p. 327.
58 Le Grand, *Statuts d'Hôtels-Dieu et de léproseries*, p. 150.
59 *Archives législatives de la ville de Reims, seconde partie: statuts*, ed. Pierre Varin, vol. 1 (Paris: Imprimerie de Crapelet, 1844), p. 138.
60 Yvonne Knibiehler and Catherine Fouquet, *La Femme et les médecins* (Paris: Hachette, 1983), p. 177.

61 See discussion of Vives's view in Chapter 5.
62 Georgina E. Brereton and Janet M. Ferrier (eds), *Le Mesnagier de Paris*, trans. Karin Ueltschi (Paris: Livre de Poche, 1994).
63 For analysis of lay nursing work in the English contemporary context, see Margaret Pelling, 'Nurses and nursekeepers: problems of identification in the early modern period', *The Common Lot: Sickness, Medical Occupations and the Urban Poor in Early Modern England* (London: Longman, 1998), pp. 179–202.
64 No. 3613, Claire Béchu, Florence Greffe and Isabelle Pébay (eds), *Minutier central des notaires de Paris: minutes du XVe siècle de l'Etude XIX* (Paris: Archives Nationales, 1993), p. 424.
65 Madeleine Jurgens (ed.), *Documents du minutier central des notaires de Paris: inventaires après décès*, vol. 1: *1483–1547* (Paris: Archives Nationales, 1982), p. 257.
66 No. 1524, E. Coyecque (ed.), *Recueil d'actes notariés relatifs à l'histoire de Paris et de ses environs au XVIe siècle, 1498–1545*, vol. 1 (Paris: Imprimerie nationale, 1905), p. 296.
67 No. 1412, *Ibid.*, p. 274.
68 No. 1245, *Ibid.*, p. 247.
69 No. 317, *Ibid.*, p. 70.
70 Coyecque, *L'Hôtel-Dieu de Paris au moyen âge*, vol. 1, p. 318.
71 *Ibid.*, p. 320.
72 *Ibid.*, p. 311.
73 *Ibid.*, p. 319.
74 'Enquête des vicaires capitulaires', in Coyecque, *L'Hôtel-Dieu de Paris au moyen âge*, vol. 1, p. 354.
75 *Ibid.*, p. 358.
76 Coyecque, *L'Hôtel-Dieu de Paris au moyen âge*, vol. 1, p. 389.
77 *Ibid.*, p. 318.
78 *Ibid.*, p. 316.
79 *Ibid.*, p. 319.
80 René Coursault, *La Médecine en Touraine du moyen âge à nos jours* (Paris: Maisonneuve & Larose, 1991), pp. 42–3.
81 C. A. Ernest Wickersheimer, *La Médecine et les médecins en France à l'époque de la renaissance* (Paris: A. Maloine, 1906), p. 324.
82 Natalie Zemon Davis, 'Scandale à l'Hôtel-Dieu de Lyon (1537–1543)', *La France d'Ancien Régime: études réunies en l'honneur de Pierre Goubert*, vol. 1 (Toulouse: Privat, 1984), p. 178.
83 Artaud, *Le Grand Hôtel-Dieu de Lyon*, pp. 317–18.
84 Davis, 'Scandale à l'Hôtel-Dieu de Lyon (1537–1543)', p. 185.
85 *Ibid.*, p. 178.
86 *Ibid.*, p. 175.
87 Artaud, *Le Grand Hôtel-Dieu de Lyon*, p. 318.
88 See the seventy-second *nouvelle* of the *Heptaméron*.
89 Coyecque, *L'Hôtel-Dieu de Paris au moyen âge*, vol. 1, p. 312.
90 *Ibid.*, pp. 319–20.
91 6/4/1536 Arrêt du Parlement, Arch. Nat. Parlement, Matinées, x1a 4900, fol. 385. in Coyecque, *L'Hôtel-Dieu de Paris au moyen âge*, vol. 1, p. 370.
92 30/9/1536 Arrêt du parlement, Arch. Nat., L 53321, expédition, 4 feuillets in *Ibid.*, p. 373.

93 30/9/1536 Arrêt du parlement, Arch. Nat., L 53321, expédition, 4 feuillets in *Ibid.*, p. 374.
94 'Enquête du promoteur du chapitre de Nôtre-Dame sur la conduite des religieuses lors de l'installation du boursier Laurent Laîné – Extrait' (Arch. Nat. L 536, côte 1, original, 16 feuillets paper) in *Ibid.*, p. 306.
95 30/11/1497 (Arch. Nat. L 533, côte 4, original, parchemin) in *Ibid.*, pp. 308–10.
96 Coyecque, *L'Hôtel-Dieu de Paris au moyen âge*, vol. 2, p. 289.
97 Alexis Chevalier, *L'Hôtel-Dieu de Paris et les sœurs augustines (650 à 1810)* (Paris: H. Champion, 1901), p. 171.
98 Coyecque, *L'Hôtel-Dieu de Paris au moyen âge*, vol. 2, p. 270 and vol. 1, pp. 191–2.
99 Chevalier, *L'Hôtel-Dieu de Paris et les sœurs augustines*, p. 168.
100 Coyecque, *L'Hôtel-Dieu de Paris au moyen âge*, vol. 1, p. 376.
101 *Ibid.*, p. 376.
102 'Enquête sur le "tumulte" du 6 novembre' (Arch. Nat. L 5368), in Coyecque, *L'Hôtel-Dieu de Paris au moyen âge*, vol. 1, p. 377.
103 *Ibid.*, p. 377.
104 *Ibid.*, p. 378.
105 *Ibid.*, p. 379.
106 *Ibid.*, p. 379.
107 Règle de Pontoise, Le Grand, *Statuts d'Hôtels-Dieu et de léproseries*, p. 17.
108 Bouvier, *Etude sur l'Hôtel-Dieu d'Orléans au moyen âge et au XVIe siècle*, p. 136. Jacques Depauw's article demonstrates the continued welfare dominance of the Hôtel-Dieu in Paris even at the end of the sixteenth century, 'L'assistance à Paris à la fin du XVIe siècle', *Bulletin de la société française d'histoire des hôpitaux*, 59 (1989), pp. 10–24.
109 Many studies, however, continue to focus solely on the ecclesiastical or lay directors, as Dinet-Lecomte has noted, 'Les sœurs hospitalières au service des pauvres malades aux XVIIe et XVIIIe siècles', p. 277. Apart from Imbert's work, other studies of conflict between administrative bodies include Xavier Martin, 'La part du corps de ville dans la gestion de l'Hôtel-Dieu d'Angers à la fin du XVIe siècle', *Annales de Bretagne et des pays de l'Ouest*, 82 (1975), pp. 149–62, and Roger Nougaret, 'Les conflits de pouvoir autour de l'assistance hospitalière à Rodez: l'exemple de l'hôpital du Pas (XIVe–XVIe siècles)' *Santé, médecine et assistance au moyen âge* (Actes du 110e congrès national des sociétés savantes, Montpellier, 1985) (Paris: Editions du CTHS, 1987), pp. 317–29.
110 Colin Jones, 'Vincent de Paul, Louise de Marillac, and the Revival of Nursing in the Seventeenth Century', *The Charitable Imperative: Hospitals and Nursing in Ancien Régime and Revolutionary France* (London: Routledge, 1989). See also discussion of the roles of new nursing orders in the Counter-Reformation hospitals in Jones, 'Perspectives on poor relief, health care and the Counter-Reformation in France', and Martin Dinges, 'Health care and poor relief in regional Southern France in the Counter-Reformation', in Ole Peter Grell and Andrew Cunningham with Jon Arrizabalaga (eds), *Health Care and Poor Relief in Counter-Reformation Europe* (London: Routledge, 1999), pp. 215–39 and pp. 240–79.
111 Karen Messing, 'Hospital trash: cleaners speak of their role in disease prevention', *Medical Anthropology Quarterly*, 12:2 (1998), pp. 168–87. Karen Messing's study of cleaning staff such as cleaners, sterilisers and launderers in twentieth-century hos-

pitals demonstrates many similar reactions. The work of cleaning staff brings them into direct contact with patients every day, yet they are excluded from the management of most hospitals. Her article documents the tensions and quarrels that arise from the contempt and disdain for their work displayed by other medical staff. It is significant that facing the same perception of their medical utility, cleaning staff react in similar ways to our case study here. Messing describes how they responded to feeling invisible in health care by making their work visible, leaving a strong smell of bleach or lights on in rooms they had cleaned as well as resorting to the collective action of chanting insulting slogans to a supervisor who treated them with contempt. Religious women developed similar strategies to make their work visible, utilising the means at their disposal to have their contribution to health care recognised.

112 For an interesting parallel history of division between nursing staff, physicians and the wider community, see Louis S. Greenbaum, 'Science, medicine, religion: three views of health care in France in the eve of the French Revolution', *Studies in Eighteenth Century Culture*, 10 (1981), pp. 373–91.

4

Female healing before the law

THE REGULATION of women's nursing activities within the Hôtel-Dieu, categorised primarily as part of their religious vocation, was not intrinsically motivated by a desire to maintain control over their medical practice. However, in the sixteenth century, important transformations were taking place which served to narrow women's medical opportunities; changes which could make a claim to any kind of religious healing authority dangerous and potentially lethal. In March 1567, Jeanne Lescallier was prohibited by the *lieutenant criminel* in the Senechalscy of Anjou from practising medicine, from making medical diagnosis and from administering any potions and brews to the sick, or she would be fined. Lescallier made no appeal against her sentence, but instead, as the physicians of Angers later complained 'nevertheless she continued at it'. They claimed that she went subtly from village to village giving her help.[1] In 1571, the syndic of the physicians in Angers, Pierre Daburon, asked that the courts again prohibit her medical practice. On 3 April 1571, Lescallier was forbidden again by the *lieutenant criminel* Pierre Ayrault 'from making or prescribing any brews, potions or other medicines to enter the human body and generally to do and prescribe nothing that relates to medicine or surgery', this time 'on pain of prison and an arbitrary fine'.[2] Now, with the apparent support of the neighbourhoods in which she practised, Lescallier appealed the seneschalsy sentence. It would not be heard before 1573 and was in vain: the arguments of Lescallier and her supporters were rejected.

Jeanne claimed that she cared for those around her out of charity using simple remedies she had gathered from years of experience, like many other women. However, unlike the majority of women in her position, Jeanne continued to pursue her right to practise her own form of medicine, and took the unusual step of contesting the Angers appeal ruling of 1573. The case was heard in 1578 before the *Parlement* of Paris which was the appeal court for decisions made at the presidial court at Angers. It was an important step. The outlay of costs and the difficulties of assembling witnesses for appeal cases in Paris were prohibitive for many. However, the complexities of sixteenth-century French law provided those who felt their convictions were in error with a number of courts before which to pursue appeals. In theory, one of the benefits of the newly created presidial courts was to allow criminal defendants to get final justice closer to their homes, at less expense and inconvenience. But litigants could still choose to appeal to the higher court of the *Parlement* if they did not receive a favourable outcome.[3] The determination of Lescallier to have her case heard and to pursue it through most of the available appeal mechanisms, makes it imperative to try to understand the motives behind her actions, and the foundations for her convictions. She was not alone in her opinion: she was apparently supported by local villagers from the parishes of Denée, Saint-Maurille des Ponts-de-Cé and Sainte-Gemmes-sur-Loire who used her services. They too asked that the judgement be amended in order to allow 'Lescallier to continue to exercise medicine, as she had previously done, and the appellants to be able to consult her in their illnesses as they saw fit'.[4] How could Lescallier and the local community argue that she had the authority to exercise medicine in the face of such organised opposition from the physicians of Angers?

This chapter will examine the existing documentation surrounding the presentation of the case before the *Parlement* of Paris. Lescallier's case was presented by René Bautru, sieur des Matras, from the presidial court in Angers, a municipal magistrate and future mayor of the town. The physicians of the Faculty of Medicine at Angers were represented by the lawyer from the *Parlement* of Paris, reputed as one of the great legal minds of his day, and a competent self-publicist, Simon Marion.[5] By analysing the opposing narratives put forward by these jurists for the legal community, we can understand how female healing was perceived by sixteenth-century law. The choice of the term narrative is important, in so far as each side attempted to construct a compelling argument to convince the *Parlement*, much as the historian Natalie Zemon Davis has argued to read explanations and tales by convicted criminals seeking pardon as persuasive fictions.[6] In Lescallier's case, each side manipulated existing stereotypes of the female healer that they believed would be pertinent and convincing within the legal fraternity, but also with reference to contemporary notions in the medical, ecclesiastical and local communities. Such documents can be instrumental in understanding the contemporary perception of female medical practices and their relationship to other contemporary discourses.

Women and charitable medical practice

The sixteenth-century discourse surrounding the right and duty of women to care for those around them was complex. Social level played a distinct role. Behaviour manuals destined for noblewomen encouraged them to show benevolent interest in the health of those living in their household and on their lands. Anne de Beaujeu advised her daughter, Suzanne, 'you must, in moving from one place to another, wherever you are, greet the simple poor people ... and graciously talk with them of their husbands, wives, children and households'.[7] Christine de Pizan had suggested that the wise princess should sometimes, out of charity, visit hospitals, the poor and sick, speaking and comforting them with a gentle touch while making her donations to the poor.[8] In his agricultural manual, the learned gentleman Olivier de Serres encouraged women to use simple herbs to treat those injured or sick in their household. 'Several Ladies and young ladies,' he explained, 'earning much praise, have knowledge of the virtues of herbs and simple plants, with which they aid their families and the poor in times of need'.[9]

Noblewomen were often involved in the management of hospitals under both ecclesiastical and municipal administration, contributing both funds and their services.[10] In Rouen, as a result of Father Poissevin's Lenten sermon in the cathedral in 1570, 'several notable ladies of this town gathered as much in deniers as in linens from the parishes and households'. Other elite women went to the Hôtel-Dieu to console the poor and sick, and brought jams and other remedies for the weakest among them.[11] Yet, while many small urban environments encouraged, and needed, women to participate in the health-care programme of the town, as Chapter 6 will examine more closely, for large hospitals such as the Hôtel-Dieu in Paris, the charitable labour of noblewomen could cause difficulties. The trend for noblewomen to visit the Hôtel-Dieu carrying alms and visiting the patients was so great that the governors were obliged to institute regulations to co-ordinate the arrival of ladies whose presence had reportedly perturbed the personnel in their tasks and even the patients in their rest. The deliberations of 1608 stipulate that ladies 'who undertake from devotion to see and observe the treatment which is given to the patients in the House, are asked to let the nuns do their tasks and to content themselves with taking care that the nuns do their duty'.[12] Although it was not the primary motivation, this stipulation created the possibility for laywomen to become participants, by their observation, in the increasing regulation of the Hôtel-Dieu's nursing staff that was examined in the previous chapter. In 1612, the hospital council had to prevent the nuns from accepting noblewomen's alms of bread, wine and meat because they created 'more inconvenience to the patients than profit, with a great deal of confusion'.[13]

During the sixteenth century, there was an increase in the publication of medical texts written in French rather than Latin, and many authors sought recompense for their work from noblewomen.[14] Indeed, as will be explored in the following chapter, physicians produced a significant literature demonstrating practical domestic medicine for the use of the lay community, particularly women. Their dedications to wealthy and influential noblewomen often highlighted the charitable work of such ladies on their lands. The physician, Jean Lyège, praised the 'incredible charity and goodness' of Antoinette de Bourbon, which she used to assist a great number of the poor, infirm and sick. 'Above all,' wrote Lyège, 'you desire those sick to be nourished and fed (to which I can attest) methodically, and according to their fever, or to the illness, whatever it may cost'.[15] Lyège even implored Antoinette de Bourbon to continue her charitable medical work: 'I beg with all the force of my heart, that God give you the grace, Madame, to persevere in this divine charity', and devoted to her his text which would help her to recognise and differentiate the symptoms and choose the treatment appropriate to any one of a variety of fevers.[16]

It was clear that there were important restrictions implied in how much medical knowledge physicians expected women to acquire, and in the ways they used it. Firstly, women were to exercise their expertise only out of a spirit of charity. An *arrêt* from the *Parlement* of Dijon in June 1594, which declared null and void a donation made by a patient with cancer to the noblewoman who had nursed him, lauded the pure spirit of charity of the lady involved, rather than condemning her interference in professional health-care work.[17] Secondly, the majority of women whose medical contribution was praised by doctors belonged to the upper levels of society or to the nobility. Jacques-Auguste de Thou recounted how, when he was an ailing child, Gabrielle de Mareuil, 'heiress of the illustrious house of Mareuil in Périgord', nursed him back to health: 'far from despairing of his health, she believed, based on the idea she had of his temperament, that he would recover'. It was unlikely that women of the wealthier levels of society would be pursued by the faculties for their medical work, and, as patrons, this very same work was openly encouraged by physicians. Thirdly, women were only to nurse the sick and not to diagnose their illnesses by themselves. Mareuil did not treat de Thou until after 'Le Grand and Le Jay, his physicians, believing him without hope, abandoned him'.[18] In so doing, noble ladies were not in competition with the medical professionals. In these three ways, Madame Scarron represented the ideal charitable carer for the surgeon and author Jacques Guillemeau. He recounted how Scarron, anxious for the welfare of a farmer's wife on her lands during a difficult birth, called the surgeons (of which Guillemeau was one) to help the woman. In doing so, Scarron assumed her medical responsibility towards the people on her lands, while recognising the superior knowledge of surgeons.[19]

Yet this same charitable medical work was not seen as favourably by physicians and surgeons when performed by women lower down the social hierarchy. In 1580, Laurent Joubert, the chancellor of the Faculty of Medicine at Montpellier, dedicated his translation of *La Grande Chirurgie de M. Gui de Chauliac* to his mother, Catherine de Genas, because of her care for the poor and ill in her region:[20]

> Who has ever seen, or read a remedy more certain and marvellous, than your unguent for sore nipples, with which you have healed an infinite number of poor women, who were almost in despair of pain and inflammation? Your unguent for burns is as admirable as it is widely used. The Gaultier cloth that you use for old ulcers of the legs is of inestimable value. And then the fortified wine ... that you have invented, and composed, of all the herbs in your garden and of wine in your vineyards, is most approved for its notable success. I will say nothing of the many good jams and distilled waters that you make, all for poor patients and for love of God.[21]

Joubert made clear that Genas made her own potions purely out of charity and not for personal profit: 'For it has been the custom of your house, to have some particular remedies, made charitably by the hands of women, for the sick poor'.[22] He underlined that Genas' work was not that of a surgeon or apothecary, since the Genas family had always lived nobly from their rents and revenues.[23]

Elsewhere, however, the same Joubert was highly critical of women's interference in medicine. 'There are some people who know nothing at all about medicine, as to discourse or reason, such as ignorant women who know not even to read or write, but who have some observations and rules'.[24] The physician Jean de Renou also complained that 'there is no miserable village in which one cannot find some old witch who meddles in setting dislocated bones, raising ... the wombs of women, and I hardly dare say it, the paralytic organs of men, by means of I know not what muffled words that they gnash between their teeth'.[25]

The comments by both authors suggested that there were class and social status boundaries about those who were suitable to possess university medical knowledge. The focus on women's illiteracy and lack of a 'suitable' medical knowledge system was clearly important to university-trained practitioners. The latter preferred medical assistance provided by women who were (relatively speaking) learned, or who at least accredited university-derived knowledge as superior.

Lescallier's case is important because her defence was constructed in a way that problematised many of the tacit understandings about the boundaries of female participation in health-care provision. Lescallier's instruction was situated as part of the charitable medical tradition encouraged by medical authors, because she held her competence from a virtuous lady 'indeed of the most illustrious in France', who conducted many works of piety, the nourishment of the poor and cure of illnesses, 'which our said Court does not find strange, given that this holy and praiseworthy vocation and of such great merit, has been ... exercised here in France by several great Princesses, the kindness and charity of whom has come to us from posterity.'[26] Lescallier's lawyer used the physicians' own discourse on charitable medical practice, which allowed noblewomen to treat the poor out of charity. The nobility of Lescallier's patron was emphasised and her own status minimised.

Matras's arguments for Lescallier highlighted the difficulties in differentiating her medical practice from that of the noble lady, such as her recently deceased mistress, if both offered their services and knowledge for free:

> as much as a good and singular nourishment is never lost, so similarly it is with charity, she who was until recently imbued with the good morals and virtuous example of her mistress to help her neighbours afflicted with various illnesses, has since employed herself to treating, aiding and gratifying them as best she can, ... by her diligence ... and good treatment, several patients afflicted by various contagions recovered after physicians had abandoned them.[27]

Lescallier's medical work neatly cast her position within the acceptable boundaries promulgated by physicians themselves. She only treated those patients abandoned by medical professionals, and thus claimed not to be in competition with the prescriptions and treatments that they might prescribe.

How, her lawyer asked, could physicians encourage the charitable medical care of noblewomen and at the same time pursue others before the law for the very same actions as a criminal activity?

> [T]he aid she gave to the sick, charitably without gain, without profit, without any hope of recognition, was of the greatest merit, doing it not to enrich herself nor to be a hindrance to the faculty, but because it was a praiseworthy thing commanded by God, and recommended by the Church.[28]

If Lescallier possessed medical knowledge that could help the sick, she would be neglecting her Christian duty if she did not provide the aid that she could offer. It was even possible, she argued, that she could be accused of cold-blooded murder:

> It would be a thing worse than murder committed in fury, to leave her neighbour in necessity, sick, without helping him, however much one might have means to do it and to prevent the contagion of the illness, the greatest good and the greatest grace that one could give to the patient, would be to give him means and hope of a prompt recovery, one could receive no more certain ease to his illness. Principally, these are poor rustic people distanced from aid, indigent, worked by hard labour and by unusual and strange illnesses, so that to leave them to suffer would be to double their pain and to mock their frailty.[29]

Rural folk against urban physicians

Lescallier's defence was depicted by Matras as having the support of her local community: the habitants of surrounding parishes who received her care.[30] Their opinion was summarised as, for the past twenty years

> they have received infinite commodities from Jeanne Lescallier, the appellant, who, for having watched them and knowing their temperament and complexion, has so dexterously aided their children and their families in all their illnesses . . . and even a large number of poor people that she treated by charity.[31]

The cost of medical services provided by university-trained physicians was a target of attack. The villagers who supported Jeanne Lescallier were depicted as convinced that the urban doctors were concerned to resolve the affair only through greed because Lescallier aided potential clients:

> nevertheless one would have it today that for the desire of five or six physicians in a large town, who have no interest here, . . . to deprive the appellants of all their goods and commodities, and should one prohibit Lescallier from medicining in the future, the said appellants would be constrained to aid themselves and to have recourse from now on to the physicians of Angers who are usually occupied and

look after the greatest [people], who would only take a step out of town with such great expense that it would be impossible for the said habitants to provide it.[32]

Lescallier's lawyer distinguished between medical services dispensed in the town and the countryside, rather than opposing providers qualified and non-qualified by the medical faculties.

In many respects, the case raised unresolved issues about the rights of the rural poor and isolated to have access to medical services. Lescallier's arguments emphasised that it was precisely because there were no doctors in the countryside that she undertook to treat the sick, which 'the laws permit . . . in the event that one cannot find a physician promptly to aid the sick'.[33] Her practice, it was argued, did not interfere with that of the physicians, since she did not provide for the townspeople of Angers. Thus 'she should be dispensed from all the laws of the town of Angers, because she does not live nor make any stay in the said town, nor takes any money, all that she does, she does charitably'.[34] Her services were only intended for the villagers and country dwellers who lived near her. If physicians did not want to leave the town to treat them, nor charge prices that they could afford, the villagers demanded that they be free to profit from the free and charitable assistance Lescallier offered them. Furthermore, the representation of rural opinions of faculty-trained doctors were highly critical. Lawyers reprised a contemporary view that villagers perceived physicians as 'men so stupid that they do not even know how to interpret the illness' and spoke of experiences with physicians who were forced 'at the first illness and indisposition that they encountered to seek out two or three medical texts'.[35] The villagers found it ridiculous that in spite of the incompetence of the physicians, the latter forbade rural people 'to use the remedies that they find at their door'.[36] Matras argued that it was their choice to decide who to consult about their illnesses, and that was why 'they intervene in this cause for the interest that they have that she be tolerated'.[37]

The power of rural people to decide on their medical intervention was a contemporary concern of physicians. The Angevin physician André du Breil, whose text appeared shortly after Lescallier's Parisian appeal, complained of the perverse obstinacy of the common people in continuing to employ and encourage empirics. He also lamented that another abuse of medical authority was those who claimed to practise out of charity and piety. This may have been a direct reference to Lescallier's case.[38] The argument of the physicians denied any awareness of medical knowledge in the general community, in order to dismiss such an assessment of medical knowledge and maintain their authority. Moreover, the rural seat of one of the professors of the Faculty of Medicine in Angers, Piau, was in Lescallier's very parish, Denée.[39] Thus Matras's accusations about the lack of help to rural folk struck close to the bone for the Angers physicians. The physicians' lawyer Marion responded by labelling the peasants idiots and emphasising 'the simplicity of rustic people'.[40] It was added that *arrêts* were made especially for the people in the countryside and small villages, to 'chase Empirics from the villages as much as the towns, for in the towns the people are more prudent, and can better defend themselves from impostors than rustics'.[41] Consequently, physicians could justify that it was their duty to help an ignorant public to have access to accredited medical services, by eliminating those not trained by the faculty or guilds:

> [T]he habitants are not capable people ... it is not for the people to approve physicians ... that is resolved in legitimately established universities and it is to them to say if this women medicates well and if she cures them.[42]

The doctors were presented as astonished by the interference of the people in a matter that they perceived as not theirs to decide: 'in truth it is absurd that an ignorant people judge the competence of a physician'.[43] The physicians justified their medical authority and pursuit of Lescallier in saying: 'there is a university in Angers whose statutes like all others in the kingdom are known to the court and in these statutes there is an article which expressly forbids doctors of medicine to tolerate and dissimulate empirics. But on the contrary, enjoins them to pursue them in law'.[44]

Empiric, charlatan or herbal healer?

The physicians' case emphasised Lescallier's lack of university medical qualifications. They advanced that the science of medicine was 'acquired by labour, by supervision and study, by the knowledge of natural causes, by anatomical dissections, and other similar means'.[45] Consequently, 'as the said appellant confesses ... to have never studied medicine, and to have no knowledge of the art and precepts of it', they could accuse her of using empirical methods.[46] Yet, although she had no medical training, Lescallier emphasised that her knowledge was derived from university medicine: 'in her youth, she was in Gascony and in Ferrara, where she saw several physicians practise, from which she retained some things of what she saw done'.[47] Furthermore, other members of the recognised medical community supported her knowledge, as indicated by the testimony that several barbers and surgeons of the parishes supplied for her.[48]

With strong justifications in her favour, Lescallier's arguments even ventured to criticise the medical profession, challenging their definition of the term physician (*médecin*). As she reasoned, 'it is not the title nor the profession, but the operation, in such a way that he who knows well how to medicine and cure is the true doctor'.[49] Since she could also heal, through 'simple domestic remedies' by what right might she not also call herself a doctor? After all, for people in the surrounding parishes, she was their 'only hope of usual aid in all their illnesses'.[50] She 'had helped a multitude of people who praised her happy practice acquired by the long time that she had employed to visiting the sick, which is the principal utility of a physician's knowledge'.[51] Even more hazardous, Lescallier's lawyer insinuated that physicians considered her a disloyal rival, precisely because she offered her services for free out of Christian charity:

> [S]eeing that she liberally offered to do her best for them, of which the physicians were advised, they have machinated against her, employing all means to destroy her, because she is lauded for her good work, and because her knowledge is free, and by the fact of a pure spirit of vengeance and without reason, have the physicians brought the said appellant before the *Lieutenant Criminel* of Angers, in order to forbid her to practise the art of medicine.[52]

Moreover, the appellants criticised the greed of doctors: 'one could as well try to reproach the abuse, trickeries and licence which physicians give themselves to abandon the sick seeing them in extremity, after having taken their money'.[53]

On the other hand, Jeanne Lescallier, it was claimed by her lawyer Matras, had knowledge of the virtues of herbs and of distillations for waters and oils:

> the medicaments that she makes with them, the care and vigilance that she takes with the sick, are the means that she uses ... she has cured a multitude of people abandoned and despaired of by the physicians.[54]

Her lawyer distinguished between her activities as a herbal healer gathering simples and those of Empirics: 'those who practise in the fields and in the villages have never been included by the *arrêts* given against Empirics'.[55] As examined in Chapter 2, *arrêts* from the *Parlement* of Paris throughout the sixteenth century condemned both male and female empirics, as well as the people who used their skills and services. The frequency with which such *arrêts* were produced (in 1535, 1537, 1566, 1575, 1577, 1579 and 1598) indicated that the problem was widespread and endemic.[56] At least one of these *arrêts*, in 1566, enjoined physicians, surgeons and apothecaries to act such that 'the poor might be treated in their illnesses at moderated prices and costs'.[57] In juxtaposing physicians' fees against Lescallier's charitable medical work, Matras was targeting a common concern among parliamentary members. Moreover, her treatments were not those of an empirical healer:

> it is not a question here of condemning a simple Empiric as they claim, but of abolishing a sort of medicine which has existed for all time, even in the first Church and between the first Christians religiously without needing other approbation, and that God has gifted some of the simplest people, to help those in need.[58]

Lescallier's work was situated in a tradition perpetuated by the people that had no place in a conflict with services offered by university physicians.

The arguments made on Lescallier's behalf were strong, and were viewed sympathetically, and the physicians struggled to provide compelling evidence in their favour. The doctors' case rested on two premises: that Lescallier had not undergone formal medical training, and that she charged for her expertise. Lescallier readily admitted she did not have university medical education, but argued that she had a valid basis for her practice through her extensive knowledge of simple herbal remedies. Moreover, she maintained that she had only ever acted out of charity and the physicians never provided any proof that Lescallier was paid for her services. Coupled with the apparent local support for her practice, the medical community's case looked unconvincing. The criminality of Lescallier's healing practices rested on her being paid, and if the physicians were not able to prove this, then legally their case foundered. There was no legal basis to prevent women engaging in charitable herbal healing, like the domestic medicine most women performed in their homes, and physicians even wrote texts to advise women how to perform this type of medicine.

Indeed, it seems that the courts were not particularly concerned by female healers, and learned men outside the medical community did not appear, in general, critical of their work. Although the courts most often found in favour of the faculties, sentences were often lenient and sympathetic to healers. When the courts were faced with cases against female medical practitioners, some of whom were charged with sorcery for their actions, their sentences were minimal. In 1566, Michelle Jacquelin, the wife of François Rousselot, a labourer at Montaillé, was only fined by the courts for having 'sent some concoctions to several people to cure them'. Jacquelin also appealed her case before the *Parlement* of Paris where her sentence was confirmed and she was forbidden to 'meddle in medicine'.[59] In 1586, Renée de Triquière, called 'la Medecine', from a clearly superior social milieu, the widow of Jean Bridet, sieur de La Forêt, came before the court to testify in a trial against another female healer. When asked the source of her own medical expertise, Triquière claimed that it had been passed on to her from her mother. The court sent her away with no more than a prohibition 'to assist further in medicine'.[60]

If many men outside of the university medical community appeared somewhat sympathetic to female healing, it was in part because it did not interfere with their own professional activities. When the lawyer René Choppin recounted the case of Lescallier in his *Traicte des privileges des personnes vivans aux champs* he did not exclude the possible utility of such herbal medicine: 'For how many learned physicians have been outdone by a simple old peasant woman, who with a simple plant or herb has given relief to patients despaired of by medicine?'[61] He understood the desire of people in the country to have access to remedies when they were sick: 'For to use the elegant terms of the Emperor Constantine, one must not blame the remedies sought out for the human body, or applied innocently in rural places'.[62] Choppin perceived Lescallier's case as a struggle for the physicians to achieve legally recognised professional authority: 'because one must not permit anyone to care for the human body, if they are not approved by the Corps'. His opinion of the particularities of Lescallier's practice was sympathetic: 'she claimed that it is not by hope of gain that she practised medicine, and that she makes no profession of taking money for the cures that she makes'.[63]

Furthermore, in each of her trials, the court left unexamined significant assumptions about female healing which authorised certain aspects of Lescallier's practice. In 1571, the *lieutenant criminel* of Angers forbade her from medical practice, but then continued 'thus she is only permitted to help the sick by simple plants and herbs and not by compositions . . . as physicians and apothecaries do'.[64] Such a proviso clearly indicated the legal community did find certain healing practices acceptable: 'the appellant is to be able to help the sick . . . by the application of herbs and little remedies'.[65] Lescallier's medical work depended in part on whether the court could establish if her practice interfered with recognised faculty medicine, presumably complex composed medicines, or consisted of those herbal simples which could be pursued without challenge. Lescallier's lawyer raised this in her appeal: 'One will not tolerate *Medicinales herbivum collectionnes* if one prevents the practice of medicine that she does'.[66]

Moreover, outside the well-established and recognised medical faculties at Paris and Montpellier, the authority and respect of regional medical faculties was significantly weaker. Angers was not a renowned medical fraternity that could impose its power on the legal system in the same way as the faculty in Paris. Even if it held local sway, it was unlikely to have much influence on the proceedings of the case in Paris. When Charles Colbert was charged with producing a royal survey on the region of Anjou in 1664, his report on the functions of the Angers medical faculty suggests that it was perceived by outsiders as a relatively insignificant faculty: 'As for medicine, there is no professor engaged and there are practically no lessons'.[67] How then were the physicians to construct a perception of Lescallier's practices as dangerous and in need of permanent curtailment? There were other currents of contemporary legal issues towards which the doctors could astutely align their plaint. Marion, the physicians' lawyer, developed a menacing argument which exploited contemporary fears about female healing and its relation to sorcery in an attempt to discredit Lescallier's case. Marion manipulated the increasingly powerful popular, and also learned juridical, preoccupation with witchcraft. In fact, just two years after Lescallier's case was heard, the number of witchcraft appeals to come before the *Parlement* reached a peak for the century.[68]

Lescallier's defence of her successful practice as due to the intervention of God was brought into question. Lescallier had never suggested that hers was the work of a mystic, but simply that

> she has always referred the cure that she made of the sick to the grace that God gave her, all the applications and brews which she has made, it has been with orisons, in the name of the father, son and holy spirit, and certainly the happiness and success of the ... cures that she has made could not be attributed to any but God, so much so that it is against all reason to want to prevent the course of ... such a salutary sort of medicine: the operation of which the said appellants do not complain, on the contrary they praise it, desire it and are content with it.[69]

Such a claim was hardly exceptional. The maxim 'I treat it, God cures it' of Ambroise Paré, the royal surgeon and a contemporary of Lescallier, was well known and Paré was even lauded for the nobility of his sentiments.[70] Yet, in the case of Lescallier, the physicians were prepared to make recourse to extremely aggressive measures. Constructing one of the most dangerous arguments against Lescallier, the physicians took up her explanation that her cures came from God:

> the miracle by special grace of God attributed and conceded to some people even before the incarnation of Jesus Christ, even to the Saints who the Catholic Apostolic and Roman Church have canonised, is a most arrogant thing for the said appellant to want to attribute to herself, a thing so excellent that the Saints themselves with words alone and touching, without using herbs, drugs or medicines, cured the sick.[71]

The doctors chose to orient their argument in a hazardous direction for Lescallier: 'consequently there is no science humanly acquired nor divinely infused, from which it follows that she cannot heal at all, or that she heals by sorcery'.[72] To understand how Lescallier's statements were interpreted, we need to examine first how the Catholic Church accepted female religious healing.

The Catholic Church and female healing

In the late fifteenth century and early sixteenth century, an array of women were recognised as religious healers by the Church. Many women who were perceived by their local communities as holy women performed medical work as part of their spiritual activities. The Blessed Jeanne-Marie de Maillé (1332–1414) was recorded as performing 39 miracles in her lifetime, as well as 13 after her death. Her tomb near the convent of the Cordeliers in Tours became a local pilgrimage site, and was sufficiently religiously significant to warrant desecration by Huguenots in 1562. Medical work was among her miracles. Maillé's supporters deposed on her miraculous healing of those suffering from leprosy and deafness, as well as her ability to restore speech to the mute, sound to the deaf and the use of limbs to the crippled. Although her case for saintly status was not determined by Church officials until the nineteenth century, Maillé's reputation for an ability to intercede before God on behalf of patients existed in her own lifetime and was amply sustained by the local community to warrant ecclesiastical investigation and authentication some five centuries later.[73]

Sainte Jeanne de Valois, divorced wife of Louis XII and founder of the Annonciades order in Bourges, was locally renowned for her attentions to the poor and the sick of the town. Miraculous medical cures accredited to her divine intercession continued throughout the sixteenth century, despite the religious conflicts, and in 1618 the archbishop of Bourges was able to compile a list of some 130 authenticated miracles.[74]

For other women, their ability to procure divine intervention for patients only occurred after their death. Blessed Philippe de Chantemilan was one such holy woman. From a noble background, Philippe was born around 1412 in the county of Forez. She swore to a life of virginity from a young age and lived piously as a chambermaid to Anne de Norry. Chantemilan's religious devotions were permitted in the household: Norry was the sister of the archbishop of Vienne, and Chantemilan's brother Jean was the archbishop's equerry. In later years, she led a more itinerant life, travelling on pilgrimage to Rome and visiting local hospitals and prisons as part of her ritual devotions. She died of the plague at the age of 39 in 1451 and was buried in Vienne's St Maurice church, near to the episcopal palace.

Chantemilan's medical work was one of a number of spiritual acts of devotions she undertook in her lifetime, along with visiting prisoners and the poor. It is not evident from accounts of her life that she claimed, or was perceived, to practise a kind of thaumaturgic healing: her medical work was the type of charitable labour that many contemporary women might perform. Chantemilan visited and nursed in local hospitals, tending the ill and plague-stricken, and she travelled to Lyon to work with the women who served at the Hôtel-Dieu there. When her sister-in-law was abandoned by doctors with no hope of recovery, Chantemilan acted as a sicknurse, and through this work, and her prayers, the patient recovered. In these activities, Chantemilan's medical work distinguished her not as a remarkable healer, but as a pious, humble and charitable woman.

However, although Chantemilan made no specific claims to divine powers of healing in her lifetime, such claims were certainly proclaimed after her death. As her cult grew and documentation for her saintly status was prepared, no less than 60 miracles were authenticated and attributed to her intercession in the twenty years following her death. To summarise, the intercession of the Blessed Philippe de Chantemilan resulted in the resuscitation of sixteen dead, the delivery of eight women in labour, sight to two blind people, a return to their wits for four victims of rabies, and cure of eleven patients from assorted illnesses, among other miracles. Those who deposed in the ecclesiastical proceedings were mostly from local areas, including nearby towns such as

Lyon and Valence, who had sought out her divine intercession in prayer or travelled to the site of her grave in Vienne.[75]

Locally supported cults of female saints or blessed and venerable individuals accredited some women (and also men) with power to heal. In the Touraine region, the chapel of Sainte Catherine de Fierbois was a significant local site for divine healing throughout the later middle ages and into the sixteenth century. The extant manuscript recorded some 245 miracles attributed to St Catherine of Alexandria that took place between 1375 and 1536. The 238th miracle, for example, concerned Jehanne Cazaude, who had given birth to twelve children and prayed to St Catherine for a painless delivery during her next pregnancy.[76] Certainly there were local traditions across France involving women who were blessed by God, in life and death, with the power to heal, as well as ecclesiastical support for them.

In the cases of the holy women cited so far, their divine medical work was non-specific. The ill and their friends sought intercession for a range of complaints. Other saints were reputed to have healing powers specific to a complaint. For some, the connection related to details of their lives: how they had been martyred or a disease they had suffered. St Margaret, for example, was commonly prayed to by women in labour. She had predicted, before being decapitated, that women who had read or carried her book would have a smooth delivery.[77]

Patronage of saints as healers was by no means an unusual part of medical care. Municipal councils, which funded public health programmes, could pay for surgeons, physicians, and fees for people to undertake pilgrimages all as part of their health care strategies. In Lille where the municipality re-organised health-care and poor relief services much earlier than in France, women and couples who cared for sickly foundling children took them on pilgrimages to cure them of a variety of illnesses. This type of spiritual therapy was seen by the municipal authorities as service above and beyond their usual duties, and was paid an extra sum. In 1501, the council paid '40 sols to a woman for the expenses that she undertook to take a poor foundling child to Saint-Quentin in Vermandois, to say three novenas for the child', and remunerated another woman who, 'at the command of the councillors, took a foundling on pilgrimage to Saint Morant, in the town of Douai'.[78]

Accreditation of a holy woman's healing abilities came from multiple sources. The local community created the possibility for official Church recognition of a woman as a saintly healer by praying for her intervention or visiting a pilgrimage site associated with her cult. In officiating over the procedures of saintly status, ecclesiastical authorities were often ratifying the choices of the local populace as to whom they perceived to be holy, and to be effective divine medical intercessors. If the local Church authorities recorded and authenticated miracles for sainthood documentation, they could only choose which were valid from those presented to them by the community.

On the other hand, there were many factors at stake in the decision about who might become a saint, blessed or venerable. The specific inclinations of local Church authorities and the pope, or the pressure that could be brought to bear on the papacy by religious orders, monarchs or other groups, could all play a part.[79] David Gentilcore has also noted that class was a factor: poor women did not usually become saints.[80] Sainte Jeanne de Valois was the former wife of a reigning monarch. Philippe de Chantemilan was of elite status and had intimate connections to the household and family of the archbishop of Vienne. Such circumstances, as well as her piety, humility and charity, would have undoubtedly influenced the perception of her holy status among both church officials and the local population. Concepts of sanctity and divine healing were thus dynamic, and both local popular ratification as well as that of the Church hierarchy could influence perceptions held by both groups.

The criticism of the Catholic Church during the Reformation, and its responses, were to have a profound impact on women's religious healing. One of the areas that the Counter-Reformation Catholic Church examined was sainthood. The papacy looked to establish standardised canonisation procedures. Some of the evidence presented so far suggests that the reformation movements and the new regulation of sanctity had little impact on pre-existing healing cults such as that of Sainte Jeanne de Valois, which continued well into the seventeenth and eighteenth centuries. However, the tightening up of official procedures for sanctification did have an impact on the religious healing activities of women in the later sixteenth century.

After 1523, no new saints were created for 65 years. There were only six more formal canonisations until the end of the century. The papacy responded to criticism of its procedures and regulated the creation of saints, although unofficial cults continued to surround local healing and holy figures. Peter Burke's analysis of Counter-Reformation saints suggests that the ideal candidate was male, Italian or Spanish, noble and clerical.[81] No French woman in the sixteenth century was recognised with miraculous healing powers or as saintly, by the Counter-Reformation Church.

At the Council of Trent, church officials also sought to establish firmer Church rulings on who could access divine healing, either by their intercession to God or by their determination of the source of an illness as natural or supernatural. Since Tridentine Catholicism reaffirmed the principle of immanence, what was the difference between the Church's veneration of relics or processions, and the laity's invocation of rites and incantations? 'Neither the priest or his hierarchical superiors were prepared to deny the reality of an interventionist God who sanctified the Christian people through ritual observance, who, within the confines of the village church, worked the physical miracle of changing bread into Christ's body every morning.'[82] As Marvin R. O'Connell argues, the difference was a matter of degree, not of kind. However, the Tridentine Church recognised the ordained priest as the only individual who could perform sacred rituals. Now it was the priest, as exorcist, who was the Church's official source to determine whether a disease was supernatural in origin.

This ruling placed women (and men) who claimed God's help in their religious healing in a difficult position. The power of their divine intercession rested on the determination that the illness was supernatural. If it was natural, then herbal, domestic, guild or university medicine would cure it. Only if it were supernatural would divinely inspired healing have effect. Women who claimed, like exorcists, to determine whether the nature of an illness was supernatural were not recognised by the Church, but were now likely to be accused of witchcraft in the secular courts.[83]

Such healers frequently tried to define their medical powers and authority by creating an aura of mystery, differentiating their skills from both physicians and herbalists in the local community. Even if diviners used conventional herbal medicine as the basis of most of their cures, they claimed its efficacy as based on magical dynamism and divine help, not the natural properties of the plant.[84] For the diviner, the remedy's efficacy derived from his or her own mystical powers bestowed by God. In 1577, Barbe Dorée admitted that she placed a pigeon on the stomach of a patient and uttered what may seem to us an innocent and even well-meaning phrase: 'in the name of the Father etc., of Saint Anthony and of Saint Michel, can you heal this illness'. She further advised that a mass be celebrated for the following nine days in the local church.[85]

Even at the end of the sixteenth century, religious healers continued to practise in their local communities despite the Tridentine Church's position that the only recognised living religious healer was the exorcist. Some might claim to be born on divinely significant days of the year. Barbe La Grosse Gorge, from Jarville, explained her healing powers: 'that having been born on Good Friday during the reading of the Passion, she had this ability to cure sick people, especially those bewitched'.[86] Claudette Clauchepied, examined in 1601, claimed in an almost identical statement that having been born the same day, she had the gift of knowing illnesses and divining if they stemmed from diabolical or divine causes.[87] Matthew Ramsey observed similar beliefs persisting in the nineteenth century, where healing powers could be hereditary, determined by such factors as birthdate, order of birth or the way one was born.[88] But if the laity in sixteenth-century France did not fully understand the Tridentine proscription on religious healing, it nonetheless affected people's lives. In the redefined Church seeking to regulate and control the sacred, the claims and practices of the three female healers cited above were unacceptable within established religious orthodoxy. All three healers – Dorée, La Grosse Gorge and Clauchepied – would be charged with witchcraft for practising their forms of religious healing.

By the late sixteenth century, the idea of religious healing seemed almost ridiculous, and certainly unacceptable, to medical men. The physicians Du Breil and Sonnet de Courval, who composed tracts against empirics, were both Catholics. Learned men, they were perhaps more likely to understand the subtleties of the Tridentine Church's position on healing than most. Both fervently disapproved of popular saints and miracles and the women who claimed 'sacred magic, natural and supernatural, black and white'.[89] Du Breil specifically warned his readers to be wary of healers who claimed to work for God, but might really be performing evil: 'They have not received it [their healing talent] as a gratuitous gift, or by infused grace of the holy spirit: for God is never the author of evil'.[90] Du Breil and Sonnet de Courval saw no place for religion in the secular art of medicine.

Healing and witchcraft

Suggesting that Jeanne Lescallier's work equated to witchcraft was one way that the physicians could discredit her herbal healing. The physicians' lawyer, Marion, presented Lescallier's practices in a way that was designed to construct her as a witch according to the recognisable stereotypes of the time: 'the said appellant Lescallier, is commonly known as Jeanne the diviner, who involved herself in divining the future, finding lost objects and making medicine, about which the Judges of the region have received several complaints'.[91] To contemporaries, the diviner was not just someone who could predict the future. The art of divination also concerned detecting medical conditions caused by sorcery, as well as the person from whom the spell originated. The diviner claimed to possess mystical abilities and remedies to cure such supranormal illnesses.[92] The most hazardous of all the physicians' allegations was that Lescallier had treated a lawyer from Angers, by using

> a brew composed of very strange things, she asked for a live crow, which she had dismembered, and said that it was necessary to place half of it on the head of the patient, and have the other half boiled until it was consomme, then crushed, with some mistletoe, together with the brain of a man, and distilled all of it in a chapel, then gave it to the patient over nine days.[93]

The patient died afterwards. All the remedies which Lescallier used, the physicians claimed, came from witchcraft:

> to which arts of sorcery women for their weakness and fragility are much more subject than men, to exercise their vengeance, of which we find several examples in the ancient authors, even by *arrêts* of our court, there have been several women of Auvergne executed for witchcraft.[94]

Lescallier's lawyer repeated what he had already said, that if it was God who 'had given her the grace to heal people, then one must not envy her for that'.[95] Matras's summation of the people's response to these accusations of sorcery, argued clearly that

> if Lescallier had never been sought out for or suspected of such acts, if no person had even been found who complained of receiving the least displeasure from her, neither in her person nor in her goods, if for twenty years she had cured a multitude of people abandoned and despaired of by physicians, if she had helped a world of poor people who hadn't had the means to have themselves healed, if all the parishes even the most noble rendered a testimony of her integrity, of the goods and commodities that they have received and can receive from her, what malicious confusion to name good evil, life death, such a happy and commodious fact of medicine imposture and witchcraft.[96]

The willingness with which the physicians were prepared to deploy potentially fatal allegations in order to discredit Lescallier's medical expertise, and to eradicate her practice once and for all, may well attest to her power and authority within the local community. Marion, their lawyer, drew on the contemporary legal understandings of the problematic relationship between women, healing and diabolical power in an attempt to destroy her defence. Lescallier's case was heard immediately before the *Parlement* experienced its heaviest period of witchcraft appeals in the century, almost twenty a year between 1580 and 1625. In contrast, between 1565 and 1575 there were on average no more than five to six sorcery appeals a year.[97] As Robert Mandrou has observed, from 1580 on, more than thirty treatises were devoted to the subject of diabolical temptation, written by both theologians and judges discussing their own procedures.[98] The procedure of sorcery trials did not follow ordinary legal doctrine but were conducted according to the system established by the increasingly influential treatises of these famous demonologists.[99] For Marion to align Lescallier's case with witchcraft was to place it astutely in a category of heightened preoccupation for Parisian jurists.

How did contemporary jurists understand the relationship between magical healing and witchcraft? One of the most widespread and influential works on witchcraft, published just after Lescallier's trial, may help to elucidate their position. Jean Bodin, a member of the magistracy in Laon, published his treatise on witchcraft, *La Démonomanie des sorciers* in 1580, although he never convicted a witch himself.[100] However, his rather dramatic and obsessive condemnation of witches was popular with a widespread literate public, and underwent ten re-editions between 1580 and 1600 alone.[101] As Mandrou has argued, Bodin's work was a watershed moment in the history of witchcraft trials. His text helped to clarify judicial thought on demonic behaviour and practices, by establishing the legal procedure and criteria for witchcraft trials. Prior to the publication of Bodin's influential text in 1580, judges had few guides as to the legal procedure of such matters.[102] The *Malleus Maleficarum*, first published in French in 1517, was ecclesiastical in origin.[103]

Bodin was to distinguish at several levels between charitable medical practices and those that were malefic.[104] Firstly, he distinguished between medical ingredients that were diabolical or harmless. Secondly, Bodin explained that the words uttered at the same time as the treatment could be inspired by the Devil, even if they seemed ostensibly Christian in sentiment. Barbe Dorée, whose magical healing incantation was cited earlier, eventually confessed during her trial that she treated her patients with the help of simple remedies and phrases that Satan had taught her. So that, as Bodin explained, even though their content appeared harmless and even Catholic in origin, it was the Devil not God who had encouraged her to say the phrases and the resulting cures were thus diabolical not divine.[105] Bodin also reported the case of Jeanne Harvillier, from Verbery, near Compiègne, who was condemned to the stake in 1578 because she 'had begged the Devil to heal her patient'.[106]

The witch was the healer who placed her faith in the Devil, not God, for her remedies. Bodin was only able to cite a small number of witchcraft trials in France to support his arguments. Among them was Jeanne Lescallier's case. In this respect, Bodin was inaccurate, for Lescallier had not been pursued in the courts for sorcery. Yet he used her case to serve as an example of the difference between malefic and harmless healing ingredients:

> it was demonstrated that the means with which she cured were against nature, such as the brain of a cat, which is a poison, the head of a crow, and other similar things, which show well that there was no virtue by good oils and salutary unguents, as do some good and charitable people towards the poor: but by means against nature, or by charms.[107]

Pierre de Lancre, a councillor of the *Parlement* of Bordeaux, was charged by Henri IV with the mission against witches in the south-west of France. In his works published in the early seventeenth century, he distinguished four types of healers: some individuals had a gift for healing through special divine grace and others through their extraordinary sanctity might cure through prayer; however, some healers feigned a divine healing gift; and worse still were magicians and witches who used spells, incantations and rituals. To Lancre, the power of these superstitious practices stemmed from the Devil.[108] We have seen how no French woman in the later sixteenth century was recognised by contemporary ecclesiastical authorities for having a divine healing gift, or the capacity to heal through prayer, because of their exceptional sanctity. Lancre's typology of healers left women who claimed religious healing ability with a choice of being frauds or witches.[109]

The healers who were prosecuted for witchcraft tended to be women and men who did claim to work some form of magic in their healing. But most witchcraft cases were not brought forward typically by elite jurists versed in contemporary demonology, as Lescallier's appeared to be by Simon Marion and the physicians, but instead by local communities. Matras, arguing for Lescallier and the local community, drew on a different understanding of witchcraft – one which did not take its notions of diabolical healing from the works of demonologists. Diviners' cases were brought before court as witchcraft often because the local community identified failed white-magic cures. Indeed, despite the physicians' claims, witchcraft trials were one way in which the local community *could* demonstrate their ability to recognise charlatans among their midst and prevent their practice. A witness said about the diviner Barbe la

Grosse Gorge, from Jarville, that 'having drawn from people all that she could in money and victuals, she abandoned them in that state'.[110] In the trial of Claudette Clauchepied, her own assistant admitted that 'she was a trickster because she never accomplished any of the pilgrimages that she promised to do'.[111] Communities sought retribution and a stop to the activities of such white-magic healers. They could report the failed practices as suspect religious beliefs to local ecclesiastical authorities to be examined, or as fraudulent medical charlatanism to a local body of physicians. Where local communities did pursue concerns through the legal system, jurists informed about contemporary demonological theories might perceive their complaints as witchcraft accusations.

This is not to say that local communities did not have witchcraft beliefs of their own, but rather that these were different to those held by the legal fraternity. Understandings of sorcery and magical healing differed markedly between popular ideas, and juridical notions.[112] As Delcambre has argued for neighbouring Lorraine, diviners believed they held their powers from God, completely separate from the practices of the witch, and those who consulted them shared that opinion. Jurists and theologians, however, believed that any claim to be able to treat a diabolically caused illness was sinister.[113] The witchcraft of the clerics and judges was based and founded in the framework of satanic religion as reported in demonological treatises.[114] There, the art of divination was a presumption of witchcraft, even if capital punishment could not be pronounced unless the diviner admitted to making a pact with the Devil. If many diviners were successfully prosecuted as witches, it was because they eventually admitted that they were acolytes of the Devil.[115] It is significant to note that in Lescallier's case, the local community identified her as a successful healer and did not complain of her activities as incompetent or diabolical. Here it appears to be the intellectual elite (Marion and the physicians) creating witchcraft accusations for the ears of other elite jurists.

In the neighbouring regions of Lorraine and the Franche-Comté, white-magic healing formed an important part of witchcraft prosecution at the end of the sixteenth century and into the seventeenth. Monter's evidence suggests that there demonologists assumed all magical cures were achieved with diabolical aid, thus any practitioner who admitted to magical healing was seen by judges as a potential witch, even though to the accused magical healing and witchcraft might be two separate concepts.[116] However, as Briggs has pointed out, the relationships of courts in Lorraine and the Franche-Comté to official policy were different to those of courts in France, where fairly formal procedures about the prosecution of witchcraft cases were in place.[117] To examine how such understandings of white magic and healing translated into legal practice, we must examine the evidence for France.

The obsessed demonologist Jean Bodin did not represent the opinions and fervour of the *Parlement* of Paris.[118] Indeed, Bodin even complained of the laxity of his fellow jurists in pursuing cases. Robin Briggs has concluded from the evidence of Soman and Mandrou that the *Parlement* of Paris was somewhat sceptical about sorcery.[119] Lescallier and her supporters never claimed that she used white magic and divination, but derived her remedies from a partial understanding of learned medicine and herbal recipes that she made from experience. Once the procedures for legal prosecution of witchcraft were established, the *Parlement* of Paris was to recognise only three proofs of sorcery and the case of Lescallier provided none of them. There could be, firstly, material proof such as signed pacts with the Devil or mysterious diabolical powder; secondly, freely obtained admission of the fact, without torture; and lastly, an incontestable eyewitness to an act of witchcraft.[120] Moreover, Lescallier's case did not come before the *Parlement* to be judged as an appeal to a witchcraft conviction from her local court. To contrast Lescallier's case with a contemporary witchcraft conviction that the *Parlement* did ratify on appeal demonstrates these differences.

In 1586, Marie Martin came before the Court from Neufville le Roy in Picardy. In the remaining interrogation statements, she admitted that 'she gathered herbs on St Jean's eve to cure people and animals that she had bewitched to languish', though she added 'not to die'. Although she, like Lescallier, used herbal remedies, Martin confessed that her recipes were concocted both with diabolical assistance and to reverse enchantments she had herself placed upon them, sometimes using a diabolical powder. Martin also claimed that an evil spirit, Cerberus, encouraged and assisted her in her diabolical healing work. Thus, in contrast to Lescallier, Martin openly testified to her former diabolical practices during her appeal case at the *Parlement*.[121]

It is not clear that Simon Marion and the physicians ever really intended to have Lescallier tried as a witch, or simply hoped to discredit her medical work. Marion was unable to furnish clear proof of diabolical activities to a *Parlement* that appears to have been ambiguous about the relationship of sorcery and healing. The fact that communities could and did instigate proceedings against ineffective diviners and healers made their clear support for Lescallier and recognition of her beneficial medicine all the more pertinent. But the diabolical claims made by Marion certainly helped in having her appeal rejected and sufficient doubt cast on her practice that the legal fraternity were likely to be sympathetic to the physicians' cause. The 1578 ruling once more rejected Lescallier's case on the basis that other empirics with less worthy intentions ought not be encouraged to practise. Lescallier came away from the *Parlement* with an almost reluctant ruling which acknowledged her personal expertise, suppressed the fines and costs of the court, but conferred ultimate medical authority on the physicians: 'however much the appellant may have great and long experience ... the law says that it must not be permitted to anyone to apply and prescribe medicaments if they are not approved by the law and by men'.[122]

Lescallier's appeal documents are an important resource for understanding sixteenth-century perceptions about women's healing capacities and their limitation under secular and ecclesiastical law, and about the power of the populace to determine their own source of medical assistance. Her case is unusually rich in demonstrating the complexities of contemporary opinions, within the medical, ecclesiastical, legal and local communities, about the authority and criminality of female healing, and how far they were prepared to recognise it publicly. The legal defence for Lescallier presented a women and community able to articulate their right to choose their own medical service, and employed acceptable contemporary discourses, of women's natural herbal knowledge and charity, to enable Lescallier to continue her medical work. In contrast, the medical community, striving to establish their jurisdiction over authoritative medical practice, depicted the country folk as medically ignorant and credulous, but they had little legal basis to prevent women engaging in charitable herbal healing. In order to criminalise Lescallier's healing, the physicians were obliged to delve into the potentially explosive realm of witchcraft, manipulating the growing contemporary legal preoccupation with acts of sorcery.

Notes

1 Bibliothèque Nationale Manuscrit Baluze 222 (Baluze 222), *Playdr de M. Matras et Marion sur une femme qui exercoit la medecine en lannee 1573*, fol. 10r.
2 *Ibid.*, fol. 11r.
3 John A. Carey, *Judicial Reform in France before the Revolution of 1789* (Cambridge, Mass.: Harvard University Press, 1981), p. 23. Charles Colbert's survey of administration in Anjou written in 1664 was scathing of its judicial processes. He complains about 'la multiplicité des degrés de juridiction, y en ayant en aucuns lieux ... jusques à quatre et cinq où les sujets de S.M. sont obligés d'aller poursuivre auparavant que d'avoir définitivement la justice' as well as 'la quantité presque infinie de différentes

justices et de justiciers de toutes manières qu'elles produisent et qu'elles répandent partout qui, par leurs conflits, leurs jalousies et leurs contestations, déshonorent la dignité de leur ministère et, par les vexations et chicanes qu'ils font aux parties pour subsister, les dévorent et les consomment.' Charles Colbert, Rapport sur l'Anjou, in *Archives d'Anjou: Recueil de documents et mémoires inédits sur cette province*, ed. Paul Marchegay, vol. 1 (Angers: Charles Labussière, 1843), p. 143.

4 Bibliothèque Nationale manuscrit français (BN ms fr) 21737, *Arrest notable qui defend a une femme d'Anjou d'exercer la medecine, 18 avril 1578*, fol. 305v. As Xavier Martin reports, fire in 1744 at the palais de justice d'Angers destroyed much of the local judicial archives for this period. See Martin, 'Aspects de la sorcellerie en Anjou, 1570–1640', in *Histoire des faits de la sorcellerie* (Angers: Presses de l'Université d'Angers, 1985), pp. 71–110.

5 Marion published a series of his speeches to the court in Paris, 1598: Lescallier's case was not among them. See discussion of the career of Matras in Xavier Martin, 'Aspects de la sorcellerie en Anjou, 1570–1640', and that of Marion in Olivier Martin, *Les Manuscrits de Simon Marion, et la coutume de Paris au XVIe siècle* (Rennes: Imprimeries Oberthur, 1922).

6 See N. Z. Davis, *Fiction in the Archives: Pardon Tales and their Tellers in Sixteenth-Century France* (Stanford: Stanford University Press, 1987).

7 *Les Enseignements d'Anne de France Duchesse de Bourbonnois et d'Auvergne à sa fille Susanne de Bourbon*, ed. A.-M. Chazaud (Moulins: C. Desrosiers, 1878) (Marseille: Lafitte, 1978), pp. 69–70.

8 Christine de Pizan, *Le Livre des trois vertus*, intro. Charity Cannon Willard, text by Willard and Eric Hicks (Paris: Champion, 1989), p. 38.

9 Olivier de Serres, *Théâtre d'agriculture et mesnage des champs d'Olivier de Serres, Seigneur du Pradel* (Rouen: Jean Berthelin, 1646), p. 548.

10 See further discussion of this work in Chapter 6.

11 Charles de Robillard de Beaurepaire, 'Notes extraites des premières registres de l'Hôtel-Dieu de Rouen', in *Extrait du Précis des travaux de l'Académie des Sciences, Belles-Lettres et Arts de Rouen* (Rouen: H. Boissel, [1870]), pp. 9–10.

12 Alexis Chevalier, *L'Hôtel-Dieu de Paris et les sœurs augustines* (Paris: Champion, 1901), p. 253.

13 *Ibid.*, pp. 253–4.

14 For further details on the role of women in patronage of medical texts see Chapter 5.

15 Jean Lyège, *Raison de vivre pour toutes fièvres, congnues premierement par leurs differences, causes, signes, & symptomes, auec les prognostiques d'icelles* (Paris: M. Vascosan, 1557), fol. Aii r.

16 *Ibid.*, fol. A iii v.

17 M. Verdier, *La Jurisprudence de la médecine en France*, vol. 2 (Alençon: Malassis, 1762), pp. 554–5.

18 'Mémoires de Jacques-Auguste De Thou depuis 1553 jusqu'en 1601', in J.-A.-C. Buchon (ed.), *Choix de chroniques et mémoires relatifs à l'histoire de France* (Orléans: H. Herluison, 1875), p. 565.

19 Jacques Guillemeau, *Les Oeuvres de chirurgie* (Rouen: Jean Viret, François Vaultier, Clement Malassis, Jacques Besongne, 1649), p. 311. The first edition was published in 1612.

20 Laurent Joubert, *Chirurgie de M. Gui de Chauliac* (Lyon: Estienne Michel, 1580), p. 28.
21 *Ibid.*, p. 28.
22 *Ibid.*, p. 29.
23 *Ibid.*, pp. 28–9.
24 Laurent Joubert, *La Médecine et le régime de santé, des erreurs populaires et propos vulgaires* (Bordeaux: Simon Millanges, 1578) ed. Madeleine Tiollais, vol. 1 (Paris: L'Harmattan, 1997), pp. 163–4.
25 C. A. Ernest Wickersheimer, *La Médecine et les médecins en France à l'époque de la Renaissance* (Paris: A. Maloine, 1906), p. 23.
26 BN ms fr 21737, fol. 302v.
27 *Ibid.*, fol. 302v.
28 *Ibid.*, fol. 303r.
29 *Ibid.*, fol. 303v.
30 *Ibid.*, fol. 302r.
31 *Ibid.*, fol. 304r.
32 *Ibid.*, fols 304r–v.
33 *Ibid.*, fols 303r–v.
34 *Ibid.*, fol. 303r.
35 Baluze 222, fol. 1v.
36 *Ibid.*, fol. 1v.
37 *Ibid.*, fol. 1v.
38 Du Breil, *La Police de l'art et science de medecine* (Paris: Leon Cavellat, 1580), pp. 60 and 89.
39 Martin, 'Aspects de la sorcellerie en Anjou, 1570–1640', p. 86, n. 21.
40 Baluze 222, fol. 7r.
41 BN ms fr 21737, fol. 307v.
42 Baluze 222, fol. 10v.
43 *Ibid.*, fol. 11r.
44 *Ibid.*, fol. 11r.
45 BN ms fr 21737, fol. 306v.
46 *Ibid.*, fol. 307r.
47 *Ibid.*, fol. 306v.
48 Baluze 222, fol. 4r.
49 BN ms fr 21737, fol. 303v.
50 *Ibid.*, 304r.
51 Baluze 222, fols 3r–v.
52 BN ms fr 21737, fols 302v–303r. The text says literally 'in order to forbid her not [sic] to practise the art of medicine', which is likely to be a scribal error.
53 *Ibid.*, fol. 303v.
54 *Ibid.*, fols 305r–v.
55 *Ibid.*, fol. 304r.
56 Verdier, *La Jurisprudence de la médecine en France*, vol. 1 (Alençon: Malassis, 1763), p. 76.
57 Verdier, *Jurisprudence*, vol. 1, p. 683, cited in Olivier Martin, *L'Organisation corporative de la France d'ancien régime* (Paris: Sirey, 1938), p. 376.

58 BN ms fr 21737, fol. 304r.
59 Alfred Soman, 'Trente procès de sorcellerie dans le Perche 1566–1624', *L'Orne littéraire*, vol. 8, 1986 in Soman (ed.), *Sorcellerie et justice criminelle: le Parlement de Paris 16e–18e siècles* (Aldershot: Ashgate, 1992), p. 52.
60 *Ibid.*, p. 53.
61 René Choppin, *Traicte des privileges des personnes vivans aux champs* in *Les Œuvres de Me René Choppin* (Paris: P. Ménard, 1663), p. 57.
62 *Ibid.*, p. 57.
63 *Ibid.*, pp. 57–8.
64 Baluze 222, fol. 1r.
65 *Ibid.*, fol. 11r.
66 *Ibid.*, fol. 2v.
67 Colbert, *Rapport sur l'Anjou*, p. 126.
68 Soman, 'The *Parlement* of Paris and the great witch hunt (1565–1640)', *The Sixteenth Century Journal*, 9:2 (1978) in *Sorcellerie et justice criminelle*, p. 34.
69 BN ms fr 21737, fols 304v–305r.
70 H. Brabant, *Médecins, malades et maladies de la Renaissance* (Brussels: La Renaissance du livre, 1966), p. 245.
71 BN ms fr 21737, fol. 307v.
72 *Ibid.*, fol. 307v.
73 *Les Petits Bollandistes vies des saints de l'Ancien et du Nouveau Testament*, ed. Paul Guérin, vol. 4 (Paris: Bloud et Barral, 1872), p. 40.
74 *Les Petits Bollandistes*, vol. 2, pp. 264–8.
75 *Vie et miracles de la bienheureuse Philippe de Chantemilan*, ed. Ulysse Chevalier (Valence: Jules Céas, 1894).
76 AD d'Indre et Loire, 1 J 1165 Les déclarations faites à la chapelle de Sainte Catherine de Fierbois, près de Sainte-Maure en Touraine, de 245 miracles arrivés de 1375 à 1536. The Bibliothèque Nationale copy (BN ms fr 1045), is an earlier version of the text, including 237 miracles from 1375 until 1470, and has been published as Yves Chauvin (ed.), *Livre des miracles de Sainte-Catherine-de-Fierbois* (Poitiers: Société des Archives historiques de Poitou, 1976).
77 Pierre André Sigal, 'La grossesse, l'accouchement et l'attitude envers l'enfant mortné à la fin du moyen âge d'après les récits de miracles', *Santé, médecine et assistance au moyen âge* (Actes du 110e congrès national des sociétés savantes, Montpellier, 1985) (Paris: Editions du CTHS, 1987), p. 28.
78 M. de la Fons de Mélicocq, 'Dépenses faites par la ville de Lille pour les enfants trouvés', *Bulletin du comité historique des monuments écrits de l'histoire de France*, 3 (1855–56), p. 479.
79 For discussion of concepts of late medieval sainthood and community dynamics, see Aviad M. Kleinberg, *Prophets in their Own Country: Living Saints and the Making of Sainthood in the Later Middle Ages* (Chicago: The University of Chicago Press, 1992). For typologies of sainthood, see André Vauchez, *La Sainteté en occident aux derniers siècles du Moyen Age: d'après les proces de canonisation et les documents hagiographiques* (Rome: Ecole française de Rome, 1981), and Pierre Delooz, 'Towards a sociological study of canonized sainthood in the Catholic Church', in Stephen Wilson (ed.), *Saints and their Cults: Studies in Religious Sociology*,

Folklore and History (Cambridge: Cambridge University Press, 1983), pp. 189–216.

80 David Gentilcore, *From Bishop to Witch: The System of the Sacred in Early Modern Terra d'Otranto* (Manchester: Manchester University Press, 1992), p. 170.

81 Peter Burke, 'How to be a Counter-Reformation saint', in Kaspar von Greyerz (ed.), *Religion and Society in Early Modern Europe, 1500–1800* (London: Allen and Unwin, 1984), p. 49.

82 Marvin R. O'Connell, 'The Roman Catholic tradition since 1545', in Ronald L. Numbers and Darrel W. Amundsen (eds), *Caring and Curing: Health and Medicine in the Western Religious Traditions* (New York: Macmillan, 1986), p. 131.

83 For background, see Richard Kieckhefer, 'The holy and the unholy: sainthood, witchcraft and magic in late medieval Europe', *Journal of Medieval and Renaissance Studies* (1994), pp. 355–85.

84 Estienne Delcambre, *Les Devins-Guérisseurs dans la Lorraine ducale: leur activité et leurs méthodes* (Nancy: Société d'archéologie lorraine et Musée historique lorrain, 1951), pp. 72–3.

85 Verdier, *La Jurisprudence*, vol. 1, pp. 257–8.

86 Delcambre, *Les Devins-Guérisseurs*, p. 14.

87 Jean-Claude Diedler, *Démons et sorcières en Lorraine: le bien et le mal dans les communautés rurales de 1550 à 1660* (Paris: Messène, 1996), p. 20.

88 Matthew Ramsey, *Professional and Popular Medicine in France, 1770–1830: The Social World of Medical Practice* (Cambridge: Cambridge University Press, 1988), p. 244.

89 Du Breil, *La Police de l'art et science de medecine*, p. 43.

90 *Ibid.*, p. 45. Alison Klairmont Lingo, 'Empirics and charlatans in early modern France: the genesis of the classification of the "Other" in medical practice', *Journal of Social History*, 19 (1985–86), p. 590.

91 BN ms fr 21737, fol. 305v.

92 Delcambre, *Les Devins-Guérisseurs*, p. 43. For comparative studies, see also Keith Thomas, *Religion and the Decline of Magic: Studies in Popular Beliefs in Sixteenth and Seventeenth Century England* (London: Weidenfeld and Nicolson, 1971).

93 BN ms fr 21737, fol. 308r.

94 *Ibid.*, fol. 308r.

95 *Ibid.*, fol. 306v.

96 Baluze 222, fol. 3v.

97 Soman, 'The Parlement of Paris and the great witch hunt (1565–1640)', p. 34.

98 Robert Mandrou, *Magistrats et sorciers en France au XVIIe siècle: une analyse de psychologie historique* (Paris: Plon, 1968), p. 137.

99 Robert Muchembled, *Sorcières: justice et société aux 16e et 17e siècles* (Paris: Imago, 1982), p. 101. For an overview of the writings of European demonologists, see Lynn Thorndike, *A History of Magic and Experimental Science*, vol. 4 (1941) (New York: Columbia University Press, 1959). The microfiche collection *Sorciers, demonologues, magistrats, théologiens et médecins aux XVIe et XVIIe siècles*, ed. Robert Mandrou (Paris: Microeditions Hachette, 1975) is also particularly useful.

100 Soman, 'Decriminalizing witchcraft: does the French experience furnish a European model?' *Criminal Justice History*, 10 (1989), in *Sorcellerie et justice criminelle*, p. 11.

101 Mandrou, *Magistrats et sorciers*, p. 129.

102 *Ibid.*, pp. 122, 126.
103 Evidence for late medieval witchcraft trials suggest that proportions of men and women accused and convicted were fairly even in France, but became increasingly femininised in the sixteenth and seventeenth centuries. See Robert Favreau, 'La sorcellerie en Poitou à la fin du Moyen Age', *Bulletin de la Société des Antiquaires de l'Ouest*, 18 (1985), pp. 133–54, see especially p. 138 and fn. 29. Henri Carré, 'Quelques mots sur la sorcellerie dans les provinces de l'Ouest au XVIe et XVIIe siècle', *Bulletin de la Société des Antiquaires de l'Ouest*, 7 (1925–27), pp. 631–74.
104 Soman, 'Decriminalizing witchcraft', p. 11.
105 Jean Bodin, *De la démonomanie des sorciers* (1580) (Paris Jacques du Puys, 1587), fol. 272v.
106 *Ibid.*, fols aiijr–v.
107 *Ibid.*, fols 142v–143r.
108 Ramsey, *Professional and popular medicine in France*, p. 231.
109 Nuanced understandings of the gendering of witchcraft specifically in France can be found in Stuart Clark, 'The "gendering" of witchcraft in French demonology: misogyny or polarity?', *French History*, 5 (1991), pp. 406–37 and Robin Briggs, 'Women as victims? Witches, judges, and the community', *French History*, 5 (1991), pp. 438–80.
110 Delcambre, *Les Devins-Guérisseurs*, p. 48.
111 *Ibid.*, p. 48.
112 Muchembled, *Sorcières: justice et société*, pp. 123–8. For discussion of the differences between popular and learned witchcraft, see, for example, R. Briggs, *Communities of Belief: Cultural and Social Tension in Early Modern France* (Oxford: Clarendon Press, 1989). Muchembled's theories of acculturation and absorption of elite beliefs by the populace have been widely debated: see arguments for and against in *Religion and Society in Early Modern Europe*, ed. Greyerz, pp. 56–78.
113 Delcambre, *Les Devins-Guérisseurs*, p. 217.
114 Muchembled, *Sorcières: justice et société*, p. 128.
115 Delcambre, *Les Devins-Guérisseurs*, p. 217.
116 E. William Monter, *Witchcraft in France and Switzerland: The Borderlands During the Reformation* (Ithaca: Cornell University Press, 1976), pp. 175–85.
117 Briggs, *Communities of Belief*, p. 13.
118 For discussion, and personal contexts of, demonologists like Bodin, see *The Damned Art: Essays in the Literature of Witchcraft*, ed. Sydney Anglo (London: Routledge, 1977).
119 Briggs, *Communities of Belief*, p. 12. For a slightly later period, Andrews argues that local seigneurial and baillaige courts were in small towns and villages and had sparse police forces, unlike the magistrates of Châtelet or the *Parlement* of Paris. Provincial judges were probably inclined to compensate for their weakness in policing by severity in punishment. His survey suggests *Parlement* reversed many decisions taken by local courts and tended to give more lenient sentences. This evidence appears to correlate with some of the findings of Soman and Mandrou, and conclusions of Briggs, for sixteenth-century witchcraft. Richard Mowery Andrews, *Law, Magistracy and Crime in Old Regime Paris, 1735–1789, vol. 1: The System of Criminal Justice* (Cambridge: Cambridge University Press, 1994), pp. 492–3.

120 Soman, 'Les Procès de sorcellerie au Parlement de Paris 1565–1640', *Annales: Economies, Sociétés, Civilisations*, 32 (1977) in *Sorcellerie et justice criminelle*, p. 807.
121 Louis Le Caron, *De la Tranquilité d'Esprit, Livre Singulier, plus un discours sur le procès criminel faict à une sorcière condamnée à mort par Arrest de la Court de Parlement* (Paris: Jacques Du Puy, 1588), pp. 159–200.
122 BN ms fr 21737, fols 308v–309r.

5

The book trades: female medical practice in print

THE SIXTEENTH CENTURY, with the introduction and widespread use of the print medium, saw an extraordinary transformation in the meanings and modes of publication.[1] Increasingly, publishers in the search for profits became more flexible about the texts they published, searching for new markets to which they could sell printed books. Popular medical literature and household manuals were just two areas which they exploited in the drive for profits, and they were to have important ramifications for women's medical knowledge and practices within the household. Moral commentators had traditionally advised women that domestic medicine, maintaining the health of their family and household, was a primary concern. Now, in the sixteenth century, learned authors from both the university medical and lay community made clear to a wider public readership, through their printed works, that women had a vital role to play in primary medical care. It was a role, however, which was frequently problematised in contemporary literature, suggesting an often uneasy alliance between the medical ideal and the practicalities of everyday life.

Medicine in print: new authors and disciplines

The advent of the printing press created opportunities for a wider body of people to become authors. Print offered greater access to those excluded by status, profession, religion or region, to name only a few, from the exclusive circles who had previously produced and circulated scribal texts among themselves. Printers and publishers also searched for new and different authors whom they could market to ever wider audiences. Increasing emphasis was placed on experience as an essential part of knowledge, rather than accepted wisdom in the works of the ancients. Some contemporary craftspeople published practical manuals explaining the skills of their trade. Hope Glidden cites the example of Bernard Palissy whose 1580 *Discours admirables de la nature des eaux et fontaines* pitted Theory against Practice in a debate over the source of knowledge, questioning the precedence of textual authority over the author's personal experience.² Plurality, insisting on diverse and individual voices, became necessary to a new subjective knowledge that could only be gained by historically bound, personal authorial experience.

Among these new authors were surgeons and apothecaries. They used publications to celebrate the importance of their medical work, and to increase their public prestige. Urbain Hémard, surgeon to the Cardinal d'Armagnac, despaired of surgery's status as a mechanical art and urged fellow surgeons to publish useful studies of their art like his *Recherche de la vraye anatomie des dents*.³ Others, such as the surgeon Jehan Breche, recommended that surgical professionals disclose their knowledge to distinguish themselves from the many non-professionals who plagued the medical professions. In 1545, Breche argued that 'surgeons must and are held to know and understand natures and causes, and give reason to what they do. Otherwise they are without art and method, and do no more than those mad old weak-minded women, who meddle in curing fevers'.⁴ The surgeon Claude Dalechamps published his translation of Galen into French with the desire to increase the knowledge of his counterparts: 'the reading of this book is not only useful, but also necessary to surgeons'.⁵ Distinguishing their learning from those unqualified by any recognised medical system and pride in their skills and knowledge of Latin and Greek may have been reasons why surgeons chose to declare their knowledge in vernacular print.

Yet other medical writers advised fellow professionals to guard closely the secrets of their expertise in order to prevent 'outsiders' (both male and female) from accessing their knowledge. Some were particularly concerned that medical knowledge was now accessible to the general public, through French-language publications. As Alison Klairmont Lingo has argued, many saw printing in the vernacular as a threat to their monopoly on approved medical knowledge. When the collected works of the eminent Protestant surgeon Ambroise Paré were to appear in French in 1575, both the medical faculty and some surgeons tried unsuccessfully to prevent its publication. The subsequent text included the 'response of M. Ambroise Paré, first surgeon of the King, to the slander of some physicians and surgeons concerning his works'.⁶ Republished again in 1579, the widespread popularity of Paré's works was undeniable. Then, in 1582, Paré's works were translated into Latin and published in a scholastic in-folio edition.⁷ The publication was steeped in significance: the humble barber–surgeon had been accepted into university-approved medical discourse. But it was all relative. Depending on where one was placed in the broader medical spectrum, the same vernacular Paré editions could be used by others as a source of approved authority. Louise Bourgeois, the most influential midwife in the period and wife of a surgeon, claimed to have learnt her craft from the study of Paré's works as a way of indicating that she had knowledge of learned medicine.

Some surgeons and apothecaries also published their own studies of their medical work as a form of resistance to domination by physicians. Although the latter complained about surgeons' and apothecaries' publications, physicians were not adverse to contributing their own printed works (in both French and Latin) concerning surgery and pharmacy, rather than about their own activities. Some physicians' texts critiqued the practices of guild medical providers, sparking heated debates between guild and university practitioners. Some physicians argued that they translated texts that would be useful for surgeons or apothecaries to know for their work.[8] More often than not, guild practitioners saw such publications as interference from physicians trying to impose their knowledge on those lower down the medical hierarchy.[9]

A second consequence of publishers' eagerness to print original work was an expansion of medical literature targeted specifically at the general public. It could be written by medical professionals as well as lay members of the community. Not all of it was entirely concerned with medicine; much was joined to almanacs, or astrological and magical information. The steady rate of reprints of this kind of literature throughout the sixteenth century suggests a wide sector of the general population were interested in improving their medical knowledge and learning different medical techniques and practices.

One of the first and most widespread handbooks to appear that included discussion of medical practices was the 1494 *Le Grand Calendrier et compost des bergers*.[10] Popular medical instruction was included because: 'the thing which the shepherd most desires in the world is to live long, and that which he fears most is to die young, . . . [it is] to know and do things possible and required [to live] long, healthily and joyously that this present calendar teaches'.[11] The early sixteenth-century Parisian edition included anatomy: 'the name of the bones of the body and the number of them, and there are in sum two hundred and forty eight', and as to surgery, provided a list of the appropriate veins to be bled for differing illnesses. Humeral theory was used to indicate 'signs by which shepherds know man to be healthy and well disposed in his body' as well as other signs which 'show a surplus of bad humours to be purged'. Finally there followed a discussion of healthy diet and lifestyle.[12]

The *Grand Calendrier* is just one example of the sort of medical knowledge that could be gained from popular printed texts. Alternatively, the many versions of the *Petit Albert* and *Grand Albert*, attributed to Albert the Grand, circulated knowledge of the medicinal virtues of a variety of plants as well as more 'magical' recipes such as that designed to determine whether the (evidently male) reader's wife was faithful. These early but enduringly popular texts included recipes which were in many ways akin to the kind of healing and divining white magic which was, as the previous chapter has demonstrated, increasingly problematised over the sixteenth century. Another recurrent theme of interest to all at the time was that of the plague. Klairmont Lingo's study of publications concerning the plague in sixteenth-century France observes the self-conscious and defensive way in which many authors presented their texts. She argues that, because many were apothecaries, barbers and surgeons, they were conscious of lacking the skills in scholastic disputation of their university-trained counterparts.[13] Paul Slack, observing a similar defensive stance in popular medical literature in England, suggests that it is a trope: an attempt to tantalise readers with information that was previously hidden from their view.[14] Both theories are likely to hold value, and fear of the plague supported the publication of at least eight different texts on the subject in France during the period.[15]

Popular texts provided one sort of information that literate women, or those with access to a literate reader, might employ to develop a knowledge of domestic medicine. Dietetic medicine and preparation of medicinal waters were both the duties of the good wife in her home. *La Grand Propietaire* [sic] *de toutes choses*, 'very useful and profitable for keeping the human body in good health, containing ... preservative remedies', translated into French by Jean Corbichon and first published in 1556, also included detailed discussion of the medicinal value of the trees and plants treated in its seventeenth book. Almond oil, for example, 'kill worms in the stomach, and bring on periods in ladies, and does good to those who are deaf and removes dirt in the ears when one drips it warm inside them'.[16] Elsewhere the *Grand Propietaire* instructed how to prepare herbal waters by distillation, in a chapter on 'the virtues and properties of artificial waters'.[17] Other medical texts which were exclusively aimed at housewives would also appear in the period, teaching them how to care for their families, but the majority of these texts were published by authors who preferred to remain anonymous. In 1558, there appeared *La Pratique de faire toutes confitures, condiments*, *distillations d'eaux odiferantes et plusieurs autres receptes tresutiles.*[18] Equally without mention of their authors were the *Régime du vivre tresutile et necessaire, contenant la propriété des herbes* in 1556 and *La Pratique pour faire toutes sortes de confitures, condimens, distillations, compostes, cottignac, hypocrats, pugmens, tyzenne... Et un souverain remede contre la peste* in 1590.[19] The resort to anonymity bears witness to the poor consideration that domestic medicine was accorded by physicians, even if there existed a clear interest among readers for such knowledge.

Given the participation in printed medical debates of not only guild-regulated medical practitioners but also of the general public, increasingly over the sixteenth century physicians themselves did begin to record their medical knowledge and practices in print. Some produced their works in French, like Jean Lyège with his 1557 *Raison de vivre pour toutes fièvres*.[20] Alternatively, several physicians translated the Greek and Latin works of their predecessors, with the specific claim of bringing that knowledge to the use of the wider (literate) community. Such were the claims of Claude Valgelas, who in 1559 translated Hierosme de Monteux's *Commentaire de la conservation de santé, et prolongation de vie*; the physician to the royal children, Guillaume Chrestian, 1559 translator of Jacques du Bois's *Livre de la nature et utilité des moys des femmes*; and the surgeon Claude Dalechamps, who translated Galen in his 1566 *De l'usage des parties du corps humains*.[21] Dalechamps argued that such works could be beneficial to all the general public: 'I do not want to enumerate how much this book will be useful to physicians, surgeons, philosophers, and generally to any person desirous to learn the miracles of God'.[22]

The physician Philibert Guibert was perhaps one of the most prolific generators of university-acquired medical knowledge to the general population in the early seventeenth century. His texts were small and affordable, including the twelve-page manual, *Le Médecin des pauvres*, which offered some curious advice on 'prayers and orisons against toothache, cuts, rhumatism, fever, ringworm, colic, burns, and evil spirits'[23] and the 23-page *Le Médecin charitable*. Guibert's 1625 *L'Apothicaire du médecin charitable* promised to teach readers 'to make in their houses composed medicines with great ease, with little cost or time'. Finally, in 1629 he reprinted these texts in his comprehensive 688-page manual *Les Oeuvres charitables de Philibert Guybert*.

Guibert's *Oeuvres charitables* was a best seller, republished eleven times in the four years between 1624 and 1627. It was also a blatant attack on the practices and utility of apothecaries. Guibert provided details on how to compose common pharmaceutical compounds and advised the public to buy directly from spicers, bypassing the need for apothecaries altogether.²⁴ Guibert's information was by no means original, but the notion of publicising apothecaries' skills and practices in such a way certainly was. Guibert, professor of pharmacy at the Parisian medical faculty, continued to pursue his aggressive policy, despite the outcry from apothecaries. At the same time as faculty physicians were preparing a new *Antidotarium* to replace the twelfth-century classic by Nicolas of Salerno, which stipulated what drugs apothecaries ought to keep in their boutiques, Guibert produced his *Prix et valeur des Médicaments*, outlining what drugs apothecaries stocked and (his idea of) what price they should be. Then, there was his *Apothicaire charitable*, which listed more details of composed remedies that the general public could make for themselves. Philippe Albou argues that Guibert's texts undoubtedly had an impact on contemporary mentalities about the public's own responsibilities for, and limits of, preserving health.²⁵ But if physicians considered that they were empowering the public to take charge of their own health, it rarely extended to revealing their own medical knowledge. It was the same Guibert who, as discussed in Chapter 1, refused to open his medical cabinet to the notaries charged with producing an inventory after his wife's death in 1631, on the grounds that it contained drugs and compositions that could not be divulged. The matter was only resolved by calling two physicians from the faculty to estimate the cabinet's value, but its contents were never revealed.²⁶

The physician André du Breil, in his text against empirics, complained that the publication of medical texts contributed to the problem of unlicensed practitioners. It was now too easy for people to learn and imitate the practices of physicians by books published in French, with the result that all sorts of people were undertaking medical work including scholars, priests, barbers and noblewomen.²⁷ Even if not all physicians were in favour of sharing their university-acquired knowledge with the entire population, many realised that it was at least one way of controlling how the general population could perceive, and practise, medicine. As Natalie Zemon Davis has argued about Laurent Joubert's 1578 explanation of the *Erreurs populaires* of doctors right down to the common people, the Chancellor of the Medical Faculty at Montpellier intended 'to use the press and the vernacular as a means of control over medical practice and over the people', although, as she notes, physicians themselves were among the most interested readers of such texts.²⁸

Could women participate too as new authors and as creators of new medical knowledge in print? Only rarely. Many women did not necessarily require literacy for their medical or health care work, and so it was unlikely that many were capable of producing such texts, unless they were dictated. If women did not publish medical texts themselves, it was more likely to result from their lack of opportunities than from any institutional bar from the book trades on their publication. It seems likely that publishers would have been interested in medical texts from a female perspective, which would have constituted a marketable novelty.[29]

In 1609, a midwife, Louise Bourgeois, published her own account of gynaecology and obstetrics in *Observations diverse sur la sterilité, perte de fruict, foecondité, accouchements et maladies des femmes et enfants nouveaux naix.*[30] She insisted that her experience as a midwife, both to the women of her neighbourhood and later to the queen, Marie de Medici, would rectify the errors of physicians.[31] Bourgeois emphasised her occupational identity to invest some value and authority in her work as that of an individual historical writer influenced by personal experience. In 1609, Pierre de l'Estoile bought her first work *Observations* and recorded in his diary: 'I have bought today a new work (timely and worthy of this century), printed in octavo by Saugrain, in fact by Boursier [her married name], midwife of the Queen, treating illnesses and deliveries of women'. L'Estoile accredited Bourgeois with authority because 'this I imagine to be much more authentic and collectable, ... this woman can know a lot of the little secrets of nature that she has learnt at the barber's basin'.[32] To his mind, it was the combination of her own experiences and her association with the trade of her husband, a barber–surgeon, which rendered her expert in medical matters.

Born in 1563 in Paris, Bourgeois married in 1584 the Tourangeau, Martin Boursier, attaché to the army of the King, student of Ambroise Paré and later surgeon to the King.[33] Bourgeois tells us that she learned her craft, after the birth of her children, through studying the works of Paré and, as she wrote, 'my husband who had remained twenty years in the household of the late master Ambroise Paré, first surgeon of the King, could teach me a great deal'.[34] After extensive experience among both poor and later noblewomen in Paris, Bourgeois was recommended by local ladies at court and physicians, to the pregnant Marie de Medici. In her *Recit véritable de la naissance des messeigneurs et dames les enfans de France* (1625) Bourgeois demonstrated her determination and tenacity to surmount the intrigue and factionalism leading to the important appointment, which situated her as the most powerful and influential midwife of her generation.[35]

Bourgeois was also the first midwife to disseminate her medical practices and knowledge in French and in print. In 1609 she published her *Observations*, which dealt with the issues to which she had most claim to authority: obstetrical and gynaecological matters of which she had proven experience.[36] Despite this, Bourgeois expected criticism of her public discussion of female matters. She sought to convince her readers that she wrote frankly of her practices and observations for the public good.[37] Bourgeois knew she would be attacked for her bold public language and used the metatextual material of her work to construct her defence. On the frontispiece was her portrait where she, like her male counterparts, boldly looked out upon her audience. Lianne McTavish argues that portraits such as those of Bourgeois and her male counterparts were important at a time when visual evaluation of the character and ability of a practitioner were commonplace. Understanding obstetrical authority in the early modern period, as she rightly observes, must incorporate such visual aspects.[38] Bourgeois made little apology for usurping the didactic role of the learned physician. 'To the Scandalmonger', she argued, 'If you, envious, have the audacity to attack my writings, let me know in what place you have done better than I say'. Drawing upon her justification of authority by experience, she continued: 'My practice is not a language,/These are true effects'.[39] Bourgeois was here positioning herself as a practitioner by experience rather than textual authority alone.

The *Observations* were indeed popular with readers, undergoing many reprints and even translated into Latin. François Rouget observes that by her use and control of language, Bourgeois's texts educated, moved and entertained readers at the same time, thereby achieving the aim of early modern literature: to mix the useful with the agreeable.[40] Bourgeois followed up her successful entry into public discourse with other works: the autobiographical *Recit véritable*, mentioned earlier, and the 1626 *Instruction à ma troisiesme fille, qui a choisi & esleu l'art de Sage-femme*.[41] In this work, Bourgeois offered further explanation for her own belief system and understanding about the medical corps. She advised her daughter, 'Do not hide the good remedies that you know from physicians and wise people, otherwise they will value you as little as a charlatan ... One must speak freely of what one knows and give it reason'.[42] One senses that Bourgeois may have experienced ridicule at her own medical writings. Other more practical recommendations to her daughter also address aspects of criticism levelled at contemporary midwives. She advised her daughter never to accept pregnant women into her own home, lest she be accused of collusion in aborting a foetus or killing an illegitimate child at birth.

Bourgeois's *Recueil de secrets choisis et eprouvez pour diverses maladies, principalement celles des femmes, & pour leur embellissement*

(1635) is perhaps one of her most interesting ventures into print because she did not limit herself to issues only concerning female health. Here, Bourgeois gave advice and remedies for epilepsy, rabies, toothaches, headaches and chest problems, fevers, plague, kidney and liver problems among others, and it was only in the third section (of five) that she approached the issues that she could claim her authority by occupational experience as a midwife; that is, illnesses of women, illnesses that occur before and during pregnancy, remedies for labour and remedies for after the delivery.[43] Bourgeois claimed in the preface that she had not sought to make public her knowledge outside of her own specialty, but had been asked by others to respond to a genuine public need. Through this conventional justification, she attempted to avoid accusations that she had willingly entered other medical areas where she had no claims to expertise.

Women as patrons and readers of medical texts

Louise Bourgeois provides us with one example of how women could contribute their own medical experience to a printed medical discourse. Other women could participate in creating and supporting the publication of medical texts as their patrons and readers. Elite women were often cited as the patrons or dedicatees of works by medical men. Did these authors expect women to engage with their works?

Dedications of several medical texts demonstrate a range of reading expectations of their authors. In addressing Diane de Poitiers, Claude Valgelas suggested in his dedication that his primary interest was her patronage power. On the other hand, Guillaume Chrestian in his translation dedicated to her indicated that Diane's interest in medical literature, particularly reproductive medicine, was well known.[44] Similarly, Jean Lyège expected that Antoinette de Bourbon would appreciate his medical text dedicated to her, because of her keen charitable interest in nursing the poor and sick.[45] Claude Valgelas specified, first to Diane de Poitiers, the highly influential mistress of Henri II, reputed for her interest in medical matters which will be explored in Chapter 7, then to Louise Dansezune in almost identical prefaces, that his text was 'of an inestimable utility, and necessary not only to physicians, but also to all people who would have cure of bodily health'.[46] But were physicians really encouraging women to deepen their medical knowledge by reading such texts? Some probably were. Claude Dalechamps marvelled in 1566 at the intense medical interest of Jacqueline de Monbel in his translation *De l'usage des parties du corps humains*. Acquiring 'not only ordinary things common to the sex and condition of ladies', he remarked, she 'aspires to the most arduous and rare sciences' and had asked him once to dissect the eyeball of an ox, in order that she might examine its structure.[47] However, the fact that Dalechamps marvelled at Monbel's intelligence and interest in medical science suggests that she was an exception rather than the rule. We should note too that it was manual surgery, not theoretical medicine, that Monbel investigated under his tutelage.

The very fact that Valgelas' dedications to Diane de Poitiers and Louise Dansezune in successive editions of his work were almost identical suggests that the dedication to the archetypal charitable lady quickly became a cliched and generic genre, rather than a real indication of a growing desire of doctors to see noblewomen integrated into the university medical world. The dedication of Sébastien Colin to Antoinette d'Aubeterre, dame de Soubize, in his work *Lordre et regime qu'on doit garder et tenir en la cure des fievres*, was followed by a second preface, in Latin, 'to the reader'.[48] The physician Thomas Sonnet de Courval complained that such literature caused some ladies to be 'so presumptuous and wandering in their senses that there is no Physician in the world more learned and experienced than them: How many great ladies are there whose cabinets are all stuffed with makeup, unguents, distilled waters and a great number of drugs, which they use without experienced knowledge, nor judgement to the ruin of the poor patients . . . ?'[49] It was clear that there were limits as to the extent of medical knowledge that medical men expected literate noblewomen to acquire, let alone women generally.

Were other women reading medical literature? Monica H. Green has contributed two important studies in this field, investigating the possibilities of access to medical texts for laywomen, female practitioners and religious women in medieval Europe.[50] She finds that lay and religious women had very limited possibilities to access learned medical culture, because it was mostly transmitted in manuscript circulation and in Latin. The evidence of medical book ownership by women is relatively low, and mostly concerned regimens, herbals and simple recipe collections.[51]

Women's opportunities for education and literacy may have been slightly better in the sixteenth century, but they did not permit most women to read Latin or the specialist medical literature of the universities.[52] Although some elite women owned large libraries, medical literature does not generally appear to be a significant feature in them.[53] Nor does it appear so for women of a slightly lower economic and social status. From my survey of 94 women owning books in Paris (1493–1597) and Amiens (1503–83), total collections were typically very small. A collection of four to five books, mostly books of hours, was usual for 'bourgeois' women. Those few women whose libraries were exceptionally large and contained works in both Latin and French were widows who may have inherited at least part, if not all, of the former collection from their husbands. These libraries may have then contained some medical texts – though we have to debate whether women had the skills to read them. We might question whether women even wanted to read university medical texts. It is possible that they might not have been interested in the academic debates and theoretical approaches of the texts. Practical manuals suited to solving medical problems that they were likely to face in everyday life, such as the regimens and herbal collections that Green found in their holdings, were probably of greater relevance to their lives. Some sixteenth-century women held works for which notaries did not record details because they were not considered financially significant. It is possible that some of these were recipe and remedy chapbooks or manuscripts. Evidence for contemporary European countries suggests that women did keep recipe and remedy books, and many were passed on to female relatives in a matrilineal tradition.[54]

Women and domestic medicine

We have seen that there were popular handbooks produced with female medical practice in mind, and that indeed where women held medical works, they were generally of this variety. This section of the chapter will seek to determine how women's domestic medical work was perceived by contemporaries, both the university medical and lay communities. Where histories of medicine acknowledge the role of women in primary and domestic medicine, it is commonplace to conclude that we cannot understand women's specific medical practices in the home because they were passed on orally (or tacitly, that women still do what they have always done, and therefore their health-care work cannot be historicised).

Women at all levels were involved in treatment of the sick, and the maintenance of health, within their family or household. We have seen how, even at the highest social levels, noblewomen were encouraged by moral and medical commentators to provide charitable medical help to their families and surrounding territories. Families in the country were less likely than urban dwellers to have access to the services of guild or university-trained medical practitioners, and so may have practised higher degrees of self-medication. Poorer families too might have abstained from purchasing medical help outside the home. The services of local medical practitioners such as bonesetters could sometimes be more expensive than a surgeon.[55] The very poorest families might have been more exposed to the work of guild and university-trained providers than other families if they were able to qualify for assistance from religious or municipal poor relief systems.

Domestic medical practices could be accumulated from a wide range of experiences such as observation of the work of other practitioners, university, guild, religious, empiric among them; from the advice of those around them, neighbours, community members and relatives; by their own observations of their bodies, and perhaps from the pictures and texts of medical works. Even illiterate women might understand a medical text if they could access someone who could read it to them. Late medieval recipe books often had a section listing dishes for the sick. This included both culinary therapy: specific foods which were intended therapeutically for certain illnesses, as well as dishes which were nourishing for those ailing or weak such as children, the elderly or convalescents.[56] The institutions through which this domestic medical knowledge could be transmitted were numerous, including the local community, and particularly the household. Transmission of the information was often verbal, but the existence of manuscript remedy books would suggest that written records could also be significant in the transmission of familial medical knowledge.

Moral commentators had no doubts that the health of the family and household was women's primary concern. Women had a 'natural' duty to care for those in their household and family. The medieval *Mesnagier de Paris* instructed his young wife that she should watch over her husband, not just in sickness but also to maintain his health. The householder provided her with recipes of drinks and soups for the ill.[57] His suggestions for preventative medicine included preparing a calm and clean environment for her husband to return to. She should 'provide him always with clean linen'.[58] She was to keep the house free of fleas and mosquitos, and he offered remedies to eradicate them both. The householder's message was clear: women were primarily responsible for maintaining their family and household in good health.

Should a family member become ill, it fell to the woman, as a wife or mother, to care for the patient. Translated into French in 1542, *Livre de l'institution de la Femme Chrestienne* of the humanist Jean-Louis Vives instructed the elite married women to whom his treatise was directed to watch over their husbands personally in sickness and not to leave it to the care of servants:

With your own hands treat his body and wounds, cover his limbs to keep them from the cold: Give him food and drink yourself, and do not employ your domestics who have no great love for him.[59]

Vives then developed his argument through the tale of the exemplary wife, Clere, married to invalid Bernard Vauldeure, one of Vives's relations. Not only had Clere 'prepared meats for him, dressed his wounds' but she took pleasure in dressing his intolerably pustulous legs 'as though she smelled musk or some other sweet smell'.[60] Vives's extreme example, similar to those religious works composed for active nursing nuns seen earlier in Chapter 3, nonetheless reinforced the contemporary view that it was women who nursed the family in sickness.

Catherine des Roches, in her 1583 humanist manifesto for women's education, the *Dialogue de Placide et Severe*, had the enlightened father Placide encourage health-care education for women, albeit for limited application:

> She who was the disciple of the learned Hierophile, shows well that she learnt Medicine for the wellbeing of others. There are some today who only aid their little children, ease the pains of their neighbours, cure their servants using certain domestic remedies that Experience has taught them.[61]

Des Roches was careful to argue that women should not extend their medical knowledge by reading medical texts, but merely to draw on their experience to aid those in their immediate household.

Yet while early modern moral commentators such as Vives and Des Roches had no doubts that women ought to concern themselves with maintaining the health of their household, they provided few practical examples of solutions to everyday illnesses women might encounter. Here we will explore the published sixteenth-century literature: firstly depicting women's relationship with physicians in the domain of domestic medicine, and then two manuals written to instruct the housewife and farmwife how to treat those in her care. These texts demonstrate how the participation of the housewife in medicine could be understood and delimited by a variety of authors.

Marguerite de Navarre and domestic medicine

Marguerite de Navarre's play *Le Malade* provides a unique female perspective on the interaction between the university medical community and the good housewife. The work, one of several evangelical plays, was composed between 1530 and 1543, and remained unpublished in her lifetime.[62] The plot focuses on four characters: the patient, his wife, the physician and the spiritually enlightened chambermaid who finally convinces the patient that a cure for his ills will come through faith alone.

Physicians such as Laurent Joubert highlighted the interference of women in medical care as a significant contest of authority:

> There are people who know nothing at all about medicine, as to discourse or reason like ignorant women who do not even know how to read or write; but have some observations and rules, knowing how to make a soup, jelly, restorative, barley water, who make a bed well, cover a patient, know some little remedy for mange, burns, ... worms, suffocation of the womb ... From that, they think they know everything.[63]

André du Breil was particularly concerned that women held community power about when and which doctor was to be called. There were, in his view,

> a multitude of bad, shameless, impudent, lying women who reign today and hold court everywhere: they call themselves sicknurses, hiding behind the title of wise women, or matrons, who are usually called upon to assess an illness and to give their advice, as to whether to seek a doctor, and if he is needed according to them, which physician, surgeon or apothecary should be called or consulted in their opinion, and which is the most learned, appropriate and experienced.[64]

His text revealed a perception that women in local communities held patronage power over medical practitioners, and advised and referred patients, sometimes receiving money for their referral.

Marguerite gives expression to this type of conflict in her sixteenth-century play. How might a lay female author perceive women's domestic practices? Marguerite portrays lively and animated characters whose knowledge and practices correspond with our understanding of contemporary medical practice derived from learned medical texts. As Jean Liébault would recommend some decades later, dietetic and herbal medicine is the first resource for medical care for the Wife. She first advises her husband to eat to restore his health.[65] Marguerite highlighted here a number of important points in contemporary perception of women's medical practices. Women made use of food products to which they had immediate access: 'if only you would drink, only five treads of eggs, you will soon see your story change and you will be surely cured'.[66] 'And with a herb, I know which, I will make you a *cathaplume*', promises the Wife.[67] Although the Wife mispronounces the word *cataplasme* (poultice) Marguerite's pun presents a woman using the practices, if not the terminology, of contemporary medicine.

When the Patient rejects her practices in favour of the Physician, the Wife is critical of his choice. 'Their step is dangerous', she argues, 'Do you think that their great science can know all things?'[68] Marguerite depicts a woman who doubts the authority of learned medicine and who is proud of her practices through experience and botanical knowledge: 'Between us poor little women, we have some experience and we know the little herbs as well as them.'[69] Repeatedly, when the Wife offers treatments, confident in her knowledge of the medicinal property of herbs, it is followed by a justification for medical authority through experience: 'It's my custom'.

Marguerite portrays an attitude of condescension by the Physician towards the Wife and her medical knowledge. 'Be silent, mad woman that you are', he responds to one remedy she offers.[70]

> I've never seen an illness, however difficult the cure, that some woman cannot thoughtlessly procure a thousand remedies for: and if it happens, by chance, that some can be cured of it, one hundred thousand (ignorant of their temperament) are killed by this herb.[71]

He refuses to elaborate his apothecary's script to her, on the grounds that she is not learned: 'You understand neither *goumes* or herbs, why, you cannot name them'.[72]

Yet the Wife does not demur in the face of his learned textual authority. She confidently claims upon the arrival of the Physician that his visit will be useless: 'Monsieur, I say that I make a good brew with the shit of a white pigeon, which costs not a *blanc*, and can do no damage'.[73] Here, Marguerite is indeed an accurate source of contemporary views on women's practices. Pigeon carcasses and their faeces feature commonly in accounts of women's medical broths discussed in trials as empirics and witches. As the Physician responds, 'you are not wise, . . . for making this soup is prohibited in Languedoc.'[74]

Furthermore, the Wife equally attacks his learned medical practice when he recommends phlebotomy for the Patient's ills and again offers her own alternative. 'Monsieur, I've seen some cured perfectly without bleeding, just by drinking a brew of poppy juice'.[75] When, through faith, the Patient's condition improves, it is to the Wife that the Physician turns to find an explanation: 'You've given him some herb, tell me which, do not hide it'.[76] Even though he will not share his knowledge with her, the Physician expects her to divulge her remedies to him. The Wife does not miss the moment to point out the irony of the situation, 'given that you call me mad for this much'.[77] Even the Chambermaid, to whom the Physician turns next for explanation of the patient's cure, is not afraid to critique learned medicine in her reply.

> Physician: We have learned doctors who frequent the schools: They provide us with protocols which we must heed.
>
> Chambermaid: But, if they say silly things, are women wrong to doubt?[78]

For the purposes of the religious message, in the end, both Physician and Wife are condemned as 'false doctors'. However, Marguerite's portrayal of the interaction of medical providers does not seem nearly as one-sided as scholars have previously suggested.[79] Although the Physician clearly treats the Wife and her knowledge with haughty disdain (until he thinks she may have cured the patient), Marguerite depicts the Wife as a valid provider of domestic medical treatment, who is confident of her abilities. She certainly acknowledges his university learning but does not devalue her own knowledge as consequently less worthy. The Wife constantly treats her knowledge as a valid 'other' to that of the Physician. Marguerite's contemporary portrayal of the confident and even critical attitude of an experiential medical provider towards their university-taught counterparts reminds us yet again that we cannot assume the universal dominance and authority of the formally trained community in medical matters.

The housewife according to Olivier de Serres

In 1600, Olivier de Serres, Seigneur de Pradel, published his exhaustive manual for the country household, the *Théâtre d'agriculture*. Within its many subjects of interest was the instruction of the housewife in medical treatment for everyday complaints since as he explained 'It is more appropriate to women than men, for their natural temperament is charitable'.[80] Teaching women rudimentary medical knowledge, Serres the non-physician argued, was necessary since

> the solitude of our habitation, which distances us from Physicians, Surgeons and Apothecaries which the towns enjoy... constrains us to seek a Physician in necessity... who is often far away and they arrive too late at the house.[81]

Since, Serres explained, country living meant university-acquired medical assistance was difficult to obtain, 'intelligent people try... to help themselves at the onset of illnesses and those of their children and servants, while waiting for more ample remedies from the Physician'.[82] Serres' arguments supported much of the legal defence for Jeanne Lescallier's charitable domestic medicine which her lawyer had used in court in the 1570s, discussed in Chapter 4. In particular, his concern was the immediate treatment of a wide range of typical country mishaps, such as falls, injuries and burns.[83] Furthermore, he envisioned a range of other sicknesses that were simply unnecessary to be treated by a member of the corporative medical community and to which a woman could apply her medical knowledge with no opposition from 'the learned physician'. These sicknesses 'of little importance' included the 'minor languor of women and children, not meriting to send for a Physician'.[84]

Since the reality was that women would be performing simple medical work in the home, what then was the housewife to be taught of medical knowledge? Serres promised to teach her the secrets of university-acquired medicine, hitherto inaccessible to women, from texts translated from the Greek and Latin known only to a few. Perhaps this was partly a sales pitch to attract readers. It was Serres, the leisured gentleman, who would expose this new world of knowledge to the housewife: providing 'a list of remedies to the most common illnesses, drawn from books and from experience which she can use'.[85] He offered no justification of medical experience or background to explain why his interpretations would be accurate and claimed only that his 'experiments, [were] performed with fidelity, by me and many of my closest friends: about which one can be assured'.[86]

Beyond revealing remedies drawn from medical texts, Serres encouraged a recognition of dietetic medicine and the health-care control that women could exert within the household. Serres promised to instruct the housewife how to make jams which could comfort and revive the ill.[87] He furthermore gave detailed instruction on distilling procedures by which women could prepare medicinal waters, 'showing our mother of a family how and to what extent she can apply herself in these cares, without delving into the . . . subtleties of master distillers and abstracters of quintessences'.[88] Even though he envisaged a limit to their medical knowledge and practice, Serres nonetheless furthered public recognition of a primary medical role for women.

Serres' medical discussion for women was carefully balanced between the power of faculty-trained physicians and the housewife. At every opportunity, he emphasised her supplementary role in deference to the 'Physician'. The remedies he listed were to be used, only 'in waiting for more ample remedies from the learned Physician'. However, Serres was vague about when she was to call the physician, repeating his advice that his remedies were only 'for the comfort of her family, at the onset of illness, she might patiently wait the arrival of the learned Physician when in need'.[89] He also recommended that the good housewife ought to buy drugs from an apothecary and

> make a little cabinet, in which, like the boutique of an Apothecary, she will place remedies for common illnesses: so that in necessity she finds them close to her, without being constrained to send for them hastily in town at the Apothecary's. So she will make provision of all the drugs that she sees that she will need.[90]

Serres tacitly acknowledged that the housewife had authority enough to treat minor ailments within her household, and it remained her decision which illnesses or injuries warranted the physician.

Serres also distinguished the different practices that learned doctor and housewife had in the treatment of illness and the meanings behind them. For example, for headaches, he prefaced his remedy by saying 'the search for the causes we leave to the learned Physician to purge the body, according to its needs: waiting for that, the mother of the family will use these remedies'.[91] Similarly, for 'eye soreness' he stipulated that 'it is the duty of the judicious Physician discerning the particular humours causing the illness of the eye, to evacuate them by appropriate purgings'.[92] Serres differentiated between treatment of the illness's symptoms, to which the housewife could apply herself, and determining the causes of the illness which was the task of the learned physician. For nasal problems, he clearly stated, 'as for the internal [symptoms], always the cause must be removed, and this by the advice of the learned Physician, and against the external, she will employ these remedies here'. Thus, Serres situated medical aims (and illness) within a hierarchical value system. While treatment of the external, obvious symptoms of an illness could be undertaken by the 'untrained' housewife, diagnosis of its causes required university training in learned medical sciences to unlock and interpret its hidden meanings.

The *Théâtre d'agriculture* shows how the learned gentleman could perceive women capable to be enlisted in support of learned medicine. Serres' justifications for providing women with university-acquired medical knowledge, and his careful and repeated clarifications of the limited supportive practices of the housewife, suggests that he anticipated resistance to such a move. His perception of the housewife as the passive recipient of learned medical knowledge and practices reveals a lack of recognition (or an unwillingness to recognise publicly) that women might already have medical knowledge of their own. Unlike other contemporaries, Serres made no recognition of women's healthcare practices or epistemologies, even if to condemn them in favour of what learned science could teach them.

The farmwife according to Liébault

L'Agriculture, et maison rustique de M. M. Charles Estienne, & Iean Liébault, docteurs en medecine, first published in 1564, represents another way to recognise women's role in medical care. Unlike Olivier de Serres, however, Jean Liébault, who composed the medical section of the text, was a university-trained physician. His receptivity to non-university-acquired medical practices and his emphasis on 'experience which is the mistress of all arts and sciences'[93] suggests that the elite university community did not universally condemn experiential medical epistemologies and practices.

Like Serres, Liébault argued that the farmwife must know what he termed natural medicine for 'her own family and others, when misfortune strikes . . . for to have the physician at all hours, without urgent need is not to the profit of the household'.[94] Somewhat curiously for a member of the university medical community, Liébault argued the good housewife had a duty to be economical, and offered no argument that a physician's costs were justified because of his expertise. Liébault in fact provided much less justification generally for revealing learned medical knowledge to women, than did the non-physician Serres.

Liébault specified that his aim was to discuss 'medicinal herbs, which the farmwife should know about, to provide remedies for the illness of her people. And in this regard, it will not be strange if we use some words of the culture more usual and familiar to women, leaving more ample and exact descriptions of them to those who make a profession of it'.[95] Here then was a physician arguing that women had a vital role to play in the management of health and illness in conjunction, rather than competition, with physicians. Liébault's arguments were highly favourable to Jeanne Lescallier's claims for charitable domestic healthcare argued before the courts just a few decades later.[96] Liébault, unlike the Angers medical faculty, did not appear to feel personally or professionally threatened by unpaid female medical work but argued that the farmwife could use 'natural remedies with which she will aid her people in their illnesses, . . . leaving more complex remedies to the physicians in towns'.[97] It is clear that both Serres and Liébault saw tacit limits to the type of illnesses treated by the farmwife. Each text restricts the list of remedies provided to everyday complaints, such as headaches and toothaches, minor accidents such as black eyes, or stable medical conditions such as epilepsy and asthma. Neither provided treatment for more serious injuries or illnesses.

For the modern reader, it is sometimes difficult to distinguish what basis some of Liébault's suggested remedies seem to have in learned medical practices. For example, to relieve the pain of toothache, the author recommended 'carrying around the neck the tooth of a man wrapped in a knot of taffeta'.[98] Similarly, he assured his readers that 'If you cut the feet of a large greenfinch or toad, during the waning of the moon, . . . and when you apply it around the neck of one who has scrofula, it is a sovereign remedy'.[99] It is possible that Liébault was trying to adapt remedies which he thought readers could understand, with which they were familiar or could easily obtain ingredients. Rather than instructing general readers in learned medical truth he seemed on occasion to endorse selected popular remedies which corresponded with university-acquired medical logic.

Like Serres, Liébault too recommended that the rural household maintain a medicinal garden. He explained how to grow herbs and also discussed the preparation of medicinal oils and waters, including illustrations to aid the reader. Liébault offered instruction in drying herbs and disputed the practices of apothecaries. He also recognised the potential of dietetic medicine and provided a detailed list of the medicinal value of all plants and trees within the garden and orchard. The cabbage provides one such example: 'The good housewife at all times will have cabbage in her garden for the nourishment of her family, and in times and necessity of illness she can help her household. For the first brew of red cabbage with butter or oil without salt, cleans the stomach, kills a cough and renders the voice better. If sugar is added to the brew it will be most singular for asthmatics'.[100]

Our physician was also not averse to praising the medical work of (elite) women, disproving modern perceptions that elite medical practice sought specifically to exclude the practices of women: 'There is a herb . . . which Mademoiselle de Ville-neufve . . . had distilled . . . which is singular for urinal difficulties and kidney stones: I have tried it several times'.[101] Liébault even admitted that physicians had learnt from women's medical practices: 'the farmwife learns many remedies for illnesses: one must not doubt that we have learnt a lot of remedies by the experience and observations of these sort of women'.[102]

The texts of the gentleman author Serres and the physician Liébault served to recognise and endorse ideas about dietetic medicine, culinary therapy and the nutritional benefits of certain foods that were already held in the general population. Louis XI paid one Perrette la Mauvaise to prepare for him medicinal yoghurts and cheeses that were reputed to improve intestinal wellbeing,[103] though no household manual recommended that the housewife use her dietetic expertise for financial gain. Elite women's letters contained many references to the exchange of medicinal preparations and foods. When her sister, Claude de Foix, was ill with a cold, Anne de Laval wrote to her sending fruit from her garden. Some foods were considered fortifying. Hearing of her pregnancy, Anne sent her 'peas in their pods, which is food for a pregnant woman'.[104] Diane de Poitiers, the powerful mistress of King Henri II, encouraged the wetnurse of the royal children to maintain her health through drinking beer and cider. In the Hôtel-Dieu in Orléans, the provision of meals exposed beliefs about the medicinal properties of meats in particular. Governors and female nursing staff agreed that grievously ill patients should receive lighter meats such as poultry and veal, which were perceived to be more suited to the delicate invalid than the heavier meats such as beef, mutton and pork given to other patients.[105]

Given the general community's understanding of dietetic knowledge and culinary therapy already, what influence did texts like that of Liébault have on them? We have to consider whether academic ratification for certain of their remedies had any impact on the general populace. After all, even if some of their remedies were dismissed as nonsense, what other sources of medical supplies did they have regular access to? In the trial and appeals against Jeanne Lescallier's charitable household medicine discussed in Chapter 4, the local community who used her services argued that it was unjust for physicians to forbid them 'to use the remedies that they have at their door'.[106] It is possible that Liébault's public acclamation of domestic medicine may have had more of an impact upon the elite medical community itself. Literate in the vernacular, which cannot be said for the majority of the French population, medical men had more access to these texts than did the general population. Contrary to his aim to transmit learned medical knowledge to the people, Liébault's dietetic medical exploration probably did more to reveal (and approve) popular understanding to the learned medical community. Learned medical texts ratified female domestic practices.

There were other ramifications from the publication of these new medical texts. The publication of herbal medical knowledge by physicians such as Liébault also impinged upon the pharmaceutical authority of guild medical practitioners, the apothecaries. The physician Sébastien Colin critiqued apothecaries as overcharging and incompetent practitioners in his 1553 *Déclaration des abus et tromperies que font les apothicaires*.[107] Pierre Braillier responded with his *Déclaration des abus et ignorance des médecins*, in 1557.[108] The publication of domestic medical texts, including herbal compositions and distillations, signalled the willingness of physicians to make public the knowledge of those lower down the medical hierarchy, as they defined it. After all, it was not their university-acquired learned theoretical expertise they were revealing in such publications, it was the knowledge and skills of apothecaries. Liébault even ventured to critique the practices of drying herbs used by apothecaries and offered his preferred techniques to his lay male and female readers. Philibert Guibert, discussed earlier in this chapter, was following a well-established tradition when he produced his texts exposing the practices of apothecaries in the early seventeenth century. Such publications indicate the complexity of contemporary distinctions that medical practitioners could make between medical knowledge suitable for the greater literate public and that which was to be closely guarded and transmitted in Latin among fellow members of the university-approved medical corps.

Herbal medicine and pharmaceutical knowledge

Medical faculties and their product, the physician, had little to do with herbal medicine or pharmaceutical knowledge before the middle of the sixteenth century. In 1578, Nicolas Houël, a Parisian apothecary, opened on rue de l'Arbalète, a 'House of Christian charity' where he proposed to instruct orphan children in the art of pharmacy and to provide free medication to the poor. Attached to the house would be an apothecary's garden of medicinal plants. The Faculty of Medicine in Paris, who had little control over Houël's establishment, strongly opposed the project.[109]

But apart from publications such as Liébault's, physicians felt the rising influence of Paracelsian chemical theories, which could not be ignored. Paracelsus himself had proposed that physicians should 'learn of old Women, Egyptians, and such-like persons; for they have greater experience in such things than all the Academians'.[110] However, Paracelsianism as it was later understood by the faculties developed elaborate occult alchemical, magical and cosmological influences to its chemical theories, and had very little relationship to women's herbal and culinary practices. The faculty at Montpellier which had established a chair in botany some time before the Parisian faculty, was always more open to the Paracelsian influences that the rigidly Galenist Paris Faculty. In 1593, Henri IV established a Royal Garden for the Montpellier faculty, appointing Pierre Richer de Belleval as its director.[111]

By the early seventeenth century, physicians began to argue for the integration of dietetic medical arts such as distillation, and herbal remedies into the learned university medical sciences.[112] In particular, Guy de La Brosse, a physician in the king's retinue, sought 'the re-establishment of plants in medicine'.[113] In 1616, he proposed the establishment of a botanical garden that would form part of a teaching institution where medical students could learn the art of distillation and the preparation of herbal remedies, both simple and complex, as well as those prepared chemically. Previously physicians had perceived such arts as either the affair of the housewife or of the guild-trained apothecary, and not worthy to be incorporated fully into university medical practice and epistemologies. Indeed, La Brosse's plans met with resistance from the Faculty of Medicine in Paris. La Brosse was equally critical of the faculty's traditional approaches and unwillingness to explore and exploit the medicinal properties of plants. On the frontispiece to his 1628 *De la nature, vertu, et utilité des plantes*, in which he discussed the possibilities for the use of plants in medicine, La Brosse pointedly critiqued the conservatism of the medical faculty in Paris and argued for new medical epistemologies and practices. The page featured four portraits – of Hippocrates, Dioscorides, Theophrastus and Paracelsus – each accompanied by mottoes. Under Dioscorides was 'From experience to knowledge' and Theophrastus 'in vain is Medicine without plants'.[114] Significantly, La Brosse's encouragement for the use of plants in medicine drew its authority from the ancients, not the housewives who were probably its greatest practitioners. In 1626, La Brosse was appointed the first intendant of the Parisian *Jardin médicinal des plantes* when it was finally approved, and by 1634, it could boast a range of over 1,500 different plants.[115]

Brosse's aim to improve learned medical science by the incorporation of botanical studies had other, detrimental, effects on women's medical authority. Like the publications of Serres and Liébault, Brosse's efforts gave learned recognition to herbal preparations and distillations that transformed the perception they were given in learned discourse and moved them decisively away from knowledge within the domestic setting to knowledge of the written domain. Once they became valued as sources within learned medicine and incorporated into its practices, women had few claims to being unique providers of, and thus authorities in, dietetic, nutritional and herbal remedies. Indeed, by 1608, Jean de Renou speculated in his *Institutionum pharmaceuticarum* whether there even was an oral tradition among women about domestic medicine, or whether it was a fantasy created in the minds of credulous authors.[116] Physicians were never interested in replacing women as primary domestic carers. They were realistic enough to understand that economics and circumstances would continue to produce situations where women conducted medical work in the home. However, it was to be the ancients, and the newly modernised medical faculties, who were to be consulted as herbal or primary-care experts. Now physicians could produce authoritative texts to instruct women how best to carry out medical work in the home.

Notes

1 For an overview, see particularly Elizabeth L. Eisenstein's *The Printing Press as an Agent of Change: Communications and Cultural Transformations in Early Modern Europe* (Cambridge: Cambridge University Press, 1979).
2 H. H. Glidden, *The Storyteller as Humanist: The Serées of Guillaume Bouchet* French Forum Monograph 25 (Lexington, Kentucky: French Forum, 1981), p. 112.
3 (Lyon: Rigaud, 1582). This was the only work of its kind. Alison Klairmont Lingo, *The Rise of Medical Practitioners in Sixteenth-Century France: The Case of Lyon and Montpellier* (PhD, University of California–Berkeley, 1980), pp. 33–4.
4 Preface (attributed to Jehan Breche), *Les Troys premiers livres de Claude Galien de la composition des medicamens en general* (Tours: 1545) in Paul Dorveaux, *Notice sur la vie et les œuvres de Thibault Lespleigney apothicaire à Tours (1496–1567)* (Paris: H. Welter, 1898), p. 72.
5 Claude Dalechamps, trans., *De l'usage des parties du corps humains Livres XVII, escriptes par Claude Galien, & traduicts fidellement du Grec en François* (Lyon: Guillaume Roville, 1566), p. 9.
6 Alison Klairmont Lingo, 'Print's role in the politics of women's health care in early modern France', in Barbara B. Diefendorf and Carla Hesse (eds), *Culture and Identity in Early Modern Europe (1500–1800): Essays in Honor of Natalie Zemon Davis* (Ann Arbor: The University of Michigan Press, 1993), p. 207. See also MMLVIII, *Index Chronologicus Chartarum pertinentium ad historiam Universitatis Parisiensis ad ejus originibus ad finem decimi sexti sæculi*, ed. C. Jourdain (Paris, 1862) (Bruxelles: Culture et Civilisation, 1966), p. 393.
7 *Opera omnia latinitate donata*, trans. Jacques Guillemeau (Paris: Jacques du Puy, 1582).
8 Klairmont Lingo, *The Rise of Medical Practitioners*, pp. 34–5.
9 See Vivian Nutton, 'Humanist surgery', in A. Wear, R. K. French and I. M. Lonie (eds), *The Medical Renaissance of the Sixteenth Century* (Cambridge: Cambridge University Press, 1985), pp. 75–99.
10 (Troyes: 1494).
11 François Lebrun, *Se soigner autrefois: médecins, saints et sorciers aux XVIe et XVIIIe siècles* (Paris: Temps Actuel, 1983), p. 23.
12 *Le Grand Calendrier et compost des bergiers* (Paris: Alain Lotrian, early sixteenth century).

13 Alison Klairmont Lingo, 'The problem of the plague: new challenges to healing in sixteenth-century France', *Proceedings of the Western Society for French History*, 5 (1977), p. 120.
14 See Paul Slack, 'Mirrors of health and treasures of poor men: the uses of vernacular medical literature of Tudor England', in Charles Webster (ed.), *Health, Medicine and Mortality in the Sixteenth Century* (Cambridge: Cambridge University Press, 1979), pp. 237–73.
15 Howard Stone, 'The French Language in Renaissance Medicine', *Bibliothèque d'Humanisme et Renaissance*, 15 (1953), p. 318.
16 *La Grand Propietaire* [sic] *de toutes choses. Tresutile et profitable pour tenir le corps humain en santé. Contenant plusieurs diverses maladies, & dont ilz procedent, & aussi le remedes preservatifz* (Paris: Jean Ruelle, 1556), fol. cxlvij v.
17 *Ibid.*, fol. ccxv r.
18 (Lyon: B. Rigaud & J. Saugrain).
19 (Paris: Norment & Bruneau, et Lyon: B. Rigaud).
20 Jean Lyège, *Raison de vivre pour toutes fièvres, congnues premierement par leurs differences, causes, signes, & symptomes, auec les prognostiques d'icelles* (Paris: M. Vascosan, 1557).
21 Jacques du Bois, *Livre de la nature et utilité des moys des femmes, & de la curation des maladies qui en surviennent*, trans. Guillaume Chrestian (Paris: Guillaume Morel, 1559); H. de Monteux, *Commentaire de la conservation de santé, et prolongation de vie*, trans. Claude Valgelas (Lyon: Ian de Tournes, 1559).
22 Dalechamps, trans., *De l'usage des parties du corps humains*, p. 7.
23 Lebrun, *Se soigner autrefois*, p. 23.
24 Philippe Albou, 'Histoire des Oeuvres charitables de Philibert Guybert', *Histoire des Sciences Médicales*, 32:1 (1998), pp. 11–26, p. 13.
25 *Ibid.*, p. 22.
26 Françoise Lehoux, *Le Cadre de vie des médecins parisiens aux XVIe et XVIIe siècles* (Paris: A. et J. Picard, 1976), p. 443.
27 André du Breil, *La Police de l'art et science de medecine* (Paris: Leon Cavellat, 1580), p. 118.
28 Natalie Zemon Davis, 'Proverbial wisdom and popular error', *Society and Culture in Early Modern France* (Stanford: Stanford University Press, 1975), p. 238. Paul Slack concludes similarly in his 'Mirrors of health and treasures of poor men', p. 272.
29 For women publishing generally see my *Women and the Book Trade in Sixteenth-Century France* (Aldershot: Ashgate, 2002).
30 (Paris: A. Saugrain, 1609).
31 Davis, *Society and Culture in Early Modern France*, p. 217.
32 8 janvier 1609, *Journal pour le règne de Henri IV*, vol. 2 (1958), p. 416 cited in Nicole Pellegrin, 'L'androgyne au XVIe siècle: pour une relecture des savoirs', in Danielle Haase-Dubosc and Eliane Viennot (eds), *Femmes et pouvoirs sous l'Ancien Régime* (Paris: Rivages/Histoire, 1991), p. 42.
33 Louis Dubreuil-Chambardel, 'L'enseignement des sages-femmes en Touraine', *Bulletin et mémoires de la société archéologique de Touraine*, 48 (1909), p. 52.
34 Bourgeois, *Observations diverses sur la sterilité, perte de fruicts, foecondité, accouchements, et maladies des femmes et enfants nouveaux naiz* (1609) (Paris: Abraham Saugrain, 1617), p. 108.

35 See further discussion in Chapter 7. See also the modern edition: *Récit véritable de la naissance de messeigneurs et dames les enfans de France, Instruction à ma fille et autres textes*, eds Francois Rouget and Colette H. Winn (Geneva: Droz, 2000).

36 See also Wendy Perkins, 'The relationship between midwife and client in the works of Louise Bourgeois', *Seventeenth-Century French Studies* (1989), pp. 28–45; and her monograph *Midwifery and Medicine in Early Modern France: Louise Bourgeois* (Exeter: University of Exeter Press, 1996).

37 Bourgeois, *Observations diverses*, fol. Aiiir.

38 Lianne McTavish, 'On display: portraits of seventeenth-century French men-midwives', *Social History of Medicine*, 14:3 (2001), pp. 389–415, pp. 414–15.

39 Bourgeois, *Observations diverses*, n.p.

40 François Rouget, 'De la sage-femme à la femme sage: réflexion et réflexivité dans les *Observations* de Louise Boursier', *Papers on French Seventeenth-Century Literature*, 49 (1998), pp. 483–96, p. 495.

41 *Instruction à ma troisiesme fille, qui a choisi & esleu l'art de sage-femme, & qui peut servir à toutes autres, où se peut voir plusieurs choses remarquables sur divers sujets, mesmes pour les accidens qui arrivent par aucuns sages-femmes, & par le choix indiscret des nourrices, & par l'indiscretion de plusieurs ieunes femmes grosses. Et l'erreur qui peut arriver sur le iugement de la grossesse d'une femme* (1626).

42 Bourgeois, *Instruction à ma fille*, dans *Observations diverses* (Paris: Jean Dehoury, 1710), p. 153.

43 Bourgeois, *Recueil de secrets choisis et eprouvez pour diverses maladies, principalement celles des Femmes, & pour leur embellissement, Loüise Bourgeois, dite Boursier, Sage-femme de la Reyne Marie de Medicis* (Paris: Laurent d'Houry, 1710).

44 *Commentaire de la conservation de santé*, trans. Valgelas and *Livre de la nature et utilité des moys des femmes*, trans. Christian, p. 104.

45 See also Chapter 4. Jean Lyège, *Raison de vivre pour toutes fièvres*, sig. Aii r–v.

46 *Commentaire de la conservation de santé*, trans. Valgelas (1559), fol. A2 r and (Paris: Simon Calvarin, 1572), fol. Aij v.

47 *De L'usage des parties du corps humains*, trans. Claude Dalechamps (Lyon: Guillaume Roville, 1566), pp. 9–10.

48 Sébastien Colin, *Lordre et regime qu'on doit garder et tenir en la cure des fievres* (Poitiers: Enguilbert de Marnef, 1558).

49 Thomas Sonnet de Courval, *Satyre contre les charlatans, et pseudomedecins empyriques* (Paris: Jean Milot, 1610), pp. 123–4.

50 Monica H. Green, 'The possibilities of literacy and the limits of reading: women and the gendering of medical literacy', in her *Women's Healthcare in the Medieval West: Texts and Contexts* (Aldershot: Ashgate, 2000), pp. 1–76; 'Books as a source of medical education for women in the Middle Ages', *Dynamis*, 20 (2000), pp. 331–69.

51 Green, 'The possibilities of literacy', p. 45. Although she found that women in France had disproportionately high levels of medical book ownership, I think the limitations of her survey sample (smaller than that of her other European samples and almost all the women were noble or had received their books for noblewomen, p. 14) probably explain this anomaly. My evidence does not suggest any preponderance for medical book ownership by women in sixteenth-century France.

52 For an overview of women's education and literacy in sixteenth-century France, see my *Women and the Book Trade*, Chapter 1.
53 Diane de Poitiers did hold at least four French medical texts in her library, although this does not necessarily indicate that she read them. Melinda Lipinska, *Des femmes médecines depuis l'antiquité jusqu'à nos jours* (Paris: G. Jacques, 1900), p. 184.
54 Linda Pollock, *With Faith and Physic: The Life of a Tudor Gentlewoman, Lady Grace Mildmay, 1552–1620* (New York: St Martin's Press, 1993); Jennifer Wynne Hellwarth, '"Be unto me as a precious ointment": Lady Grace Mildmay, sixteenth-century female practitioner', *Dynamis*, 19 (1999), pp. 95–117.
55 See evidence for Tours in Chapter 6.
56 See Terence Scully, 'The sickdish in early French recipe collections', in Sheila Campbell, Bert Hall and David Klausner (eds), *Health, Disease and Healing in Medieval Culture* (New York: St Martin's Press, 1992), pp. 132–51.
57 *Le Mesnagier de Paris*, eds Georgina E. Brereton and Janet M. Ferrier, trans. Karin Ueltschi (Paris: Le Livre de Poche, 1994), pp. 761–9.
58 *Ibid.*, pp. 295, 297.
59 Book 2, Chapter 3, Jean-Louis Vives, *Livre de l'institution de la femme chrestienne*, trans. Pierre de Changy (Paris: Jacques Kerver, 1542) (Havre: Lemale, 1891), p. 168.
60 *Ibid.*, p. 171.
61 *Les Secondes Oeuvres de mes-dames des Roches de Poictiers, mere et fille* (Poitiers: Nicolas Courtoys), fol. 38v.
62 Marguerite de Navarre, *Théâtre profane*, ed. Verdun L. Saulnier (Paris: Droz, 1946), p. 4.
63 Laurent Joubert, *La Médecine et le régime de santé, des erreurs populaires et propos vulgaires*, Livre I (Bordeaux: Simon Millanges, 1578) ed. Madeleine Tiollais, vol. 1 (Paris: L'Harmattan, 1997), pp. 163–4.
64 Du Breil, *La Police de l'art et science de medecine*, p. 66.
65 Marguerite de Navarre, *Théâtre profane*, p. 14.
66 *Ibid.*, p. 16.
67 *Ibid.*, p. 15.
68 *Ibid.*, p. 15.
69 *Ibid.*, p. 15.
70 *Ibid.*, p. 23.
71 *Ibid.*, p. 23.
72 *Ibid.*, p. 23.
73 *Ibid.*, p. 20.
74 *Ibid.*, p. 20.
75 *Ibid.*, pp. 22–3.
76 *Ibid.*, p. 27.
77 *Ibid.*, p. 27.
78 *Ibid.*, p. 30.
79 See, for example, Saulnier's introduction to Marguerite de Navarre, *Théâtre profane* and the assessment of Evelyne Berriot-Salvadore, *Les Femmes dans la société française de la Renaissance* (Geneva: Droz, 1990), p. 243.
80 Olivier de Serres, *Théâtre d'agriculture et mesnage des champs d'Olivier de Serres, Seigneur du Pradel* (Rouen: Jean Berthelin, 1646), p. 802.

81 *Ibid.*, p. 802.
82 *Ibid.*, p. 802.
83 *Ibid.*, p. 802.
84 *Ibid.*, p. 802.
85 *Ibid.*, pp. 802–3.
86 *Ibid.*, p. 803.
87 *Ibid.*, p. 764.
88 *Ibid.*, p. 803.
89 *Ibid.*, p. 803.
90 *Ibid.*, p. 803.
91 *Ibid.*, p. 810.
92 *Ibid.*, p. 812.
93 *L'Agriculture, et maison rustique de M. M. Charles Estienne, & Iean Liébault, docteurs en medecine* (Paris: Nicolas de la Vigne, 1640), p. 26.
94 *Ibid.*, p. 36.
95 *Ibid.*, p. 184.
96 See discussion of Lescallier's case in Chapter 4.
97 Estienne and Liébault, *L'Agriculture, et maison rustique*, p. 36.
98 *Ibid.*, p. 44.
99 *Ibid.*, p. 40.
100 *Ibid.*, p. 156.
101 *Ibid.*, p. 51.
102 *Ibid.*, p. 149.
103 Emile Aron, *Louis XI et ses guérisseurs* (Chambray: CLD, 1983), p. 159.
104 *Les La Trémoille pendant cinq siècles: Charles, François et Louis III, 1485–1577*, vol. 3, ed. Louis de La Trémoille (Nantes: E. Grimaud, 1894), pp. 87–8.
105 Pierre Bouvier, *Etude sur l'Hôtel-Dieu d'Orléans au moyen-âge et au XVIe siècle* (Orléans: Paul Pigelet, 1914), p. 76.
106 Bibliothèque Nationale Manuscrit Baluze 222, *Playdr de M Matras et Marion sur une femme qui exercoit la medecine en lannee 1573*, fol. 1v.
107 Klairmont Lingo, *The Rise of Medical Practitioners*, p. 29.
108 Tours, Cherchellé, 1553. E. Giraudet, *Histoire de la ville de Tours* (1873), vol. 2 (Brussels: Culture et Civilisations, 1976), p. 79.
109 Jules Guiart, *Histoire de la médecine française: son passé, son présent, son avenir* (Paris: Nagel, 1947), p. 126. For a study of Nicolas Houel's attempts to obtain Catherine de Medici's patronage for his garden, see Sheila Ffolliott, 'A Queen's Garden of Power: Catherine de' Medici and the Locus of Female Power', in Mario A. Di Cesare (ed.), *Reconsidering the Renaissance* (Binghamton, NY: Medieval and Renaissance Texts and Studies, 1992), pp. 245–55.
110 Paracelsus (1656) p. 88. in Allen G. Debus, *The French Paracelsians: The Chemical Challenge to Medical and Scientific Tradition in Early Modern France* (Cambridge: Cambridge University Press, 1991), p. 9.
111 Henry Guerliac, 'Guy de la Brosse and the French Paracelsians', in Allen G. Debus (ed.), *Science, Medicine and Society in the Renaissance: Essays to Honor Walter Pagel*, vol. 1 (London: Heinemann, 1972), pp. 184, 196. See also Louis Dulieu, 'La diétetique et la nutrition à Montpellier à travers les âges', *Monspeliensis Hippocrates* (1969), pp. 5–16.

112 A precursor to Guy de La Brosse's vision was Jacques Gohory: see E.-T. Hamy, 'Jacques Gohory et le Lycium philosophal de Saint-Marceau-lès-Paris (1571–1576)', *Nouvelles Archives du Muséum*, 4e série (1899), pp. 1–26.
113 Guy de la Brosse, *De la nature, vertu, et utilité des plantes* (Paris: Rollin Baragnes, 1628), p. 755.
114 Guerliac, 'Guy de la Brosse and the French Paracelsians', p. 184.
115 *Ibid.*, p. 189.
116 Louis de Serres' translation into French (1624) cited in H. Brabant, *Médecins, malades et maladies de la Renaissance* (Brussels: La Renaissance du livre, 1966), p. 198.

6

Nursing, caring, curing: women's work in municipal child care

THE PURPOSE of this chapter is to investigate the roles, responsibilities and perceptions of women who were paid for their work as care-givers and medical service providers in municipal childcare arrangements. The focus here will be child-care arrangements in the later sixteenth century, a time when management of hospitals, foundling and orphaned children's welfare and poor relief services was becoming centralised under a bureau of lay administrators. If, as shown in Chapter 3, the medical status of the work performed by religious women was largely ignored by ecclesiastical and lay governors of hospitals, for what medical services would councils employ townswomen, and how was their practice perceived?

Women and municipal health care

There has been a great deal of research into the creation of municipal poor relief services, which included child care, in France during the sixteenth century. It was in this century that many towns developed a centralised relief body to co-ordinate their welfare and charity to the community, incorporating hospitals, relief payments to the poor and injured, and care of foundling or orphan children.[1] Physicians, surgeons, apothecaries and midwives were increasingly involved in the medical care provided in municipal health-care programmes. They could be attached to hospitals and paid an annual salary to treat patients weekly: others were paid on a case-by-case basis.[2] Town councils also developed co-ordinated procedures such as cleaning and quarantine arrangements for dealing with epidemics like the plague.

Women were involved in these urban medical endeavours in many ways. Donations from elite and bourgeois women supported many of Poitiers' hospitals, particularly after the middle of the sixteenth century.[3]

Some had personal connections to the hospitals. The father-in-law, husband and then nephew of Guillemette Leproust had administered the Hôpital des Champs in Poitiers for fifty years. In 1586, she promised to provide its plague-stricken patients with an annual sum of 30 écus for the hospital's upkeep.[4] Jehanne de Tongrelou, a merchant's widow, governed the almshouse of Nôtre-Dame-la-Grande from 1535 until 1542, and donated many of her household utensils to it. Later records indicate she was still involved in the running of the almshouse at least until 1549.[5]

Other women dedicated themselves to collecting linen for the hospitals in Poitiers: this was always a significant expenditure for hospitals in terms of finances and labour for its laundering. Some women donated linen directly to the hospitals, such as the wives of a local apothecary and a surgeon in 1568. More women, from elite, middling and lower social levels, were involved in Poitiers' annual drive to collect linen among the parishes. The council's records of this well-established system indicated that the collectors of linen for Poitiers' hospitals were assumed to be women.[6] Apart from the pious donations of wealthy women, hospitals also benefited from religiously motivated women who wished to serve as servants to hospitals. In 1550, Catherine de La Cour, a Franciscan tertiary, obtained permission from the council in Poitiers to serve the plague-stricken without payment. She was to be given the same food as the poor, was to clothe herself at her own expense and to lead an 'honest and religious life' for the privilege.[7]

Across France, women were involved in these municipal healthcare programmes. In Poitiers selected townswomen were responsible for transporting sick indigents to the hospitals, in the years before this became the responsibility of the hospital caretakers. In 1564, two women were paid 4 sols for bringing a poor girl 'having the fever, who was sleeping on a dunghill behind the walls near Pont-Joubert' to the hospital. Toinette Moinarde was paid for bringing a poor beggarwoman from in front of the church of St Pierre to the hospital. This piecemeal work performed by women was integral to maintaining public health in the town.[8] In times of plague, the sterilising work of women laundering and cleaning the houses of plague victims, as *héridesses*, however undesirable, was essential to quarantine measures in towns. The 1597 plague regulations in Dijon discussed 'priests, surgeons, porters, gravediggers and *héridesses*' as the key personnel for its public health programme.[9]

As well as their work as midwives, we know that women were paid to treat particular illnesses on a case-by-case basis. Alison Klairmont Lingo has observed that in Lyon women were paid especially for treating syphilis and skin diseases.[10] Both male and female practitioners were paid by the Lyon city council to heal the pox, as were Françoise Page and Marie Rodillon, and women's payments were equal to those of male practitioners.[11] As hospital beds were in short supply, the Poitiers council paid women to care for patients in their homes. In 1544, a poor woman received alms for caring for a passing Italian suffering from dysentry. Barbe Gracieuse received 20 sols for caring for three patients in her Poitiers home in 1584.[12]

Municipal health care in Tours

The evidence of Tours provides a useful case study as to women's involvement in health-care services for foundling and orphan children. This silk town in the Loire valley was once one of France's major centres with well-established administration and infrastructure due to Louis XII's residence nearby at Plessis-lès-Tours. Later at the end of the sixteenth century, it would come into national focus once more as the capital, briefly, of Henri IV in the 1590s. A mid-sized provincial city of about 16,000 in the early sixteenth century, doubling by the seventeenth century, Tours was both a loyal royalist and Catholic town.[13] In 1547, an act of the bailiff of Touraine united local hospitals under a central administration.[14] In 1552, poor relief, hospital management and child care were centralised under the municipal Aumône Générale. Although some records remain from this period, they are comprehensive only from the 1580s onwards. Overall, a study of the receipts, deliberations and original pauper letters for the extant years 1580–83, 1585–87, 1589, 1591 and 1592, some 2,465 documents, allows us to examine municipal poor relief management in Tours exceptionally well over the decade of the 1580s. This study focuses then not on the early establishment, conceptual basis and teething problems of municipal child care, but upon a fully functioning Catholic poor relief system at work. Run by municipal governors elected to a council, they managed according to their own description left in the account books, 'the almshouses and hospitals of Tours, foundling children left at the doors of the hospitals, churches, boutiques and other places in the town of Tours, sent to wetnurses at the expenses of the poor'.[15] Needy passers-by, the poor and sick were issued *la pitance* consisting of meat (beef, mutton or veal).[16] Beyond this, the town's hospitals also catered for a population of sick, poor and dying. On a weekly basis, the major adult hospital St Gatien averaged about 55 *pauvres malades* in the year 1582–83 (the accounting year ran from 24 June), for which 4 large loaves a day, and 12 pounds of

beef and of mutton per week were supplied.[17] At the same time La
Madeleine children's hospital held about 22 children. Of course, as will
be discussed below, many more foundlings and orphan children were
cared for in the houses of townspeople.

In Tours, the town's health-care services clearly relied on the work
of townswomen, as well as physicians, apothecaries and most commonly
surgeons. The town council particularly favoured the surgeon for most
cases where the poor applied for money to pay for medical procedures,
in part surely because they could pay him smaller sums than those
quoted by the poor as the fees of local bonesetters and stonecutters.
Local women ran the hospital and almhouse St Gatien on a daily basis.
In 1578, Flourentine Desfossés was its keeper. One male 'master servant'
and two female servants were also employed, as well as the surgeon and
a chaplain. If remuneration indicated their respective positions in the
hierarchy of authority, Desfossés (13 écus per year) ranked behind the
surgeon (23 écus), but above the chaplain (8 écus 20 sols) and master
servant (12 écus). The female servants, Silvine Bellenger and Jehanne
Morin, each received 5 écus for their annual wages.[18] As in Lyon, women
were paid to treat cases of pox. In the same year, one Marguerite Bussière
was paid by the council 2 écus for her work curing a patient of 'the
Naples' sickness'.[19] In 1585, female servants working in the Sanitas
hospital on the outskirts of Tours, where cases of plague were treated,
were each paid 1 écu a month. This sum, which matched that of the
garde of the largest hospital, St Gatien, seven years earlier, probably
reflected some inflation but also both the risks of the work and its
instability. In times of epidemics, the council paid women, as well as
extra porters and surgeons, in daily, weekly and monthly rates to work
as long as the crises lasted.[20]

Child-care work and its value in Tours

Townswomen were generally paid as specialist healers for particular
ailments, or as nursing staff under the supervision of surgeons, but
there was one domain where women were the only medical providers employed: children's health and illnesses. In 1564, Marguerite
Bricard nursed three children with ringworm for 50 sous.[21] In 1581, 'La
Chemanière' was paid for curing six children from La Madeleine of
ringworm.[22] Sick children, whether they had ringworm, pox or were
just labelled 'ill', seemed to have been seen by the council as the concern
of women. Moreover, many more women were paid to nurse, care for
and maintain the health of foundling or orphaned children. Children

who were abandoned, orphaned or whose mothers were ill could be distributed to respectable married women and widows in neighbouring parishes who were contracted to 'nurse at the breast' the infants, or 'feed/nurse and maintain in all things' the weaned child.[23] Perhaps surprisingly, the bulk of the Tours relief business was not occupied with distributing alms to the poor, but concerned child-care arrangements. More than half the cases that came before the relief council for consideration involved wet- or dry-nursing, and the rest were a combination of regular payments for those poor individuals or families on the relief rolls (for six months at a time) or for one-off support as a result of an illness, injury or some other pressing need.

We can gain an understanding of how the council perceived women's work as carers for children who were sick, malnourished or simply too young to survive without care, by examining their child-care arrangements. In his study on child abandonment in ancient and medieval western Europe, John Boswell concludes that 'in Renaissance cities the infants disappeared quietly and efficiently through the revolving doors of state-run foundling homes, out of sight and mind, into social oblivion, or, more likely, death by disease'.[24] Historians have analysed the sixteenth century very closely as a time in which the growing spirit of humanism encouraged town councils to re-organise local poor relief services in France, services that included provisions for child care.[25] Although there have been some early general studies of foundling facilities and hospitals in France,[26] most cover a large time frame and therefore lack detail on the changes specific to child-care arrangements in the sixteenth century. Did women's child-care work change in the sixteenth century as a result of the new administrative structures and concepts of humanism?

Formal child-care arrangements were not a new initiative in the sixteenth century, even if their administration by town councils generally was.[27] Many medieval urban environments had in place well-organised establishments at least as early as the fourteenth century, for which records are still accessible. In all of these systems, local women were paid to wet- and dry-nurse infants and small children. The hospital order of Saint-Esprit, first established in Montpellier by a certain Frère Guy before 1180, encompassed both the sick and abandoned children in its care. By the thirteenth century, Saint-Esprit houses had spread across France, to Marseille, Bergerac, and Troyes, as well as to other countries.[28] In Toulouse, the ordinance of Charles V in August 1379 outlines its hospice's role as 'receiving poor orphan children, providing them with nurses, preparing them until the age of 14 for a manual profession'.[29]

Extant account records for the Saint-Esprit hospital in Marseille demonstrate a strictly regulated welfare organisation for poor and foundling children at least as early as the turn of the fourteenth century. Accounts recorded the name and address of each nurse, the name and age of the child given to her, payments made and the return or decease of the child. For example, in 1306 'we had delivered a female child to dame Hugone d'Aubagne, who lives in rue des Pilliers, above Sainte-Catherine, and she has a husband named Isnard Guigou, and she is paid 4 sols a month'.[30] Regulations of 1399 fixed the length of wetnursing to a strict 22 months.[31] Not only are the written records well maintained, but they reveal that the administrators took care to observe the children's welfare by surveying the nurses. In 1434, the records state 'We have paid Brémone, at 6 sols a month ... We removed the child the first day of May, for she nursed her badly'.[32]

These child-care systems were not then new initiatives to late medieval France. Leah L. Otis's study of the municipal wetnursing system in fifteenth-century Montpellier gives no indication of it being a newly established system in that period but rather an enduring functional framework. Although there was no institutional establishment to care for children as there would be in later periods, the Montpellier municipality maintained careful records of its wetnursing networks through what were apparently quite substantial records, although not all remain today.[33] Similarly, a study of the accounts concerning child care of the municipal council of Lille suggest that the early sixteenth-century developments were just that: developments of a pre-existing system, rather than innovations in child care.[34] Much like hospital nursing, women's work as child carers underpinned the organisation under different managing groups. What altered was that responsibility for child-care services moved from these religious organisations to the town councils and specialised services for foundlings, orphans and the children of poor parents were provided accordingly. Such a process was not smooth: in many areas there was conflict and confusion between hospitals and town councils over who was primarily responsible for infant and child care.[35]

In the years with which this study is concerned, at least 185 children can be documented in the records at Tours. In the accounting year running from 24 June, we have remaining records for 1580–81, 1581–82, 1582–83, 1585–86, 1586–87, 1590–91 and 1591–92. The average number of children documented in the system for each of those years was 54.[36] Most of these were ongoing cases, with a small proportion of new cases added to the books each year, and some cases leaving the books through the death or return of the child. It is possible to trace the year of entry into the system for 118 different children (with the rest commencing municipal support before 1581 or during the gap years of 1583–84 and 1587–89).[37] This constitutes an average of 17 new children (both orphans and foundlings) added to the system annually (118 cases in 7 years of documented entries) and suggests that there were about 36 cases of ongoing child care each year.

The role of the nurse was often not only to breastfeed the infant; it was a much more extensive health-care role. She was expected to have medical knowledge to treat run-of-the-mill childhood ailments, maintain the child in good health and to teach the child the first elements of its moral education. The town council in Tours appeared to pay women for their care-giving skills relatively well and their wages even rose over the decade of the 1580s. While the majority of women were initially paid 6 écus a year for caring for a child (either wet- or dry-nursing – no distinction appears to made in the records), by 1590 and 1591 the rate is more typically 8 écus a year. Amounts for child care were commonly expressed in council deliberations and receipts as year-long rates, which were normally paid quarterly. This rate – of 6 écus or 360 sols in the early and mid-1580s, and 8 écus or 480 sols in the early 1590s – appears reasonably generous if compared to the wages that the council paid to domestic servants in its hospitals. In 1583, a typical (female) pay for a domestic servant was 150 sols a year, and in the 1590s, 260–80 sols a year.[38] The relatively high annual payment directed to nursing women suggests then that care of the foundling children of Tours was considered a worthy expenditure of the council's funds – particularly given the relatively large number of children (compared to cases of poor relief) with which the council was concerned. If the council was prepared to direct typically 240 sols to each case of poor relief (individual or family), then they accorded double by the 1590s to the women paid to nurse an orphan or foundling child.

If women were relatively well paid for their care-giving work, was this a reflection of how the council valued their skills? To explore this, we need to understand how the council selected the women who cared for children. Children were generally distributed to married women and widows in neighbouring parishes. The children of very poor or sick mothers could also be placed for short periods with widows and families in the neighbourhood. Often it is difficult to determine who were the women who cared for children. Their identities, circumstances and work habits are often obscured behind the names of male relatives – most commonly husbands and sons, or sometimes male neighbours

– who collected payments on their behalf. It is only by following through the history of such cases for a number of years that one discovers an incidental mention of a woman's name included alongside that of the male recipient of her payment.[39]

Wetnurses and carers for the children of Tours were chosen by the council according to a number of criteria. Firstly, although men often collected payments from the governors for these activities as husbands, sons or relatives of carers, it was women, as wives or widows, who cared for children. No single or widowed man appears to have cared for a foundling or orphan. Secondly, many of those widows or families chosen as carers were poor themselves. By paying a poor widow to nurse a child, the council managed two pressing needs with one payment. As we have seen, the payments made to women and families who cared for children were more substantial than those given to people receiving regular poor relief. Furthermore, while the average poor relief payments rarely lasted longer than a year, a wetnurse or carer who maintained the child in good health might be paid for as long as five or six years for their work. The council in Tours prioritised child care, not only in terms of the number of cases supported, but also in the proportion of its funds allocated to provide long-term carers and stability for the children.

The council also tended to send children to outlying parishes around Tours. Sixteenth-century recommendations for wetnurses often insisted that she be a country woman used to fresh air and simple foods.[40] The council appears to have followed this policy, sending children to rural areas near Tours. Children were most commonly sent to the north of the town, to the viticultural parishes (now communes) of Neuillé Pont Pierre, Rochecorbon and St Georges sur Loire, but also as far away as Chanceaux, Parçay and St Pierre de Vouvray. A number of families in the rural areas to the east of the town were paid to care for children, at St Pierre des Corps primarily but also at Montlouis sur Loire and even the nearby town of Amboise. Far fewer children were sent to families in the west, at La Riche, or to the fertile but damp parishes of Nouzilly or St Venant at Ballan-Miré to the south of Tours where the river Cher was prone to flood.

Not surprisingly, given the parishes in which most carers lived, the majority of those whose profession was noted in the governors' records (as husbands living or dead of care-givers) were listed as day labourers or vinegrowers, often interchangeably according to the season. The relatively unskilled, piecemeal and seasonal work of such men made them particularly vulnerable to economic hardship and to fluctuate in and out of poverty. Most of those receiving poor relief generally through the council were similarly classified as day labourers. Caring for a child then could provide an important, steady form of income to the household. Other occupations of the husbands of care-givers reflected the cloth-trade economy of Tours, with cloth-dyers, silk workers, trimming merchants, drapers and silk weavers among them. Finally, several who were involved in the council's medical service provision in the town's hospitals and almshouse also became carers for children. Catherine Boyer, the wife of the administrator of the St Martin almshouse, nursed four different children over the period from 1580 to 1592. Some infants were nursed on a short-term basis of a few weeks before a permanent carer was found, but others remained with the family for more than 12 months.[41]

Being female, poor and in an outlying parish were not the only criteria for work as a carer, however. The council also valued experience, sometimes sending children to the same woman and occasionally even while they nursed another child. Sainte Alliot, the widow of Lyenard Collart, then wife of Mathurin Courangon, cared for four different children over the eleven-year period.[42] Of course, children might be sent to the same woman when the first child had died or was returned to the orphanage, because she was in continued need of assistance, but it seems unlikely that, on these grounds alone, the council would have doubled her payment by sending her two children to manage at once, when there were more families in need than could be sent children. The widow Jehanne Geipoulleau also nursed two children for the council at the same time in 1580: the eighteen-month-old Blaise and four-year-old Denyse.[43] Moreover, Alliot remarried during the period, a time at which it might be expected that her financial status improved somewhat, and yet she continued to care for, and be sent, children. Such evidence suggests that Alliot may have been poor, but was also recognised by the council for her care-giving work.

Nursing a child was not without its dangers for women and their families. Hospital accounts recorded compensation given to wetnursing women who contracted illnesses from an infected child. Thus, René Garnyer was paid 2 écus by the administrators of the poor relief and hospitals of Tours to help him care for Michelle Rouille his wife 'of pox which came of having nursed a child sick of the illness'.[44] Equally, in February 1581, Jacques Myet and his wife Jehanne Marche were paid the same sum, 'ill of the sickness of the pox for having taken a child sick with the illness to breastfeed'.[45] The work of the wetnurse carried thus a risk not only to the woman, but also to her husband and children who all lived under the same roof.

Although this evidence suggests that the council frequently paid poor women or families to care for children as a way of solving two problems at once, there was a rationale as to which women or families were selected. Clearly, there were communally recognised definitions of what constituted appropriate child-care knowledge. The governors recognised a community of mothering peers who were capable of caring for children. This community was composed only of women, and only of those who had borne children. By following this policy, the administrators validated a discourse of maternal authority, not as an innate faculty of being a woman, but recognising that women learned and accumulated child-caring skills through experience themselves. Naomi J. Miller has recently argued that 'the pervasive powers of influence associated with maternity in early modern society extended not simply to actual mothers, but to other female caregivers as well, whose standing was variably and yet inextricably linked with strengths as well as the shortcomings of maternal authority'.[46] While maternity undoubtedly did provide a 'touchpoint' for female positions of authority, as can be seen in Chapter 8, I would argue that, in the context of medical care of its children, the governors in Tours promoted the opposite position: authority to give care to children rested on the basis of specific bodily experiences and did not credit similar influence to other women without these defined practices with children. Bodies and subjectivity mattered. The parturient bodies of these nursing townswomen validated to the governors the women's abilities and knowledge. In turn, the poor relief council's legitimisation of particular women's experiences of childbirth as a valid criterion for child-care work, contributed to how such women understood themselves and gave meaning to their lives.

The Tours administrators left no explicit documentation as to how it judged a woman's ability to care for a child. However, there were checks and balances on women's behaviour in the surrounding community. Neighbours could presumably act as witnesses to women's poor behaviour, since they were often called upon in other instances to attest to the good behaviour of municipal poor-relief recipients. Parish curés formed another network of supervision. When in September 1582 a poor child Susanne, nursed by Jehanne Geipoulleau, died, another child was immediately put in her place. When, less than a year later, that infant Blaise died in the care of Geipoulleau, he was also immediately replaced by another abandoned infant girl, Guyanne.[47] In Geipoulleau's case, there is no discussion or suspicion of ill treatment within the remaining documents. Curés acted in some ways as the verifiers of women's abilities to care for children, for it was a requirement that nurses produce for the council a letter from the curé confirming burial of the child concerned. In this way, the curé had the opportunity to oversee the care women gave to children, and to report to the council on cases of abuse or maltreatment that he perceived. A foundling child was to many a source of income and might in fact be given preferential treatment within a family. The survival of abandoned children was in the interest of those whose meagre revenues were supplemented by their care.

The council's policy maintained stability in the lives of their young charges (as well the family economy of those who cared for them). Many children remained for some years with their carers. The council typically paid a woman or couple to nurse a child for a year at a time, and paid them in quarterly instalments. Therefore, unless a child died or was returned, one receipt book contains regular payments for a child over a financial year. By tracing the name of a child and its carer across the remaining receipt books, it is possible to gain an idea of the length of time children stayed with carers. Here I have calculated the length of a child's stay with a carer from a) the entry date and date of death or return of a child (20 cases known) and b) the entry date and last known date of care for a child (from a receipt book other than the entry year) (42 cases). This amounts to 62 cases analysed. Although this data analysis is less than perfect because of the gap years where there is no extant receipt book, and is likely to be skewed towards short care periods because the full length of care cannot often be traced, the results nonetheless indicate a tendency towards long-term care patterns. Among the cases analysed, 58 per cent of children spent more than 12 months with their carers: 16 per cent of children spent (at least) 13 to 24 months with their carer, 18 per cent two to three years, 10 per cent three to four years, 6 per cent five to six years and 8 per cent six to seven years with their carer. Therefore, although this data is likely to demonstrate shorter care patterns more clearly, it indicates that at least half (58 per cent) of the children assessed spent more than a year with their carer, and almost a quarter (24 per cent) of them spent more than three years. Of course, there were always likely to be a number of children who did require long-term care, like nine-year old orphan Marin Regnault, who was cared for by Sainte Alliot and described as crippled.[48]

Marin was exceptional in the governors' records because he was older than most of the children who were supported through the municipal system. However, most children did appear to stay with their carers until at least the age of five. Although the data for children returned by carers to the orphanage of La Madeleine is small (7 cases), these children were all between the ages of four and seven. There are many records which indicate that the council continued to pay child care particularly for five- and six-year-olds, but also occasionally for children seven, eight and nine years old.

Although it is widely claimed that foundlings and orphaned children perished in large numbers throughout the early modern period, the evidence for Tours at least does not appear to support this.[49] Only 25 definite cases of death of a child are recorded in the remaining records, with six more cases where it is uncertain whether a child has been returned or died. Including these cases too, these figures suggest a death rate of only 17 per cent (31 out of 185 total cases). Although we lack data for some years, this is not likely to misrepresent the death rate of children any more than the intake rate of children and ongoing care. Such a low mortality rate for the foundling and orphan children suggests a high degree of municipal attention to the selection of competent caregivers and is testament to their nursing abilities. From those children for whom the age of death can be determined (10 of 25 cases), there seems no evidence for early infant death, but rather a broad spectrum with children ranging from six and nine months to four and six years of age.

The child in sixteenth-century thought

If valuation for women's skills as care-givers, and their removal from poor relief registers, are some of the reasons why the governors paid childcarers relatively well, these were not the only explanations. Children were themselves becoming the object of increased scrutiny in the public eye. In published literature, the sixteenth century saw a growing humanist and medical dialogue on the moral and medical welfare of children.

The medieval period was by no means devoid of literature about childhood or child care. Luke Demaitre has charted an increased specialisation occurring from 1250 to 1500, resulting in the separation of paediatrics, particularly from obstetrics and gynaecology, as its own subject.[50] The increasing publications that the sixteenth century experienced on children and child care were a continuation of this dynamic paediatric tradition.[51] Humanists were also keen commentators on moral care for children and they did not abstain from entering the more medical debate of whether breastfeeding was to be preferred over wetnursing. Physicians produced new medical literature concerned with childhood illnesses and maintenance of child health. Although the *Pedenemicon* of Gabriel Miron, physician of the children of Anne of Brittany and Claude de France, was published in 1544,[52] it was a later royal physician, Simon de Vallambert, who brought the field to some prominence in France with his *Cinq livres, de la maniere de nourrir et gouverner les enfants des leur naissance*, published in 1565. The royal surgeon Jacques Guillemeau followed in 1585 with *De la nourriture et du gouvernement des enfants*.[53]

Vallambert's text, the first of the influential paediatric publications in France, had a particularly enduring impact and set the trend for others to follow. Although it mirrored much of the style and content of Miron's earlier text, Vallambert's was written in French and had explicitly new aims and audience in mind. While previous medical writers had primarily produced their paediatric texts in Latin and directed them at a fellow medical audience, Vallambert hoped his instruction would at least 'be heard by the women of France' even if it too assumed that readers had a knowledge of Arab, Greek and Latin authors.[54] More specifically, his concerns reflected the choices made by the elite woman: how to choose a nurse, the way to nurse and govern the child before and after it is weaned, and the manner to cure the illnesses of children.

Moreover, Vallambert emphasised the importance of both childhood itself and the women involved in its care: 'The position of the midwives and nurses who handle and govern childhood is not less than the pedagogues and masters who form and instruct youth'.[55] Although Vallambert promoted firstly the knowledge of the ancients, be they Greek, Arab or Latin, as well as his more recent predecessors, he also promoted the recognition of the knowledge and practices of midwives, nurses and mothers. Further, Marie-Madeleine Fontaine has argued that compared with contemporary texts Vallambert was less critical of the remedies of 'bonnes femmes',[56] and saw them as a source for another repertoire of practices. Although it is unlikely that child carers read this or other child-rearing texts, it is more probable that the governors were exposed to their message. Children could be protected from common diseases by good health-care practices, and they were morally worth saving.

At the same time, and perhaps partly as a result of it, the separation and specialisation of municipal medical services designated children as a distinct medical and welfare concern meriting their own establishments. One of the principal reasons that child-care services were needed in urban areas was to care for abandoned or foundling children. Yet in many areas, municipal authorities were often unwilling to accept the financial burden for what appeared to contemporaries as a growing problem.[57] Furthermore, they hesitated as to whether providing care for foundlings would encourage illicit sex and increase abandonment. The abandonment of a child was a serious offence and carried severe penalties including whipping, fines and banishment.

Towns adopted a number of policies to care for foundling newborns throughout the sixteenth century. Some like the Maison-Dieu at Ballon resisted moves to take in abandoned children at the hospital. The judge who had made immediate provision with a local townswoman for one such case was forced to seek compensation from the Maison-Dieu at the court of Ballon in July 1520. When the bailiff found in his favour, the Maison-Dieu administrators refused to pay for the child's welfare and appealed the case to the seneschal of Le Mans in December of that year. The seneschal confirmed the previous judgement and ordered the hospital to take care of the child and compensate the woman who had been providing for it in the previous months.[58]

Paris was perhaps one of the most negligent and backward cities in provisions for foundlings.[59] This is all the more astonishing given its large population: foundlings must have been a constant problem. One of the major stumbling blocks for councillors in many towns seems to have been a fear that provisions made for foundlings might encourage pre-marital sex. Yet it is perhaps also Paris's size that accounts for some of the disorganised policy towards such children. Paris already had a number of institutions that cared or catered specifically for orphaned children. One of the city's oldest orphanages, at the place de Grève, founded by the confraternity of St Esprit, was a hospice open only to orphans 'born in legal marriage . . . who had neither father nor mother, nor *amys charneulx* or others who could provide for them'.[60] Indeed its statues clearly voiced some of the principal concerns for municipal officials:

> if the revenues of the said hospital were employed to nurse and care for bastard, illegitimate children, of whom it could be that there was an enormous quantity, for many people would abandon themselves . . . to sin when they see that such bastards would be cared for.[61]

Many foundlings were taken to the Hôtel-Dieu, which took orphans out of pity rather than obligation. As the Hôtel-Dieu de Paris' Sister Cecille Mareschal reported in 1531, 'swaddled infants were brought and abandoned at night in front of the two portals of the hospital. In the case that no one else took them, the sisters took them in out of pity and charity'.[62] The prioress Hélène la Petite also commented in her report that the sisters accepted children only 'out of pity, charity and compassion'.[63]

In 1536, the King's sister, Marguerite d'Angoulême, instigated the creation of the Hôpital des Enfants-Dieu, whose charges were known as *les enfants rouges* from the colour of their uniform. This hospital aimed originally to provide for those children whose parents had died while at the Hôtel-Dieu, but by 1541 it accepted all legitimate orphans from the city and suburbs of Paris. However, it refused to accept foundlings.[64] In 1545, the *Parlement* of Paris ordered the hospital La Trinité, previously a pilgrims' shelter, to become a hospice for poor male children, and soon after poor girls, les *Enfants bleus*, as they were known. La Trinité too refused to extend infant foundlings its care.[65]

The Parisian institution that took on most responsibility for foundlings then, apart from the Hôtel-Dieu, was the Couche de Nôtre-Dame, a centre for children supported by the Nôtre-Dame chapter. Already by the beginning of the fifteenth century, the system that Nôtre-Dame provided for foundlings was well established for there are testamentary donations dedicated to the 'poor children of Nôtre-Dame'.[66] In 1445, Charles VII attempted to clarify exactly what role the hôpital du Saint-Esprit in Paris played in the care of children. It declared that it 'must serve only to receive orphans born in legitimate marriage' and in doing so revealed the fate of foundlings: 'that, as for foundling and unknown children, one must continue only to take collections at a certain bed, being at the entry to the cathedral of Paris, to cry publicly to passers-by in front of the place where the children are: *Do well to these poor abandoned children*, and to use the donations coming from this collection to care for and feed these children'.[67] This cradle functioned much like a shop window: the woman in charge of caring for the foundlings placed a child in it to attract the pity and charity of passers-by who might give a donation, or even take the child home to care for it.

The Parisian system remained somewhat haphazard throughout the sixteenth century. Responsibility for foundlings technically lay in the hands of those in whose jurisdiction the child was found, but most foundlings in Paris went to *La Couche* who arranged for a wetnurse. After being weaned, most children were returned to *La Couche*. This 'institution' had no fixed location before 1570, and moved from house to house depending on which family was willing to take in the foundlings. Its management and daily operations relied on the charity of local women, usually widows. By 1552, after much complaint from the Nôtre-Dame chapter, an *arrêt* of the *Parlement* of Paris ordered all the *haut justiciers* of Paris to contribute to the financial management of the *Couche* in the region of 960 livres parisis collectively, since most jurisdictions of Paris sent their foundlings to its facilities.[68] It was not until 1570 that the *Couche* was allotted by the *Parlement* a permanent location in a house at the Port St Landry. However, even at the end of the century, only this one establishment was primarily responsible for most arrangements of wetnursing and infant child care in Paris.

Other towns also hesitated about who was to accept foundling children. After the municipal poor bureau was established in Rouen in 1534, that town's Hôtel-Dieu increasingly refused to accept foundlings, preferring to care solely for the sick. However, the bureau was unable to manage such services, and by 1538 an edict from the King demanded that the Hôtel-Dieu de la Magdelaine continue its provision of childcare services, providing 'four nurses who will stay there to receive, nurse and feed the young abandoned children newly born and brought there' – 'as a provisional measure'.[69] But it seems that this was a business the Hôtel-Dieu was keen to dismantle. Again in 1553, an edict reminded the Hôtel-Dieu that until further notice, it must 'provide nurses at the Hôtel-Dieu to nurse the abandoned newborns'.[70] Larger towns particularly seem to have suffered if they already had, as this example and that of Paris indicate, a number of institutions dedicated to child care. This created a situation where each believed another responsible for the primary provision of foundlings. In smaller urban environments with fewer facilities, one establishment and one system often served both legitimate and illegitimate children (as foundlings were often assumed to be) in need of care.

Midwives played an important role in the eyes of municipal authorities in their services, as discussed in Chapter 1. If the father of the child could be identified, he could be asked to cover the child's welfare. If he resided in another parish, the child could be passed over to that parish as its responsibility. Municipalities required the midwife delivering a single mother to refuse assistance until the mother revealed the father's name, and wrote into the oaths of local midwives that they had to procure the name of the bastard child's father 'so as to avoid so many foundlings at the expense of the poor relief of this town as we have daily'.[71] The father could then be made to pay for his own child's welfare. In Tours, the poor relief even provided the wife of one such man with a small sum to care for his bastard daughter.[72] If the father of the child was not local, they could then attribute the child, mother and their collective welfare to the appropriate town.

In Lille, there were occasions when the foundling child was individually taken around the town in the hopes that it could be identified. In 1542, the council gave 6 sols 'to a woman having carried around the crossroads banging at the drum, and for having fed it some times'.[73] In the accounts for 1527, 40 sols were given 'to a clothworker for his wine, having been the first who had advised the councillors of Lille to whom an abandoned child belonged . . . We gave him 34 sols to take the child back to Tournay, including the expenses for the child'. The town council there also recorded that 'We had published that we would give a florin to he who will give the address and knowledge of the mother of a little girl, abandoned near the porte de la Barre, by a woman from Tournay'.[74]

Throughout the sixteenth century, it appears that the Lille council observed its determination to send foundlings to other councils as their responsibility. In 1495 they sent word 'to the bailiffs and councillors of the county of Laleue, in order to make a girl, living at Sailly-sur-la-Lys, take back her child that she had abandoned in the said town of Lille, which had looked after it for some time.'[75] In 1533, 'We sent letters to the mayor and councillors of the town of Arras, to make a man residing there to come collect his children, that he had abandoned in this town of Lille'.[76] Again in 1570, 'We had two foundlings that the grand bailiff would not receive, led to the village of Lestrem.'[77]

Despite their fears regarding increased licentiousness in the population, most urban centres eventually instituted some formal provisions for abandoned children.[78] After all, one of the key arguments in humanist pedagogical literature such as that of Erasmus and Vives held that education and training of the child at an early age could shape its future path.[79] According to educational notions of the era, using the ecological metaphors of the child as a plant or tree, the child had an individuality that must be respected, but equally directed to the right path, just as a tree must be pruned and shaped into a 'suitable form' according to the needs of the community.[80] Therefore, municipal authorities reasoned that if they could take the poor indigent child early enough, through education and apprenticeship programmes, they could reduce the problem of foundlings in the future.

In Tours, most children cared for through the municipal system were foundlings and abandoned children. Of these 185 cases, 42 were specifically named on at least one record as an *enfant trouvé* or foundling, and another 69 are documented only by their Christian name with no further details. Since the council seems to have consistently recorded as much information about a child's origin as they knew, these 69 children were likely also to be foundlings. Therefore, 111 or 60 per cent of the children that the council managed were probably foundlings. The administrators at Tours did try to ascertain the origins of an abandoned child, most commonly to see if the child could be cared or its expenses covered by some other individual or council. Many of their entries included knowledge of a child's parents that had been gathered from the community: 'a small child that one says belongs to Jullian Bennoyer a cook and married man, and Denise Pelletier a prostitute'[81] or 'a child that one says belongs to a servant at Saincte Marthe'.[82] Another child named Jehan was a 'son delivered by the wife of a man who has been whipped in this town three weeks ago'.[83] When a silk worker Jehan Marchant discovered a child at the door of the cloister of St Martin's church in 1582, before the administrators accepted care of the child, they confirmed that he 'affirms not to know the father and mother of Catherine, a girl abandoned at the door of the cloister of Saint Martin, nor those who abandoned her'.[84]

Should children live through their early years, they remained with carer families until the age of five. Then, like most children in urban centres, if they hadn't been adopted by their carers,[85] they returned to a centralised institution. In Tours the children were returned to the hospital La Madeleine, which catered for all children, whether foundling, orphaned or otherwise.[86] The governor of La Madeleine was a married man who, with his wife, two female servants and a teacher, ran the child-care services. In an average year, say 1582, La Madeleine housed 23 children at a time and never more than 25. In comparison, the largest of the poor hospitals in sixteenth-century Tours, Saint Gatien, housed on average 50 to 60 adult patients (sick or poor) at any one time.[87]

Regardless of their origins, all children who received home care could be returned to the town orphanage. The council made regular investments in the health and welfare of older children at La Madeleine. It paid local women to treat childhood illnesses such as ringworm and scalp diseases. In times of plague, such as in 1582, the governors rented a country property for the children in a rural area nearby Tours, at Varenne, to 'change the air'.[88] This was a significant project, requiring the council to purchase bed and linens for the house, as well as making new clothes for the children and paying for transportation of food and supplies from Tours out to the house.[89] Children who fell ill of 'the contagion' were removed from the orphanage and treated in the private homes of country families. It seems the children were provided regularly with new sheets, clothing, bonnets, combs, hairbrushes and shoes.[90] Funding these supplies was supported by donations to the orphanage in wills, and in exchange the children might be required to process through the town at a funeral and to pray for the soul of their benefactor.[91] Provisions of food suggest that La Madeleine was prioritised over the other almshouses of Tours. In accounts for 1582–83, supplies to St Gatien, the largest almshouse in Tours, and La Madeleine can be compared. St Gatien, with an average of 55 poor or ill adult patients, received 15 large loaves of bread, 12 pounds of beef and 12 pounds of mutton a week. La Madeleine, with a child population of 24 as well as 5 adult staff, received a much higher relative provision of 21 loaves and 7.5 pounds of both beef and mutton.

Apart from the provision of food, clothing and linen, the governors mapped out an educational programme for the children of La Madeleine. A cleric was employed 'to demonstrate to the children', and accounts indicate purchases of religious books.[92] For the years of this study, only a few apprenticeship and dowry agreements remain. From these, we know that the council did arrange apprenticeships for boys with local master craftsmen – one twelve-year-old orphan was apprenticed to Jacques Foucault, a master silk worker, for six years. Silk work was, by this period, an important industry for the Tours economy, and this evidence would seem to support Natalie Zemon Davis' argument that councils may have used apprenticeship of children on the poor relief system to encourage the expansion of manufacture.[93] Girls too were taught professional skills. Françoise Mireur, to whom Jehanne Doulcette from La Madeleine had been contracted in 1570 'to learn a trade', applied to the governors in 1582 that a dowry be provided to Doulcette so that she could marry a local silk-spinner. The governors provided Doulcette with 4 écus to buy furniture for her new home on the instruction that she 'govern herself honestly'.[94]

The provision of care, time, facilities and financial resources to children was enormous at Tours. Not only did the council prioritise care to children over other poor relief recipients, but it made no differentiation in treatment and payments to carers between orphans and foundlings, or legitimate and illegitimate children. As a mid-sized city it was too large to ignore the plight of foundling children and too small to require more than one orphanage, which would have likely separated male and female children (as in Lyon) or distinguished between legitimate and foundling children, as in Paris. The evidence suggests that in Tours children were valued by the community. They could become a source of revenue for the foundling hospitals, as participants in community ceremonies. On several occasions, testators left significant sums to the hospitals in return for the prayers and procession of the foundling children at their death.[95] To the counter-reformation mind, the prayers of the poor and innocent foundling children, in their candle-lit processions, made a visible social contribution back to the town to which they owed their very survival. Moreover, they were given training that would produce workers with increased skilling and literacy, who would not then fall into the same dilemmas of poverty and indigence as their parents. Children moulded to the needs of the local community were increasingly seen as a social asset rather than burden on the town.

Women's work in child care in France

John Boswell concludes his study on child abandonment in the ancient and medieval past by arguing that, by the time of the Renaissance, children were 'reared apart from families' in impersonal institutions.[96] While it may be true that the services of child care became more closely controlled by the state by the sixteenth century, and were organised and paid for by municipal bureaux, such a statement ignores the vital ongoing contribution of women who largely nursed children in their own homes, at least until and sometimes beyond the age of five, encouraged and funded by the community purse.

Tours was no anomaly in sixteenth-century France: women were vital to all domains of municipal child care. They were obviously involved in primary infant care as wetnurses. Regional Hôtels-Dieu across France that maintained child-care services increasingly employed their own wetnurses and governesses, distinct from other hospital personnel, to care for the children brought there. For example, before the reforms to the Hôtel-Dieu in Orléans, children were sent out to nearby village women as the infants were found. However, with the reforms of 1558, the governors created provisions for children to be cared at least in the short term within the Hôtel-Dieu itself, appointing designated carers in the hospital for them. Two wetnurses were appointed to care for ten unweaned infants.[97] The governors appointed one of the nursing sisters, Jeanne Sauvoyonne, specifically to their care as 'governess of the unweaned infants and other little children below the age of five'.[98] In larger cities, the role of such institutions was most commonly to nurse a child until a suitable wetnurse could be found. In Caen, hospital regulations of 1540 clearly stipulated the number and role of carers for these children:

> that at the expense of the said Hôtel-Dieu, there will be ordinarily one nurse for the newborn children, & two others will be found when there is need, or more, if there is need. These will be outside the Hôtel-Dieu, as in the town, suburbs or in the nearby parishes, to breastfeed the little children until we have uncovered the relatives of the child, to take the child back if they have the means to feed and care for them, and not otherwise.[99]

In Rouen, a 1538 edict from the King established that the Hôtel-Dieu continue its provision of child-care services despite the introduction of new municipally controlled poor relief services.[100]

Did the women who worked as child carers feel that they had specialist knowledge or specific child-care practices? Few documents recorded how mostly illiterate poor women felt about their work. Few women who cared for children had the opportunity to have their opinions on child-care practices recorded (or were asked). Even if women could write, it is likely that they, like the nuns at the Hôtel-Dieu in Paris, would have lacked the language suitable to promote their caring knowledge to the wider community. Even as historians, it is difficult to articulate and historicise the types of knowledge and practices related to women's care-giving.[101] We have a better knowledge of the tropes of maternal authority, and its uses by both women and men, than the realities of early modern maternal practice or care-giving generally.[102] It is unquestionably easier to gain a sense of the governors' perceptions of appropriate care-giving than of the women who practised it.

Yet one rare source may illumine the question just a little. In July 1531, François I ordered an enquiry into the welfare of children in the Hôtel-Dieu in Paris. The report contained a unique insight into child-care services from the point of view of its female providers. The prioress, Hélène la Petite, had been at the Hôtel-Dieu for over fifty years. She firstly outlined the increasing difficulties due to swelling numbers of ill, poor and juvenile patients as well as the depletion in facilities to care for them. If in the past there were normally 60 to 70 children in the Hôtel-Dieu's care, either by abandonment, poverty or death of a parent, for the past ten years there had been 120 to 140 such charges per year.[103] Moreover, 'there has only been a single wetnurse all the time to cope with nursing the little children, who die for lack of breastmilk.'[104] The prioress's report is significant to our study here, because it reveals her understanding of what was required for appropriate child care.

She continued that, for lack of nurses, the nuns prepared cow's and goat's milk bottles for the infants, which, she noted, 'is not the food to raise a young infant as would be the breast of a mother or another nurse'. She argued that the nuns could not 'assist them well as they would like to do, to do well to the little ones, to clean them, pick them up, warm, cover and nurse them as they would desire'.[105] Her report promoted the need for individual care for each child and for the ability to adapt caring practices to the individual child. 'Some, without the nurse that they need, do nothing but cry and wail, which is a great vexation and torment... and the little children cannot explain their illnesses because some cannot yet speak and others are such a young age... If the little unweaned infants were treated and nursed by a particular nurse like the other little town children until the age of two, in another place which did not have such infected and corrupting air as the hospital does, it would save a great number of them each year.'[106] This report represents one of the few occasions where historians can see the perspective of women who cared for children at first hand.[107] Individualised care that recognised, and adapted experience to, the unique needs of each child was the cornerstone of what she felt was good child-care practice. As historians, we must remember that a lack of recorded evidence from the child carers themselves about quality service provision should not be interpreted as evidence that they, or their contemporaries, felt they lacked knowledge about what would be good for children, or interest in their wellbeing.[108]

Women were not only involved in child care as wet- and dry-nurses, however. They also contributed extensively to the management and organisation of establishments set up by towns for older children. In the institutions set up to house children after the age of five or seven, many were run by women, usually widows, others by married men and their wives, thus creating a family context: some were even based in the carers' own homes. I have not found one establishment that was controlled directly by a single or widowed male. The personnel of foundling and orphan hospitals therefore was in the majority female. As Davis argues, in Lyon it was women who were in charge of the foundling hospital and orphanages.[109] At Sainte Catherine, widows were expected to teach the girls to read and sew.[110] Here then was one location in which women could hold considerable community prestige and power.

Certainly the physical care and overseeing of the children was seen throughout the century as a female task. An *arrêt* of the Parisian *Parlement* in August 1552, demanding the *haut justiciers* contribute to the chapter of Nôtre-Dame's care of children in Paris, explained that the money would be given to the masters and governors of the Hôtel-Dieu de la Trinité, on the condition that they employ a woman to receive the foundlings.[111] In fact the regulations set up by the *arrêt* foresaw only women involved in the children's care: 'The said woman will make her residence there and receive the children in the form and manner that hitherto has been kept in the church of Paris, and these children brought away by her, will be sent by the administrators to honest and well known good women to raise and feed them.'[112] When in 1570 *Parlement* rather belatedly established a fixed residence for *La Couche* in Paris, at the Port Saint Landry, it was three women who were chosen to manage the facilities: 'Marie de la Croix, widow of the late Philippe le Jay, Anne Guyon, widow of the late M. Pierre d'Estampes, doctor in medicine, and Catherine Mousy, widow of the late Denis Guillebon, hitherto named by the *procureur général*, will have the governance of the food and maintenance of the foundling children; and . . . Pierre Hotman, merchant goldsmith and bourgeois of Paris will receive the deniers.'[113] Significantly, Hotman, who was to keep the books, would 'receive the deniers . . . to be distributed by him by the orders and advice of the said three women, or by two of the three'. Here then the primary administrators were women.[114]

In sickness, children seem to have been less likely to be treated by university- or guild- trained medical professionals and more often by women. Accounts drawn up by the lay administrators of the hospital indicated that they also employed townswomen to care for special cases of illness among the children. Childhood illnesses such as ringworm and scurvy were particularly considered the medical domain of women. One of the distinct services of the Parisian hospital of Saint-Esprit, catering only for legitimate orphans by the sixteenth century, was treatment for ringworm, run by a mistress who was to be 'a person of good and honest living, and of good conscience, and especially one who is pitying and charitable.'[115] She was assisted in her work by two poor orphan girls who would be trained to take over the service. Children with ringworm were always given to townswomen to cure in sixteenth-century Poitiers. Vincente Glorielle received 20 sols for curing two little girls in 1573. Fees for this service ranged from 15 sols to 3 livres, depending on the age of the child and the duration of the illness.[116] Chapter 4 has already discussed how, in Lille, women and couples who cared for foundling children also took them on pilgrimages, usually designed to cure them of a variety of illnesses. Almost all these institutions then relied on a large network of female support in the community to treat individual children with a range of caring, curing or nursing practices.

Whatever the impact at the municipal level of increased supervision and organisation of child-care services, and of distinct establishments to cater for children, the day-to-day contact with the young recipients of care continued to be provided by women throughout the century. Municipal health-care policies employed women as child carers in response to a number of contemporary notions. It was a good use of the council's resources to pay a poor woman or family who needed financial support to nurse a foundling or orphan child. The knowledge of experienced female carers to treat children in sickness and in health appeared to be privileged above that of physicians or surgeons – but it was also likely to come at a cheaper price from the council's point of view. As children were increasingly perceived to have a social value to the community in their own right, their care was prioritised.[117] Poor women in Tours and elsewhere in France stood to benefit with relatively well-paid work. The council's estimation that the women it chose were effective carers appears justified by the exceptionally low mortality rates for children in their charge. The care of children and their ongoing health was central to the concerns of all classes, but women's unchallenged primacy in health-care provision depended a great deal on the status of their charges. This is particularly clear in the correspondence of royal and elite households, as we will explore in the following chapter.

Notes

1 Natalie Zemon Davis, 'Poor relief, humanism, and heresy', *Society and Culture in Early Modern France* (Stanford: Stanford University Press, 1975), pp. 17–64. See also Marcel Fosseyeux, 'L'assistance parisienne au milieu du XVIe siècle', *Mémoires de l'histoire de Paris et de l'Ile-de-France* (1916), pp. 83–128; Jean-Pierre Gutton, *La Société et les pauvres, l'exemple de la généralité de Lyon. 1534–1789* (Paris: Les Belles Lettres, 1971); Gutton, *La Société et les pauvres en Europe, XVIe–XVIIIe siècles* (Paris: Presses universitaires de France, 1974); Jean Louis Goglin, *Les Misérables dans l'occident médiéval* (Paris: Editions du Seuil, 1976); Michel Mollat, *Les Pauvres au moyen age, étude sociale* (Paris: Hachette, 1978); Bronislaw Geremek, *Poverty: A History*, trans. A. Kolakowska (Oxford: Blackwell, 1994); for a slightly later period: Olwen Hufton, *The Poor of Eighteenth-Century France, 1750–1789* (Oxford: Clarendon Press, 1974); Cissie C. Fairchilds, *Poverty and Charity in Aix-en-Provence, 1640–1789* (Baltimore: The Johns Hopkins University Press, 1976), and Colin Jones, *Charity and Bienfaisance: The Treatment of the Poor in the Montpellier Region, 1740–1815* (Cambridge: Cambridge University Press, 1982).

2 See Klairmont Lingo for how these medical practitioners participate in municipal health-care programmes in Lyon and Montpellier. Alison Klairmont Lingo, *The Rise of Medical Practitioners in Sixteenth-Century France: The Case of Lyon and Montpellier* (PhD, University of California–Berkeley, 1980). For comparative studies of medical provision in poor relief services, see Ole Peter Grell, Andrew Cunningham with Jon Arrizabalaga (eds), *Health Care and Poor Relief in Counter-Reformation Europe* (London: Routledge, 1999). This work includes two important essays on health care within poor relief systems in early modern France: Colin Jones, 'Perspectives on poor relief, health care and the Counter-Reformation in France', pp. 215–39; Martin Dinges, 'Health care and poor relief in regional Southern France in the Counter-Reformation', pp. 240–79.

3 Jehanne de Tongrelouc, a merchant's widow, in 1536, Marie Tudert in 1587, Anne Ouvrat in 1596 all donated to the Hôtel-Dieu de Poitiers; Guillemette Leproust in 1586, Mlle de Mangouere and Jehanne Durand, a servant, in 1587 supported the

Hôpital des Champs. Marie Canuza donated her dowry worth 120 livres, in 1579 to fund municipal public health projects. See P. Rambaud, 'Le rôle des femmes au point de vue de l'assistance publique à Poitiers', *Mémoires de la Société des Antiquaires de l'Ouest*, 3 (1909), pp. xix–lii.
4 *Ibid.*, pp. xxi–xxii.
5 *Ibid.*, p. xxvii.
6 See for example the records for 1591, cited in *Ibid.*, p. xxxii.
7 *Ibid.*, p. xl.
8 *Ibid.*, p. xxxviii.
9 *Journal du Gabriel Breunot, conseiller au parlement de Dijon*, ed. J. Garnier, vol. 3, Dijon. 1864, pp. 91–6 cited in Françoise Hildesheimer, *Fléaux et société de la Grande Peste au choléra XIVe–XIXe siècle* (Paris: Hachette, 1993), p. 32.
10 Alison Klairmont Lingo, 'Women healers and the medical marketplace of sixteenth-century Lyon', *Dynamis*, 19 (1999), pp. 79–94.
11 Klairmont Lingo, *The Rise of Medical Practitioners*, p. 257.
12 Rambaud, 'Le rôle des femmes', p. xxxix.
13 Philip Benedict, 'French cities from the sixteenth century to the Revolution: an overview', in Philip Benedict (ed.), *Cities and Social Change in Early Modern France* (London: Unwin Hyman, 1989), p. 24, Table 1.2.
14 Jean-Pierre Gutton, 'Mutations et continuité (XVIe siècle)', Jean Imbert (ed.), *Histoire des hôpitaux en France* (Toulouse: Privat, 1982), p. 152.
15 Archives départementales (AD) d'Indre et Loire, H depot 4/88, fol. 117v.
16 R. Caisso, 'Les aumônes et l'hôpital des enfants exposés de Tours', *Bulletin de la société archéologique de Tours*, 39 (1981), p. 822.
17 Archives municipales de Tours (AMT), GG 4 document 25.
18 A. Giraudet, 'Histoire de l'ancien Hôtel-Dieu de Tours', *Bulletin de la société archéologique de Tours*, 2 (1871–73), pp. 152–3.
19 *Ibid.*, pp. 152–3.
20 See accounts in AMT, GG 20, Sanitas, 1563–99.
21 Caisso, 'Les aumônes et l'hôpital des enfants exposés de Tours', p. 839.
22 AMT, GG 3, Carton 2, document 839.
23 AD Indre et Loire, H dépôt 4/88, fol. 121r.
24 John Boswell, *The Kindness of Strangers: The Abandonment of Children in Western Europe From Late Antiquity to the Renaissance* (New York: Pantheon Books, 1988), p. 433.
25 Davis, 'Poor relief, humanism, and heresy', pp. 17–64.
26 J. Desnoyers, 'Recherches sur le sort des enfants trouvés en France, antérieurement à saint Vincent de Paul', *Bulletin du comité historique des monuments écrits de l'histoire de France*, 3 (1855–56) pp. 444–74; Léon Lallemand, *Histoire des enfants abandonés et délaissés: études sur la protection de l'enfance aux diverses époques de la civilisation* (Paris: A. Picard, 1885); A. Dupoux, *Sur les pas de Monsieur Vincent. Trois cents ans d'histoire parisienne de l'enfance abandonnée* (Paris: Revue de l'Assistance publique à Paris, 1958).
27 The collection of papers in *Enfance abandonnée et société en Europe XIVe–XXe siècles* (Rome, 30–31 janvier, 1987) (Rome: Ecole française de Rome, 1991) provides excellent comparative studies, though most are for later periods than the sixteenth century. For some comparative studies of welfare arrangements generally, see Peregrine

Hordern and Richard Smith (eds), *The Locus of Care: Families, Communities, Institutions and the Provision of Welfare since Antiquity* (London: Routledge, 1998).

28 B.-B. Remâcle, *Des hospices des enfans trouvés en Europe, et principalement en France* (Paris: Treuttel et Wurtz, 1838), p. 34. The Saint-Esprit hospital in Paris later changed its status in the fifteenth century to care only for legitimate children, not foundlings.

29 *Recueil des ordonnances du Louvre* vol. 6, p. 430 in J. M. de Gerando, *De la bienfaisance publique*, vol. 2 (Paris: Jules Renouard, 1839), p. 88.

30 Remâcle, *Des hospices des enfans trouvés*, p. 45.

31 *Ibid.*, p. 47.

32 *Ibid.*, p. 46.

33 Leah L. Otis, 'Municipal wet nurses in fifteenth-century Montpellier', in Barbara A. Hanawalt (ed.), *Women and Work in Preindustrial Europe* (Bloomington: Indiana University Press, 1986), pp. 83–93.

34 M. de la Fons de Mélicocq, 'Dépenses faites par la ville de Lille pour les enfants trouvés', *Bulletin du comité historique des monuments écrits de l'histoire de France*, 3 (1855–56), pp. 475–80.

35 See Annie Saulnier, 'De l'enfant à l'hôpital à l'hôpital pour enfants. Tentative d'analyse de l'élaboration d'une adaptation spécifique de l'hospitalisation pour l'enfant au tournant des XVe et XVIe siècles', *Annales de démographie historique* (1994), pp. 293–302.

36 AMT GG 3 Cartons 1 and 2 (1580–82) contain 140 cases, GG 4 Carton 1 (1582–83) 61, GG 4 Carton 2 (1585–86) 77, GG 2 (1586–87) 41, and GG 5 Carton 1 (1590–92) 57 cases.

37 1580–81 (17 new children added), 1581–82 (13), 1582–83 (5), 1585–86 (26), 1586–87 (19), 1590–91 (24), 1591–92 (14).

38 In 1590, 260 sols per year and 1592, 280 sols per year. AMT GG 5 Carton 1, documents 453 and 455.

39 An observation made also by Otis for the accounts at Montpellier.

40 See also Marie-Madeleine Fontaine, 'L'alimentation du jeune enfant au XVIe siècle', in Jean-Claude Margolin and Robert Sauzet (eds), *Pratiques et discours alimentaires à la Renaissance: Actes du colloque de Tours de mars 1979*, CESR (Paris: Maisonneuve et Larose, 1982).

41 AMT, GG 4 Carton 2 54–55, GG 2 Receptes et Despences de St Jean Baptiste 1586–87, GG 5 Carton 1 353.

42 François: AMT, GG 3 Carton 2 543–8, GG 4 Carton 1 261–4, GG 4 Carton 2 153–4, GG 2 Receptes et Despences de St Jean Baptiste 1586–87; Marin Regnault: AMT, GG 4 Carton 2 76–7, GG 4 Carton 2 154; Jacquine: AMT, GG 4 Carton 2 154; Anthoine: AMT, GG 5 Carton 1 266–72.

43 Blaise: AMT, GG 3 Carton 2 606–613, GG 4 Carton 1 183–87 and Denyse: AMT, GG 3 Carton 2 614–21.

44 AMT, GG 3, document 812.

45 AMT, GG 3, documents 849 and 850.

46 Naomi J. Miller, 'Mothering others: caregiving as spectrum and spectacle in the early modern period', in Miller and Naomi Yavneh (eds), *Maternal Measures: Figuring Caregiving in the Early Modern Period* (Aldershot: Ashgate, 2000), pp. 18–19.

47 AD Indre et Loire, H dépôt 4/218, and AMT, GG 4, documents 179 to 187.

48 AMT, GG 4 Carton 2, documents 76–7, GG 4 Carton 2, document 154.
49 See statements elsewhere in this chapter and notes by Boswell, Isabelle Robin and Agnès Walch as examples.
50 Luke Demaitre, 'The idea of childhood and child care in medical writings of the Middle Ages', *Journal of Psychohistory*, 4:4 (1977), pp. 461–90, p. 463. Philippe Ariès's contention that childhood did not exist as a concept does not appear to be supported by the distinct paediatric and child-rearing literature produced in the period. See his *Centuries of Childhood*, trans. R. Baldick (London: Jonathan Cape, 1962), pp. 128–33.
51 Demaitre, 'The idea of childhood and child care', p. 483.
52 Jean Roussel, Tours.
53 For studies of medical paediatric texts, see Evelyne Berriot-Salvadore, 'Corps humain ou corps humains: homme, femme, enfant dans la médecine de la Renaissance', Jean Céard, Marie-Madeleine Fontaine and Jean-Claude Margolin (eds), *Le Corps à la Renaissance: Actes du XXXe colloque de Tours, 1987* (Paris: Amateurs de Livres, 1990); Fontaine, 'L'alimentation du jeune enfant au XVIe siècle'. For childrearing texts, see Susan Broomhall, 'Savoir féminin puériculteur: *Le Verger fertile des Vertus* des Mesdames du Verger', *Mots Pluriels*, 11 (1999). Available on-line: www.arts.uwa.edu.au/MotsPluriels/MP1199sb.html.
54 Fontaine, 'L'alimentation du jeune enfant au XVIe siècle', p. 58.
55 Livre 2, p. 29, cited in Berriot-Salvadore, 'Corps humain ou corps humains', p. 444.
56 Fontaine, 'L'alimentation du jeune enfant au XVIe siècle', p. 59.
57 See particularly Véronique Demars-Sion, 'Illégitimité et abandon d'enfant: la position des provinces du Nord (XVIe–XVIIIe)', *Revue du Nord*, 65:258 (1983), pp. 481–506.
58 H Supplement 169, B 53 liasse, p. 48–9 in *Inventaire sommaire des archives hospitalieres: hospices de Sillé-Le-Guillaume*, Archives départementales de Sarthe, ed. J. L'Hermitte (Le Mans: Monnoyer, 1931), p. 63.
59 For a more detailed account of Parisian children's establishments, see Saulnier, 'De l'enfant à l'hôpital à l'hôpital pour enfants', pp. 293–302. Jacques Depauw's article provides an overview of welfare organisations at the end of the century: 'L'assistance à Paris à la fin du XVIe siècle', *Bulletin de la société française d'histoire des hôpitaux*, 59 (1989), pp. 10–24.
60 Joseph Berthelé, 'La vie intérieure d'un hospice du XIV au XVIe siècle: l'hôpital du Saint-Esprit en Grève à Paris', *Revue de l'hôpital et l'aide sociale à Paris* (1961), as cited in Kristen Elizabeth Gager, *Blood Ties and Fictive Ties: Adoption and Family Life in Early Modern France* (Princeton: Princeton University Press, 1996), p. 106.
61 Lallemand, *Histoire des enfants abandonés et délaissés*, p. 121.
62 'Fonds de l'Hôpital des Enfants Rouges, information de Pierre Carrel sur le sort des enfants à l'Hôtel-Dieu', 1531, fol. 10r, cited in Gager, *Blood Ties and Fictive Ties*, p. 108.
63 'Fonds de l'Hopital des Enfants Rouges', cited in Dupoux, *Sur les pas de Monsieur Vincent*, pp. 20–1.
64 Gager, *Blood Ties and Fictive Ties*, p. 110.
65 Ibid., p. 110.
66 Lallemand, *Histoire des enfants abandonés et délaissés*, p. 132.

67 Louis François Benoiston de Châteauneuf, *Considerations sur les enfans trouvés dans les principaux états de l'Europe* (Paris: Martinet, 1824), p. ix.
68 Lallemand, *Histoire des enfants abandonés et délaissés*, p. 131.
69 *Documents concernant les pauvres de Rouen*, ed. G. Panel, vol. 1: *1224 to 1630* (Paris: Picard, 1917), pp. 34–5.
70 *Ibid.*, p. 99.
71 Demars-Sion, 'Illégitimité et abandon d'enfant', p. 496.
72 AMT, GG 2, Carton 2, Receptes et Despences, 1586–7, viiixxii v–r.
73 Fons de Mélicocq, 'Dépenses faites par la ville de Lille pour les enfants trouvés', pp. 475–6.
74 *Ibid.*, p. 475.
75 *Ibid.*, p. 475.
76 *Ibid.*, p. 475.
77 *Ibid.*, p. 476.
78 For a comparative study of child-care organisation in Paris, see Gager, 'Parisian charity hospices and the care of orphans and foundlings', in *Blood Ties and Fictive Ties*, pp. 105–23.
79 Pierre Huard and Robert Laplane, *Histoire illustrée de la puériculture: aspects diététiques, socio-culturels et ethnologique* (Paris: Les Editions Roger Dacosta, 1979), pp. 70–1.
80 Rebecca W. Bushnell, 'Cultivating the mind', *A Culture of Teaching: Early Modern Humanism in Theory and Practice* (Ithaca: Cornell University Press, 1996), pp. 73–116.
81 AMT, GG3, Carton 2, document 507.
82 AMT, GG 4 Carton 1, document 13, fol. 7v.
83 AMT, GG 5, Carton 1, document 244.
84 AMT, GG 4, Carton 1, document 165.
85 This appears a consistent if uncommon feature, documented in the accounts of several child-care organisations such as those at Marseille, Montpellier and Tours.
86 Some mothers who were sick or working away from the town asked for permission to have their child placed in La Madeleine.
87 AMT, GG 4, Carton 1, document 25.
88 AMT, GG 4, Carton 1, 14, document 8v.
89 AMT, GG4, Carton 1, documents 8v–10v.
90 See accounts for 1582–83, AMT, GG 4 Carton 1, document 14.
91 AMT, GG 4 Carton 1, documents 10–13.
92 AMT, GG 4 Carton 1, document 14.
93 Davis, 'Poor relief, humanism, and heresy', pp 43–5.
94 AMT, GG 3 Carton 2, document 807.
95 See for example Marc de Fortia, Conseiller du Roy, trésorier général de France, who left 100 écus to the hospital in 1583. AMT, GG 4 Carton 1, document 349.
96 Boswell, *The Kindness of Strangers*, p. 433.
97 Archives hospitalières d'Orleans, I E 1 fol. 2 and 84 in Pierre Bouvier, *Etude sur l'Hôtel-Dieu d'Orléans au moyen-âge et au XVIe siècle* (Orléans: Paul Pigelet, 1914), p. 88.
98 Bouvier, *Etude sur l'Hôtel-Dieu d'Orléans au moyen-âge et au XVIe siècle*, p. 58.

99 AD du Calvados, c. 6824, *Arrêt des grands jours tenus à Bayeux* 1540, in François Langlois, 'Les enfants abandonnés à Caen, 1661–1820', *Histoire, économie, et société*, 6:3 (1987), pp. 307–28, pp. 307–8.
100 *Documents concernant les pauvres de Rouen*, vol. 1: *1224 to 1630*, pp. 34–5.
101 I have found the following formulations and discussion of the language, practice and knowledge of caregiving useful. Hilary Graham, 'Providers, negotiators and mediators: women as the hidden carers', in Ellen Lewin and Virginia Olsen (eds), *Women, Health and Healing: Toward a New Perspective* (New York: Tavistock, 1985); Hilary Rose, 'Women's work: women's knowledge', in Juliet Mitchell and Ann Oakley (eds), *What is Feminism?* (Oxford: Basil Blackwell, 1986), pp. 161–83; Margaret A. Perkinson, 'Socialization to the family caregiving role within a continuing care retirement community', *Medical Anthropology*, 16 (1995), pp. 249–67.
102 Miller and Yavneh (eds), *Maternal Measures*. For studies of women as mothers, see Jacques Gélis, *L'Arbre et le fruit: la naissance dans l'occident moderne XVIe–XIXe siècles* (Paris: Fayard, 1984); Valerie Fildes (ed.), *Women as Mothers in Pre-Industrial England: Essays in Memory of Dorothy McLaren* (London: Routledge, 1990); Jean-Louis Flandrin, *Families in Former Times: Kinship, Household and Sexuality*, trans. R. Southern (Cambridge: Cambridge University Press, 1979). Another useful collection of essays contains studies of both literary and historical constructions of medieval mothering: John Carmi Parsons and Bonnie Wheeler (eds), *Medieval Mothering* (New York: Garland, 1996). For wetnursing, infant feeding and babycare generally, see V. A. Fildes, *Wet Nursing: A History from Antiquity to the Present* (Oxford: Blackwell, 1988); George Sussman, *Selling Mother's Milk: The Wet-Nursing Business in France, 1715–1914* (Urbana: University of Illinois Press, 1982); Diana Dick, *Yesterday's Babies: A History of Babycare* (London: Bodley Head 1987), and V. A. Fildes, *Breasts, Bottles and Babies: A History of Infant Feeding* (Edinburgh: Edinburgh University Press, 1986).
103 Arch AP 'Fonds de l'Hopital des Enfants-Rouges', cited in Gager, *Blood Ties and Fictive Ties*, pp. 20–1.
104 Gager, *Blood Ties and Fictive Ties*, p. 21.
105 *Ibid.*, p. 21.
106 *Ibid.*, p. 21.
107 Further details of this report can be found in Saulnier, 'De l'enfant à l'hôpital à l'hôpital pour enfants', pp. 297–9.
108 See for example, those who cast the sixteenth century as a period when children suffered and died in massive numbers at the hands of unprofessional carers with little or no institutional organisation before the innovations, particularly under St Vincent de Paul, of the seventeenth and eighteenth centuries. Brian Pullan stated, for example, that the major foundling establishment in Paris was 'taken over and somewhat humanized in the mid seventeenth century by Vincent de Paul and his auxiliaries': Pullan, *Orphans and Foundlings in Early Modern Europe* (Berkshire: University of Reading, 1989), pp. 12–13. Also, Isabelle Robin and Agnès Walch depict the background to their study of foundlings in Paris in the seventeenth and eighteenth centuries in a similar way: 'For a long time, society seemed insensible to these pitiable destinies. Threatened by hunger, cold, attacked by wandering animals, these children, mostly newborns (90% less than a year old) were condemned to die... The

majority died in the cold at night. Strangely, this Christian society seems to accept the tragic and sacrilegious death of these non-baptised children. The institutional assistance remained insufficient, if not non-existent. The intervention of Saint Vincent de Paul was decisive.' Isabelle Robin and Agnès Walch, 'Géographie des enfants trouvés de Paris aux XVIIe et XVIIIs siècles', *Histoire, économie, et société* 6:3 (1987), pp. 343–60, p. 344.

109 Davis, 'Scandale à l'Hôtel-Dieu de Lyon (1537–1543)', *La France d'Ancien Régime: études réunies en l'honneur de Pierre Goubert*, vol. 1 (Toulouse: Privat, 1984), p. 178.

110 Statuts et réglemens primitifs de l'Aumône Générale de Lyon, instituée en 1533, in A. Croze, 'Etudes et documents pour servir à l'histoire hospitalière lyonnaise', *Revue d'histoire de Lyon* (1915), p. 25.

111 Lallemand, *Histoire des enfants abandonés et délaissés*, p. 131.

112 *Ibid.*, p. 132.

113 Dupoux, *Sur les pas de Monsieur Vincent*, p. 27.

114 *Ibid.*, p. 27.

115 Fossoyeux, 'L'assistance parisienne au milieu du XVIe siècle', p. 102.

116 Marie Regnauld, 1572, Jeanne Blanc, 1573, Marie Laborde, 1584, Jacquette Bernard, 1601. Rambaud, 'Le rôle des femmes au point de vue de l'assistance publique à Poitiers', p. xxxix.

117 For a comparative study in England, Margaret Pelling, 'Child health as a social value in early modern England', *Social History of Medicine*, 1:2 (1988), pp. 135–64.

7

The world of the court: women serving the royal family

THE PREVIOUS CHAPTER has already discussed the development of child-care literature as a medical field in the sixteenth century, and examined how that affected women employed to care for poor or foundling children by municipal charity organisations. This chapter will examine how these developments affected the status, employment and authority of child carers at the royal court.

Women numbered among the practitioners providing medical services to the royal family. Louis XI had employed such women in his medical retinue, though usually in the least glamorous of roles. Guillemette du Luys, a surgeoness, was paid to 'steam him . . . in the lower parts'.[1] However, most commonly, women were employed in services related to what we would term obstetrical and paediatric medicine. How did women as child carers interact with the royal family and guild-trained medical retinue at court, primarily as wetnurses and governesses of the royal children?[2]

Child-care providers at court

Child care was bound to cause conflict, particularly at the royal level. There were many vested interests in the survival of the children and potential heirs. Personnel in the children's household negotiated who had the authority to decide on a child's diet, its first schooling, the rights to discipline as well as the maintenance of a child's health and appropriate treatment during illness. The key female participants in these debates were wetnurses, dry-nurses and governesses, although on some occasions midwives played an extended role after the delivery of the child. These women interacted frequently with physicians, surgeons, apothecaries and tutors as members of the child's retinue.

At the royal level, the governess was a particularly powerful figure. She supervised household staff, including the wet- and dry-nurses, and was responsible for their care of the child as well as her own. While the wetnurse provided the physical nourishment to the child, it was the governess who supervised (and often helped select) the wetnurses, she who supervised the child's health and advised on suitable remedies as well as selecting the child's diet and appropriate exercise. The governess also had an important didactic role, teaching the child to speak, and interact in society, and also beginning its moral education. A governess had to learn to balance the advice that stemmed from parents, physicians and others about the child's diet, all of whom had different interests and investments in the child. Kings did not disdain from entering this debate. For example, Madame de La Bellière, governess of the children of Louis XI's legitimated sister, Marie de Valois, had to carefully negotiate how to accept the advice of Louis XI on his nieces' diet. In July 1477, he wrote:

> I am not a physician, but it seems to me that one must not prevent them from drinking ... if they are thirsty, but one must put a lot of water in their wine and only let them drink the little wines of the Touraine, do not give them dishes which are too salty, nor spiced meats, but boiled and well cooked meats; do not give them fruit except well matured grapes. I remember that *surins* [a type of grape] are good but there are some which are very bad and produce colic.[3]

Like all royal employees, female child-care providers relied on favour from their royal patrons, and consideration needs to be given to this motivation in understanding their activities. Moreover, a governess's relationship, and status, with university-trained medical staff was often ambiguous and as will be seen, contested. Many of the duties of a governess clearly crossed over with those of court physicians, tutors and theologians appointed to assist in the child's upbringing, as well the royal parents themselves and the evidence to be studied here testifies to the difficulties in naming any one participant as the specialist in child care at the court.

Despite their superior position in the child-care hierarchy at court, the work of the governess in the early modern period has not received much attention from modern historians, even less than wetnurses or midwives. Madeleine Foisil's careful editing and analysis of the diaries of Jean Héroard concerning the child Louis XIII has greatly increased the possibilities for understanding court child-care practices in the early seventeenth century. However, her focus on the young prince and his physician leaves the role of the dauphin's governess and wetnurses largely still to be explored.[4] The correspondence produced by monarchs, queens and attendants can provide abundant material with which to analyse child-care authority in the sixteenth century. Reading this correspondence reveals the development of distinct tensions about medical epistemologies and practices among the contributors to royal child care.

Anne of Brittany, Madame du Bouchage and the physicians of the royal children

When Anne of Brittany gave birth to her first child, the Dauphin Charles-Orlando, in October 1492, she was just fifteen. Charles-Orlando was left at the château of Amboise when both Anne and Charles VIII travelled to Lyon, from where the king departed for his Italian campaign. The King himself produced some 'Instructions of the order which is to be given at Amboise for the care and safekeeping of Monseigneur the Dauphin', in August 1494, which were given to the governors of the Dauphin's household. It laid out measures to maintain the infant's health, named one hundred Scots guards to protect the château and town, specified quarantine procedures if disease should arise in the town and commanded the governors to send news of the Dauphin at least every fortnight.[5] In August of the following year, there was news from Amboise that cases of smallpox had broken out. The king sent his physicians to the town to ascertain the degree of danger to the Dauphin. Their reply to Anne acknowledged that there had been indeed been smallpox in Amboise, but that the incidence was decreasing and they expected the spate soon over. Furthermore, the guards had so well prevented the communication of citizens from the town to the château that they did not believe the dauphin needed to be removed elsewhere.[6] However, by December of that year, the dauphin died, not yet four. His royal parents were devastated.[7]

This incident appears to have shaped much of Anne's future belief in, and interaction with, the royal physicians on matters of child care. For her next children, Anne referred more to popular custom and religious beliefs than to her physicians. She surrounded her child with wetnurses from the countryside and from her native Brittany, whose milk might fortify her child. The milk of country women was commonly believed to be of better quality than from those in towns. Entries from her accounts record several women whose milk was tested in the search for a suitable wetnurse:

> To Jehan Ornuau staying at the Lion d'Angers, 20 l.t. in recompense for the expenses that he made to bring his wife who was a nurse with her little child to the lady [Anne] at Plessis les Tours, to show her milk; and also to help her to return and take the woman back to her house. 11 August 1496.
>
> To Thomas Marin, horsemen of the stables of the King, living at Le Mans, 20 l.t. in recompense for the great expense that he made in bringing his wife and her small child to the lady at Plessis, for the reason stated above; and also to return her to her house. 12 August 1496.[8]

Anne's inventories also reveal that she kept amulets and other religious icons which she sent to her children's wetnurses in order to protect the health of both nurse and child. The inventory records that she sent rosary beads to the nurse as well as more unusual gifts. She sent the nurse of her daughter Anne in 1498 a coin wrapped in paper, black wax wrapped in a golden purse and tied with a black cord, and six lizard's tongues 'one large, two average and three little ones'.[9] However, all three of her subsequent children with Charles VIII were to die young, Charles less than a year later in 1497, François also in 1497, and Anne 1498. Their grave can still be seen in a single tomb in Tours' St Gatien cathedral.

From her marriage to Louis XII, Anne bore four more children: Claude born in 1499, Renée born in 1510 and two sons in 1503 and 1512 who did not survive. For more than ten years (before the birth of Renée in 1510), Anne's daughter Claude was her only surviving child, and Anne watched over her health and welfare with great care. When circumstances forced her to be parted from Claude, Anne maintained a regular correspondence with Claude's governess, Madame du Bouchage. Anne's distrust of physicians was such that she explicitly advised Du Bouchage on several occasions to keep her child away from their influence. For example, in June 1501, Anne wrote to Du Bouchage, encouraging the governess to inform her of any ailments in her child or wetnurse so that she could advise on how to proceed.

> I was very happy to hear the news you sent of my daughter, and the small trouble that she has had which is only from her baby teeth, just as you've written. And I think that if the nurse was a bit sick that you would not hide it from me, no more than [any illness] of my daughter.[10]

Anne was sceptical about the logic of the physicians' diagnosis and their subsequent treatment, and privileged the child-care experience of her governess:

> I was troubled by the letter that master Albert sent me, that he found my daughter a bit hot; and that if it was up to him, he would give some cassia to the wetnurse. I find it strange to give medication if he finds the nurse affected or she has a fever; so, my friend, I pray that you will send straightaway for Catherine [the nurse], and see from her milk if she has a fever, or if there is some alteration. And tell her to check her [Claude] at night if she is hot or in some way different from usual.[11]

However, although Anne criticised the practices of the royal physician Albert Dupuy, she was willing to send another of the medical retinue, Gabriel Miron, to advise Du Bouchage as to an appropriate regime for the wetnurses:

> Don't change her food, for I will send for Master Millon [Miron] who will tell you what is good to do. He left Saturday and I pray you hurry a courier to me straightaway and write in detail of my daughter and her nurse.[12]

Anne held an ambiguous attitude to the hierarchy of medical practitioners. She placed value on her own opinions as well as those of her governess, and did not bestow a particular weight on the opinions of physicians as to breastfeeding and child care.

When in 1505 Claude fell ill with a fever, the physicians wrote to Anne that it was beyond their help and that they expected Claude to die. She recovered. Anne wrote in her correspondence to Du Bouchage that the physicians were not to treat her child again. From Grenoble, Anne advised Du Bouchage:

> I have received the letter that you wrote to me and the good news of my daughter, about which I am pleased. I pray you to continue always to let me know about her, and tell master Albert, between you and him, that I no longer want him to come near my daughter, because of his eyes, and also that she will have nothing more to do with physicians, and you must keep watch over her always, as you have done until now.[13]

In subsequent letters written in the weeks following the illness, Anne continued to ask for news of her daughter's improvement and reiterated her demands that Du Bouchage protect her from physicians.[14] Yet although Anne did not accept the physicians' superiority in infantile health, and seemingly preferred her own opinion and that of her governess, she did not reject their medical competence generally. The same four physicians who figured in the retinue advising on the Dauphin's illness in 1492 – Bernard Chaussade, Olivier Laurent, Gabriel Miron and

Albert Dupuy – remained in the royal service. She was generous to the royal physicians, giving them gifts and supporting their children's education. Anne distinguished between the appropriate source of advice for different medical domains: and paediatric medicine was not, to her mind, the expertise of physicians.

However, physicians did believe that they could be expert in child care. The very same Gabriel Miron who cared for Anne's children, published one of the first child-care texts produced by a French physician. His *Pedenemicon*, published in Tours in 1544, drew from the learned texts of the classical past, his more recent predecessors in the university medical tradition as well as his own experiences as physician both to Anne's children and those of her daughter Claude, who married Francis I. This text, now extremely rare and incomplete, recently analysed by Janine Bertier, was clearly an important precursor to the better-known child-care manual by Vallambert. Bertier demonstrates how Vallambert's breakdown of chapters, citation of authors and use of anecdote and scholastic presentation all betray his debt to Miron.[15]

The fragments of Miron's text allow us to perceive the complexities of authority in early modern child care. Miron was firm that the role of the physicians in child care was purely the maintenance of the child's health and treatment during illness: he followed the creed that a physician should occupy himself with 'humours and not with manners'.[16] But the boundaries of what constituted a medical interest in child care were unclear. Bertier points out that much of the remaining text does not concern explicitly medical issues. Miron relates his discussions with the other royal physician Guillaume Cop about an appropriate sleeping regime for the children.[17] Who held authority in the everyday maintenance of a child's health was particularly difficult to determine. Miron discusses whether, how often and at what age a child should be moved among royal residences, as well as the daily organisation of the lives of the royal children.[18] He debated the value of corporal punishment: Anne found it opportune, but later François I and his mother Louise de Savoie banned its use on the royal children.[19] Miron acknowledges Anne's role as an important interlocutor in the child-care debate. He discussed her opinions, such as her preference for cow's milk rather than goat's in preparing pap and gruel for her second daughter Renée.[20] It is difficult to know, however, in what light Miron accredits her opinions, for Anne was a queen, a highly learned woman in her own right, as well as a mother. In Miron's later service to the royal children, it was not their mother Claude who stipulated care of the royal children, but her husband and his mother who were cited in the debate over corporal punishment.

In this scenario, Anne of Brittany held a personal authority in child care that developed as a result not only of her power as a reigning duchess in her own right and respect as a royal consort, but also as an experienced mother. Whereas in 1492, as a fifteen-year-old, she accepted the advice of physicians about her first child, Charles-Orlando, both her later correspondence and Miron's evidence show her to be an active participant in the maintenance of children's health and treatment during illness. Anne bestowed authority on the experience of her governess, even in times of her children's illnesses. Yet physicians were increasingly extending their own authority in this field, as the publication of Miron's Latin manual demonstrates. And while the text was ostensibly a medical treatise, it is clear that the royal physicians did not disdain from entering debates about the everyday activities of the royal children, a role which was more commonly understood by contemporaries to be that of the governess.

Diane de Poitiers, Catherine de Medici and Madame de Humières

The appointment of Françoise de Contay, Madame de Humières, to the royal children of Henri II and Catherine de Medici came through her husband. Jean de Humières had a long history as governor of the royal children. François I first appointed him to the care of the dauphin in 1525, then to the care of all three of his sons. When the dauphin died, Humières became chamberlain to the future Henri II. Then in 1546, Humières and his wife became governors of Henri's children.[21] The Humières couple, who married in 1507, had 18 children together. It was clear that from the beginning of Jean de Humières's appointment that Madame de Humières's support was an essential component of his selection. Catherine de Medici wrote in late 1546 to him, saying 'I am happy that madame de Humières has arrived there for the comfort that she will bring to the governance of my children'.[22] Her knowledge of child rearing by experience was valued by the royal couple. This was all the more evident when Humières died in 1550. His wife assumed his duties and continued her care over the royal children, now entering into correspondence with the royal couple herself.

Patronage was key to the dynamics of child care in the 1550s. The influence of Diane de Poitiers, the king's mistress, on the upbringing of the children of Henri II and Catherine de Medici was well known even to contemporaries. In 1559, Guillaume Chrestian, the royal children's physician, dedicated his translation of *Livre de la generation*, by

Jacques du Bois, to her, not the children's mother Catherine de Medici, saying 'you have care not only for the conception and birth of them, but also that they are duly fed by vigorous, healthy, well complexioned wetnurses, selected among several other women chosen, with wise and prudent governesses'.[23] Diane de Poitiers was the Humières family's greatest patron and protector. But the relationship was mutual: one of Diane's spheres of influence stemmed from her role in the care of the royal children. She often advised Henri on a particular course of action, as a mother herself. Both Diane and Henri's independent letters to the Humières's couple frequently echo a common perspective. The Humières nurtured their source of favour and Diane was frequently the first to receive knowledge of the children's health and illnesses. Diane de Poitiers's correspondence with their governess, Madame de Humières, clearly demonstrates her predominance in the royal household and the delicate balance of power and authority among the various practitioners.

In response, Catherine de Medici tried to circumvent her relatively powerless position in regard to the royal children's care by appointing her own allies to the royal household. The Medici and Gondi family alliance was well established, and she chose Marie-Catherine de Pierrevive, wife of Antoine Gondi, known as Madame Duperon, to represent her in the royal children's household. However, she was not an equal to Madame de Humières: Henri placed Duperon under Humières's orders.[24] Catherine continued to have herself represented in the household. In 1550, she convinced Henri to support her selection for a vacant position, writing to Monsieur de Humières: 'to my request, the King has accorded the place that the late Fontaines held to the wife of mademoiselle de Dannemarie'. Anne Lemaye, dame de Dannemarie, had assisted Catherine in one of her pregnancies.[25] In general, though, comparison of Catherine and Diane's correspondence demonstrates the weakness of Catherine's authority in care of the royal children.

Governesses were responsible for overseeing the appointment of wetnurses. At the highest social level, in the royal family, the role of the nurse was of vital importance and thus chosen with great care. Even the king, Henri II, offered his advice on the subject: 'Above all you must check that she has fed more than one child and that her milk is good and certain.'[26] As in the days of Anne of Brittany, wetnurses were still chosen from rural backgrounds. Henry IV's wetnurse was not to be 'aged, thin & melancholy' but 'a young woman from the fields' given 'heavy meats according to her country fashion, above all forbid from her room the physician and apothecary'.[27] Nurses needed to be chosen with care because it was believed that psychological and moral characteristics could be passed to the child through the milk. Furthermore, by the middle of the century, it was important that the nurse's religious convictions were examined for the same reasons.

The position of a wetnurse was purely functional: they were considered as good as their milk. When the royal son, Monsieur d'Orléans, sickened at the breast in 1551, Diane de Poitiers wrote to Madame de Humières, offering remedies: 'if her milk has worsened, since I have seen her, it is because she has not lived as she was used to, and it seems to me that if she is made to drink cider or beer that it will refresh her a great deal and I am of the opinion to do this, I think that the physicians are of this opinion'.[28] Catherine was more pragmatic:

> I have seen what you've written about the nurse of my son d'Orléans, who, I think, is honest and well conditioned, but we do not have a problem with her competence and her virtues as we know that she is a good nurse... my son continues too often to be ill; so, madame de Humières, I pray that I hear no more about it and that she is changed, her milk is no better for all her prudence and wisdom, one sees that by experience, I do not want, for lack of acting promptly, some problem to occur from it.[29]

But Madame de Humières delayed the decision to change the wetnurse, opting to follow Diane's, rather than Catherine's, advice. Catherine showed her displeasure and a following letter demonstrated her frustration and anger over the conflicting opinions on the matter: 'I send back my physician to not move from there until a nurse is found, already I've written that a nurse should be found in place of the retained one, and that if my son does not do well with her, that she is made to serve, and I am stunned how what I sent has not been followed, such that from now on, I pray you do it, following what I have previously written to Madame du Peron.'[30] She introduced her physician into the household, privileging his medical knowledge over the opinion of Humières, as a way of promoting her own position.

But Catherine also showed sensitivity to the delicate position of nurses who came and went at the command of their milk. She allowed the defunct wetnurse to remain in her son's retinue and advised that none should treat her differently. Showing awareness for the infighting and jostling for position that might go on, she wrote at the end of May 1551 to Madame de Humières 'since my son d'Orléans has been better since they changed him to a new nurse, you can imagine the happiness I have about it... They must not... be unkind to the other nurse for what has happened... The King and I understand that the nurse who breastfed my son remains near him or to one of my girls, just as you advise is for the best'.³¹ When Diane wrote to Madame de Humières several days later, she had retrospectively adopted Catherine's position that the wetnurse should have been changed, and admonished Humières for her delay. 'I'm very happy... that Mons' d'Orléans is better for having changed nurse. It seems that the other should have been removed sooner, given that her milk was not good.'³² In this case, both governess and physicians were drawn into the power play between royal mother and mistress: they could not rely on royal favour with certainty, and played politics with the lives of the royal children at their own peril. When the first Monsieur d'Orléans died in 1550, the constable Anne de Montmorency had written a word of comfort and advice to Humières: 'I want to assure you that they know well the continual pain and care you took until his death; and since they know that madame Claude still looks awful, I am writing to the physicians that they take good care of her, for fear that some new accident should not befall her; for your part I pray you keep an eye on it!'³³

One of the most important functions that a governess could provide to the royal family was information about the children themselves. Royal children did not normally live on a daily basis within proximity to their parents but occupied a separate household complete with its own personnel. This gave members of the children's household a further duty to report on the children's health and progress to both parents. Catherine de Medici wrote on several occasions for new portraits of her children so that she could observe their development, as in this letter to Monsieur de Humières in 1548. 'I pray, Monsieur d'Humières, that you have all my children painted, but that it be from the other side that the painters are not accustomed to portray, and send me the paintings as soon as they are made.'³⁴

On several occasions in the correspondence of Catherine de Medici to her children's governess and physicians, however, one senses a clear sentiment of frustration at her distance from the situation. In 1551, she raised a threatening tone with Madame de Humières about the delays in receiving information and in following her advice, and was compelled to add to a letter written by her secretary, in her own hand: 'do not let it happen again as this time, having to write one thing so many times, when the King or I have written something to you, do it, or otherwise we will be not be content.'³⁵ This was not a one-off incident. Again in 1552 Catherine raised her concerns about the haphazard replies she received from Madame de Humières to her enquiries and addressed an even longer admonition on the subject.

> I advise you that in this I think you have understood nothing, ... it behoves you as a due of your charge to write to me particularly, and the others [in the retinue] only by a collective letter, in which you will observe in this place what until now you been accustomed to do, letting me know by the opportunities that arrive how my children are, and you will give me more pleasure than you could imagine, ... I received a letter from Rommanerie [a physician] with yours, which makes mention of another that he says to have written earlier, but it has not reached my hands.[36]

In this situation, the balance of power shifted. Here, Catherine begged for news of her children from her own employees.

News was a responsibility to be taken most seriously, particularly if the child fell ill and the royal parents did not first hear the news from the governess. Diane de Poitiers wrote to warn Madame de Humières of her attempts to smooth out one such occasion with the royal couple: 'madame Duperon wrote to me that madame [Elisabeth] is ill with measles and I advise you that the King has been stunned that you have not advised him of it, but I told him that it must have been that your letters were lost, so you would do well to make your excuses as best you can'.[37] Although in theory the royal couple held the power to dismiss a governess as they saw fit, in other instances it was they who were disempowered to govern the welfare of their own children. Physically isolated by distance and their advice delayed through correspondence, the royal couple, and in particular Catherine, were not always able to assert their authority over the treatment of their children. It was a situation that Catherine acknowledged in her letters, sometimes advising Madame de Humières to decide a course of action in consultation with the physicians: 'for you are on the spot to know better that I would what is needed'.[38]

One of the principal tasks of the governess was to keep the child in good health. On an everyday level, this was more her responsibility than that of the physicians, who were rather called upon to offer opinions in times of illness. Humières had the difficult task of receiving and acting upon a variety of sources of medical authority, including those of the royal physicians, of Diane and of the royal parents themselves. Catherine too sent advice such as on the issue of her daughter Claude's diet in 1548: 'as to what you gave written for the food of my daughter Claude, the King and I are of the opinion that she should be given panada [boiled bread and butter] rather than the other thing, for it is healthier than pap'.[39] In 1552, she observed, 'as to my son d'Angoulême's eating, I am of the opinion not to force him, for my children are more ill from being too fat than thin'.[40]

When Madame Elisabeth caught measles in 1547, Diane de Poitiers demanded that Humières 'send for mons^r Fernel and other physicians from Paris to give order that nothing serious happen' at the same time as she offered her own remedies: 'I am sending some unicorn for him to use as will be prescribed'.[41] Diane also stipulated to Madame de Humières where the children should be lodged for their best health: 'Seeing the illnesses which have arisen, they have decided to remove them from there and have them go to Ecouen, or to the houses. It seems to me that Monsr is never better than at Ecouen, you will check which of the two places is better for his health'.[42] Significantly, Diane offered little justification for why her opinions ought to be authoritative, perhaps tacitly claiming her experience in raising her own two daughters. Regardless of the efficacy of her advice, it is clear that her powerful position and influence over Henri II could override both the learned knowledge of the physicians and experience of the governesses, in whose appointments she had been instrumental.

Yet Diane also conferred authority upon Madame de Humières's own opinions and expected her to make her own decisions: 'madame Claude has been ill at night with her cough, about which we were all unhappy; however, it is an illness which is not at all dangerous, given that madame her elder sister has had it in this way. The Queen is writing to you her opinion ... I would rather trust in your opinion than the physicians, given especially the quantity of children you have had. So, madame my friend, see to the things which are necessary and do them'.[43] Madame de Humières's experience as the mother of eighteen children gave her authority in Diane's eyes. By contrast, Henri II's letters to Madame de Humières suggests that he placed more authority on the advice of the royal physicians, as this letter indicates: 'I am very happy that there was so little in the accident which happened to my daughter Claude, and of the hope that the physicians and surgeons who are close to her give that it might be remedied with as easy means as those they advise, which, to this reason, they will continue and will take care to have an eye on the matter and see to it so carefully that it is not necessary to use harsher remedies'.[44] Significantly, Henri's letter did not refer to Madame de Humières's opinion or her role in Claude's treatment.

However, tensions between vying medical practices and epistemologies could not always be balanced. In March 1552, Henri II was forced to send the following letter to Madame de Humières, at her request, specifically delineating the authority within the royal household:

> I have heard all that you have let me know by the Sieur de Contay, your son, on the two points that he addressed to me: that you claim to have charge and authority that I have given you in the household and towards my children, and to give you a response to this, you know well that as to what concerns the facts of health, diet and governance of the food of my children, it is more suitable that the physicians that I have near to them, the best and most experienced that I have, are believed in what they say and do about it, that no other can meddle in it and I have been thinking and meaning up to now that only you, and no one other than the physicians are answerable in this charge, nor equally to order on the matter of the distribution of *deniers* and verification of the expenses that are made in the house.[45]

Although he officially conferred authority on the royal physicians, Henri, in a rather confusing phrase, seems to exclude Humières from those who were to follow their advice. Henri saw both his physicians and governess as experienced, though presumably in different ways. His letter created the possibility for her to override the physicians' knowledge with her own advice, thereby making no progress in clarifying who was to have the final say.

The circumstances of royal child care during the reign of Henri II attest not so much to the conflict between governess and physicians in the royal retinue (although there were clearly some difficulties here), but rather to the effects of royal patronage on the position of all child-care providers. Both Diane and Catherine used child-care personnel to assert their own perspectives on the issue at hand, privileging women's experiential knowledge or the learned theory of physicians, as it best fitted their particular needs. In doing so, they assisted physicians to gain ground in child-care expertise and problematised the concept of maternal authority. For Diane assumed power largely as the king's mistress but publicly claimed her authority rested on her experience as a mother and older woman. Maternal authority was ambiguous: it also validated Humières's own claims against the textual knowledge of the physicians, yet Catherine, as the children's mother but weakest royal figure, was unable to establish herself as an authority in these child-care debates by using the same rhetoric.[46]

Marie de Medici, Madame de Montglat and Louise Bourgeois

One final case study of royal child care concerns the reign of Henri IV. Françoise de Longjoue, Madame de Montglat, was an experienced mother over fifty when she was appointed by Henri IV as the dauphin

Louis's governess in 1601. Louise Bourgeois, midwife to Marie de Medici, recalled in her published writings that Montglat was publicly recognised at the dauphin's birth as his primary carer. Once the baby was born, she wrote, 'I asked the King to whom it would please him that I give monsieur the Dauphin. He said to me: "To mademoiselle de Montglas, who will be his governess".'[47] She was required to survey the child's health and education, as well as supervise the wetnurses, and maintain the household, tasks that brought her into constant interaction with Héroard, Louis's personal physician.[48] The community at Saint Germain was not only that of the Dauphin Louis, but also comprised four of Henri's bastard children, as well as the additions of the other royal children.[49]

Similar problems of interaction between various medical epistemologies and practices occurred during the childhood of Louis XIII. However, unlike the cases examined above, conflicts did not generally concern the children's illnesses. The king, Henri IV, might still intervene to provide his own diagnosis on the children's sickness to Montglat: 'Mr Erouart says that it is nothing but a cold, for my part, I think it is measles',[50] but there is no evidence in correspondence or Héroard's diary that Montglat made any claims to such authority. Yet the exceptional journal of Louis's appointed physician, Jean de Héroard, reveals that there were tensions between governess and physician. The evidence of Héroard's journal suggests that he kept a close eye on every aspect of the child's daily health. Héroard demonstrates that the day-to-day running of the household of the royal children was not entirely the arena of the governess, but was a definite interest of the child's physician as well. The journal shows him to be concerned with (though by no means always the accepted authority on) the supervision of wetnurses, Montglat's day-to-day interactions with Louis, as well as corporal punishment.

One of the best documented cases of infant feeding trouble is that of the future Louis XIII. Héroard's diary documents a parade of nurses who came and went in the child's early infancy. By 19 October 1601, Louis had two nurses to supply his demand. 'Because of the lack of milk seen several times in his nurse by Monsieurs de La Riviere, du Laurens, Vide and I assembled by order of his Majesties, were resolved that Helin wife of Lemaire, the second nurse, would give milk to Monseigneur the Dauphin to help the first nurse.'[51] Héroard's account allows the governess no involvement in the choices made about wetnurses, despite the fact that she was primarily the one responsible for the smooth management of the child's personnel.

Wetnurses and staff came and went at the whim of monarchs and mistresses. By November 1601, 'The Queen does not want Madame Lemaire to give milk at all as Madame de Montglat says'. When problems persisted, 'For lack of milk, the nurse begs Madame de Montglat to have pity on her'.[52] By the end of December 1601 the King too intervened: 'Montglat shows a letter of the King of the 22 December 1601 ordering her to let Galand, wife of Mr Charles Butel, a barber surgeon in Paris, wetnurse, and to remove Catherine Hothman.'[53] Héroard marvelled at the machinations surrounding the wetnursing positions, but the evidence of his own account indicates that he did not hold the upper hand in matters of the child's feeding. By the end of January 1602 yet another wetnurse was sent away: 'Madame Lemaire his second wetnurse, ... retired for not having been agreeable to the Queen by the persuasion of some people who were close to Her Majesty. She was a very honest woman, very kind and with lots of very good milk, and thanks be to God that Monseigneur the Dauphin was fed by her in place of the first, it was better for his health, ... God pardon those who have been the cause of this'.[54] Court politics played a key role in appointments to the royal nursery, which neither governess nor physicians could control directly, even if they too were involved in manipulating such decisions for their own ends.

But the role of the governess was by no means only to maintain the child in good health. She was also expected to teach the child his first lessons, morality and good manners. Henri IV assigned Madame de Montglat educational control of the Dauphin until seven, the age of reason. Héroard also depicts moments in the nursery when his nurses participated in the daily instruction of the child. On 13 March 1605, he wrote that Louis '[a]muses himself with a book of figures of the Bible. His nurse names the figures and letters, then he says to her: "Maman doundoun ask me". He then names the letters, knows them all, to show her that he knows them.'[55]

Montglat was also responsible for moral discipline and it was a challenging duty for which she was given the authority to discipline the child physically. October 1607 provides one such incident: 'Asks to drink; Madame reproaches him for not saying please, responds that he doesn't want to say it. Madame de Montglat tells him that he must. Dauphin: "That's only for little children", refusing, must be birched for it, says it finally after telling Madame de Montglat that she is wicked'.[56] It must be said that the evidence of Héroard's diary suggests that Monglat threatened the rod much more often than she ever used it. Like all children, Louis regularly tested the boundaries of her authority. In 1605, at the age of four, he was determined to ascertain the source of her power over him. Héroard recorded the following incident. 'At eight o'clock, rose; ... "Come here. Come get dressed". Dauphin: "No I won't". Montglat: "Well, I will whip you". Dauphin: "It's not up to you to whip me". Montglat: "Oh yes it is, it is up to me". Dauphin: "You haven't the power to whip me". Montglat: "Oh yes I have". Dauphin: "Who gave it to you?" Montglat: "It was papa..."'[57]

Montglat was the subject of criticism at court. The monarchs outwardly displayed trust in her management, as Marie de Medici wrote to her: 'I will not listen to the rumours which some would say. I rely entirely upon you'.[58] But Marie was also concerned that Montglat should not enforce her right to whip too harshly and instructed her secretary, Jean Phélypeaux, to write to Héroard suggesting that he keep an eye on her behaviour. 'Her Majesty writes to the lady Montglat that she approves that she whips him but that it be with circumspection not anger and that it should not do him any illness. Her Majesty being a bit angered by this news [the rumours] has asked me to write to you particularly... if you judge appropriate that they whip him or how you would like him to be treated in this regard.'[59] Henri IV, in contrast, wrote complaining that she did not employ enough corporal punishment. In 1607, he wrote admonishing her: 'I have a complaint about you, for what you have written to me that you haven't whipped my son; for I want and command you to whip him each time that he is obstinate or does something bad, knowing well for myself that there is nothing in the world that gives him more profit than that; ... for at his age, I was whipped well. That's why I want you to do it and that you make him understand.'[60] There were always regulators on Montglat's behaviour. She never acted in isolation but was always surrounded by witnesses to every action – as Héroard's diary demonstrates.

There were also tensions between Monglat and her successor Gilles de Souvré, Louis's tutor from the age of seven to thirteen.[61] When in 1610, several years after Louis had left the children's household and Monglat's care, it is clear that she wished to retain some control over the child. Héroard records an incident where the former and current teachers measured their respective authorities over the child. 'Madame de Montglat and Mr de Souvré talked together. Madame de Montglat goes to say: "I can say that Monsieur the Dauphin is mine, the King gave him to me at his birth, saying: 'Madame de Montglat here is my son whom I give to you, take him'". Souvré: "He was yours for a time, now he is mine". Dauphin: "And I hope one day that I'll belong to me", coldly, without looking up.'[62]

Although the physician Héroard suggested in his text that he played an increasing role in the daily care of Louis, certain decisions that had clear impact on his health and wellbeing rested almost entirely on the authority of women. It was the governess in conjunction with Marie de Medici's midwife, Louise Bourgeois, who decided when the royal children would be weaned. When discussion of the matter was raised, Marie sought advice from Montglat and Bourgeois.[63] Considering the stunning array of information that Héroard provides on other issues, it is surprising just how little detail he provides about the dauphin's or other children's weaning or the decision surrounding it. On the 6 November 1602, he simply writes for Louis: 'At eight fifteen, rose. At eight thirty, is weaned.'[64] For the Dauphin's sister, Héroard recorded in 1605, 'Madame weaned, in the morning at eight o'clock. She feeds, then her nurse says to her: "Madame, you will suckle no more, you must be weaned". She says straightaway, kissing the nurse's breasts: "Adieu breast, I will suckle no more". And she hasn't wanted to suckle since.'[65]

From the depiction of the royal nursery that was presented in Héroard's journal, Madame de Montglat's medical power as a governess appeared significantly less than her predecessors such as Madame du Bouchage, who was asked by her royal patron to keep her charges away from physicians. Héroard's diary, the perspective of a university-trained physician with a vested interest in these particular politics, judged Montglat's health-care role to be less influential even in the everyday governance of her charges, than previous governesses appear to have been. If there was little explicit tension revealed in the letters of monarchs or in Héroard's journal, it is because Montglat appears not to have intervened in the decisions that physicians saw as their business. However, the queen's midwife, Louise Bourgeois, was less willing to take a secondary role in matters she felt were her purview, and she pursued her claims to be treated as an equal participant in the medical matters of the royal family.

In her *Recit véritable de la naissance des Messeigneurs et Dames les Enfans de France* Bourgeois demonstrated her tenacity to surmount the factionalism leading to her important appointment. The question of the midwife–client relationship was of great importance in Louise Bourgeois's career. It was precisely the discontent between Marie de Medici and Madame Dupuis, whom Marie found too old, which allowed Louise Bourgeois to obtain her place. To be sure the court physicians made her sit a rigorous examination, but it was the satisfaction of Marie de Medici and their privileged relationship that permitted her to be accepted.

The choice of a midwife was of prime importance to a royal consort whose principal role was to bear an heir to the kingdom.

As she anticipated, Bourgeois and her printed works did not go unnoticed by either the medical faculties or the general public. Within the texts of those of the elite medical community, while midwives in general were incompetent, Bourgeois was either cited neutrally or as an exception to the rule. For example, Jacques Guillemeau commented neutrally that he had worked with her during the confinement of Mademoiselle Danzé.[66] So too did Jean Héroard, who recorded in his diary Bourgeois's actions during the delivery of the dauphin, Louis, at whose birth he was present. Physicians were happy to cite Bourgeois when her observations and experience led her to the same conclusions that they argued in their own works. Thus, in discussing difficult births, Jacques du Val wrote 'as says the lady le Boursier obstetrician of the Queen presently reigning, in her observations, it is rare to seek out the afterbirth inside the womb, and she boasts having delivered more than two thousand women, with whom she has never been constrained to advance her hand [into the womb] to detach it.'[67]

Bourgeois's texts revealed ambiguity about the medical community of practitioners. On some occasions, she appeared to promote a vision of a united medical world recognising formally trained practitioners. In one work addressing her daughter, she wrote: 'A Doctor of medicine is the husband of your sister, your husband is doing his training to become one, one of your brothers is a pharmacist, your father is a surgeon, and me a midwife, the medical corps is complete in our household.'[68] Bourgeois's vision of co-operation probably did not represent the exchange most midwives experienced with university-educated practitioners. Bourgeois, it should be stated, was the wife of a surgeon and also worked among the powerful and rich women of Paris. When their lives and those of their children were at stake, physicians were more likely to be called than for women of more modest origins. For example, at the delivery of the dauphin Louis, several royal physicians attended as a matter of course, including Jean Héroard who has left us his observations of her work during the routine birth. Except in emergency situations, it is doubtful that the average midwife had the same type of interaction with the university medical corps.

Yet elsewhere Bourgeois's texts reveal a reality of mistrust within the university-trained and supervised medical community. Bourgeois herself recounted the opposition she experienced from other midwives, at her examination to be registered as a midwife. The midwives, she explained, asked me about the occupation of my husband, and when they learnt it, they did not want to receive me, ... Madame Dupuis said to the other, well my friend, my heart tells me nothing good will come of this for us, since she's the wife of a surgeon, she's in league with the Physicians like fairground pursecutters; we should only receive women of artisans who know nothing of our business. She said to me that my husband must support me without doing anything, and that if I did otherwise, I'd be burnt to ashes.[69]

Madame Dupuis's fears were not unfounded, for it was she whom Bourgeois eventually replaced in the privileged position as Marie de Medici's midwife. Other midwives perceived Bourgeois as a threat and representative of surgeons and physicians (whom they seem to have perceived as a coherent bloc here), indicating their fears of control from the medical faculty. Madame Dupuis's opposition probably also had its origins in a more personal rivalry with Bourgeois. The midwives' concerns demonstrated a lack of differentiation, even within the medical sphere, between the relative hierarchy between physicians and surgeons, even if physicians were keen to maintain their superiority over their corporative counterparts.

A vision of medical harmony was no more shared by court medical providers. Physicians at the court of Henri IV had preoccupations of their own. When the king gained control of Paris in 1593 he brought with him to the court a retinue of his own physicians. Many had trained at the medical faculty of Montpellier, a substantial proportion of them were Huguenots and many were favourable to the new chemical Paracelsian medicine.[70] Paris, however, had its own supreme body of medicine, the Paris medical faculty, from which traditionally many of the royal medical retinue had been drawn. The Paris medical faculty was hostile both to Protestantism, only Catholics could attend the Paris faculty, and to the new Paracelsian medicine. As Andrew Wear writes, 'Paracelsianism ... was often part of the matrix of ideas associated with radical social and medical change'[71] and this was threatening to the Parisian medical faculty, which was characterised by conservatism and Galenism. Henri's official support for their rivals then caused tensions between the Parisian medical faculty and the physicians at court. Moreover, the numbers of the Parisian medical faculty were dwindling, from 70 to 80 practitioners in the 1550s, to only 40 in the 1590s.[72] At the same time, the power of the royal physicians, and their size as an alternative medical authority, was increasing. In the 1590s there were 25 physicians serving the king and another ten for other members of the royal family.[73]

Throughout this period, there was continual dispute and debate between the 'chemists' of the royal court against the 'Galenists' of the faculty, Huguenots against Catholics, and the superiority of the Montpellier medical faculty represented by the court physicians or the Parisian faculty. The Paris faculty sought the support of the Parisian *Parlement* to counter Henri's patronage for their competitors, and to eradicate what they saw as medical heresy. This context of internal conflict between university-trained physicians is important to how we understand the tensions surrounding female child-care providers and their relations with court physicians. As the court physicians attempted to establish themselves as a legitimate and unified force to rival the Parisian medical faculty, they were not favourable to recognition of the governesses, nurses and midwives whom the court equally patronised. Women participating in court medical procedures could only detract from the royal medical retinue's efforts to form a supreme body like the Parisian medical faculty.

In 1627, Bourgeois was the midwife to Marie de Bourbon-Montpensier when the latter died shortly after giving birth. The royal physicians conducted an autopsy, from which they published a report. Within this document the court physicians claimed that they had found remains of the after-birth still attached to the womb. Such a finding suggested a fundamental error of conduct on the part of Bourgeois and implied both her knowledge and practices were faulty. Bourgeois felt that she had been used as the scapegoat by physicians whose ignorance had blinded them to the true causes of the death. Her angry response, the *Apologie de Louyse Bourgeois dite Bourcier sage femme de la Royne Mere du Roy, & de feu Madame. Contre le Rapport des Medecins*, published as a 27-page pamphlet, is a significant document for this study, revealing the complex relationship between early modern midwives and the elite medical corps, particularly those at the royal court.[74]

The divisions among providers of medical services at court are clearly shown through Bourgeois's *Apologie*. She evidently sensed that there was a conspiracy against her among the physicians. Her very willingness to imagine so demonstrates more clearly her awareness of her uneasy acceptance by other medical practitioners, than do her other works, where she presented herself as a confident and respected figure. In the *Apologie*, the tone changed and it was a Louise Bourgeois on the defensive who responded to the accusations:

> having seen the report printed of the opening of the body of the late Madame, written by the Physicians, who attended Madame in her

illness, to justify their actions in treatment and place on me the cause of her death, I believed that it was my duty to make the truth of the facts known, concerning the birth as well as the illness, and to demonstrate that the cause of her death was not at all this portion of after-birth claimed.[75]

Bourgeois argued that there may have been contributing factors to Madame's complications in birth and clarified that the patient had not been well even before the birth.[76]

Furthermore, as to what concerned the after-birth, Bourgeois was determined to show that she was competent and knew her practice. She insisted upon the fact that the physicians who had attended the birth had approved her actions. Consequently, if they were to accuse her, they were also discrediting their own actions and knowledge.[77] Bourgeois was at pains to demonstrate her thorough medical knowledge. She detailed her understanding about the nature of the placenta, showing her theoretical and practical familiarity with this fundamental obstetrical component.[78] She clearly showed her doubts about the medical explanations provided by the physicians, citing the medical facts as they were understood at the time.

Bourgeois picked holes in the autopsy procedures, highlighting flaws in their exploration and consistency in examining the body and offered her own advice about the manner in which the autopsy should have been conducted.[79] Her defence was passionate and virulent, unsurprising given the damage to her reputation caused by this public report. 'If you had the intention of making the truth known, you should have called upon other physicians with you, in no way connected with this affair, or those of the King's household, or even some of the Physicians of Paris, so as to not to be the sole judges in an affair of such importance.'[80] In her previous works Bourgeois's tone had never been so ardent as in the *Apologie*. 'The contrariety, noticeable in your report, concerning the gangrene of the womb, which you claim to be the cause of death, makes clear that your intention, in publishing your report, was to charge me with all the blame, to put yourselves in the clear.'[81]

Louise Bourgeois was clear about the source of her authority: it rested on wide experience. To back her claims, she offered to prove her knowledge. Since her epistemology stemmed from experience, so too would her proof:

> And to certify to you even further that what I say is true, I offer to verify it at the Hôtel-Dieu on the body of women, who die in the week before their delivery, and also, I will submit to the judgement of

Physicians, and Surgeons learned in Anatomy, provided that they are not in league and united together in a most dangerous cabal in the matter of Medicine, who without passion, according to science and conscience will judge your report and mine. I am certain that I will be found without blame and you others will have wrong on your side.[82]

However, she also knew that a more convincing argument in the eyes of the physicians would be to show that even doctors themselves agreed and approved her knowledge and practices. 'I am not so wicked, nor so ignorant in my occupation, which I've practised for thirty-four years in this town, and at Court, with honour and fidelity, as I have witnessed by the happy results and books which I have composed, which have been printed various times, and translated into all sorts of languages, with acknowledgements from the greatest Physicians in Europe, who have profited from reading my books.'[83]

Furthermore, if the physicians required university examples of her words and learned approval of her knowledge, Bourgeois could provide these as well. 'Hippocrates so knowledgeable in women's illnesses, as he demonstrated in so many books that he wrote on the subject, observed in the second of the *Epidemies*, that the wife of a convoying officer, after having given birth, the fourth day expelled a piece of membrane without any bad side effect: this great person wanting to make known to all posterity that this was not dangerous nor of any consequence.'[84] Here she also deployed other physicians approved by the faculties in her defence: 'I have read in Paul of Aegina in his Surgery, that the Physician must not be surprised, if a women does not expel her after-birth, as there are some who expel it in pieces or rotting four or five days after the birth. I've been advised that a great Surgeon and Anatomist named *Aquapendente* is of the same advice, and he has seen several women expel the after-birth in pieces or rotted without dying.'[85]

Bourgeois finally addressed the underlying subject of all this discussion during the Renaissance; that is, who held the last word in the obstetrical and gynaecological domain – the midwife or the physician? After all, as she reminded them, the very Ancients whose opinions physicians valued most had conferred with midwives in what concerned women's health. Thus Bourgeois reasoned: 'to know the secrets of women's illnesses, one must visit midwives, and attend several births, like your great Master and legislator Hippocrates, who in matters of women's illnesses, consulted midwives, agreeing with their judgement'.[86] As she argued, without real and thorough experience, what use was their textbook knowledge? 'By your report, you make it clear that you know nothing of the after-birth and the womb of a woman, before and after their delivery, no more than your master Galen, who having never married, and attending few women in their confinement, meddling to teach a midwife by a book that he wrote on purpose, he showed that he understood nothing of the womb of a pregnant woman, nor even her after-birth.'[87] Here was a woman publicly claiming superior competency over her university-trained contemporaries, positioning her hands-on experience above their text-based theory.

After advocating support and co-operation between academic medicine and a re-valorised experiential field knowledge, the physicians' accusations had led Bourgeois to reconsider publicly the entire question of medical epistemology. In the *Apologie*, she was moving towards a more radical position – why try to obtain approval from those whose knowledge she perceived as inferior to her own? She was arguing that the nature of university medical knowledge built upon Galen's legacy needed to be re-visited.

Such a bold public statement did not go unnoticed or unanswered by the learned medical corps. The court medical retinue regrouped and prepared an attack upon Bourgeois. Shortly after her publication came their reply in the *Remonstrance à Madame Bourcier, touchant son Apologie, contre le Rapport que les medecins ont fait, de ce qui a causé la mort deplorable de Madame*, likely written by Charles Guillemeau. Guillemeau had originally trained as a surgeon, and became a surgeon to the king, then first surgeon to Louis XIII. However, as seen in Chapter 1, surgeons were never perceived by the physicians as their equals, and Guillemeau retrained and was received by the Parisian medical faculty as a doctor of medicine in 1626. Guillemeau was no stranger to expressing his medical knowledge in print. In 1621 he had re-edited the *Suite du traité de la grossesse et accouchement* begun by his father, Jacques Guillemeau. In taking up the fight against Bourgeois, Charles Guillemeau may have sought to defend the development of the obstetrical superiority of the surgeons and physicians which both he and his father had helped to create through their works. Moreover, Guillemeau, having just been received as a physician in his own right, was perhaps more eager to defend his newly raised position in the medical hierarchy, against intruders like Bourgeois. Finally, Guillemeau had a personal interest in discrediting her work. Bourgeois had named him among the practitioners who had attended the birth and who had approved her practice. She argued that if she was at fault, physicians like Guillemeau were too.

Charles Guillemeau's response was not a defence against Bourgeois's counter-accusations to the physicians. He chose not to treat Bourgeois as a serious interlocutor in medical discourse, and critiqued the quality of her published works. 'I read some time ago a book that you wrote, ... it is so bad that it couldn't be worse'.[88] Guillemeau established a position of power: he depicted Bourgeois as a mad woman and harshly ridiculed her attempts to enter the learned medical domain: 'all the learned men who saw your book and observed your practice, ... reject them, and it would be good and useful that France had never felt the effects of them'.[89]

Furthermore, he concentrated on the boldness of a woman seeking to correct men, justifying a rejection of her knowledge purely on the basis of her sex and occupational position: 'it is an extraordinary thing to see that a Midwife meddles to admonish Doctors in Medicine and tries to prove to them by good Physician and Surgeon authors that they are ignorant in the science that they exercise'.[90] More than once Guillemeau indicated the elite medical corps' disapproval of her public display of her knowledge, 'You should have better remained the rest of your life without speaking',[91] 'you must examine your actions ... rather than to put in public all that you have judged proper, to excuse yourself from this great and irreparable fault'.[92] Finally, he advised her: 'content yourself in the boundaries of your duty, do not meddle to reprove the Physicians: for you are in no way ... capable to form an opinion about it.'[93]

The *Apologie* was Bourgeois's last publication, although her works continued to be reprinted throughout the seventeenth century and into the eighteenth. By 1627, Bourgeois had already ceased to be influential in court medical politics. Her role as midwife to Marie de Medici had terminated long ago, although she maintained a prerogative as an advisory figure on child-rearing, with the royal children's governess Madame de Montglat. Her work bears witness to the opposition that could arise between governesses, midwives and physicians at court. Indeed, Bourgeois's final work demonstrates the very extent of the gulf between university theory and female midwifery practice that she had striven elsewhere to bring together for their mutual benefit.

This third case study of women serving the royal family and particularly its children displays different currents and tensions to those of the previous two, and it must be remembered that our sources here – texts written for public consumption (at some level) by two of the major protagonists, Bourgeois and Héroard – undoubtedly represent medical power and authority at court in ways that supported their personal objectives and positions. Nevertheless, certain conclusions can be suggested. The court medical retinue surrounding the royal family during Henri IV's reign was evidently much larger than those with whom either Madame du Bouchage or Madame de Humières was interacting. The power of the court physicians during the early seventeenth century also appeared somewhat greater than previous court medical bodies. This threatened not only other medical service providers at court, such as the governesses and midwives supervising royal children, but also medical bodies outside the court such as the Parisian medical faculty. And in reverse, the struggle for supremacy between court and faculty physicians entangled those women patronised by the royal family and led court physicians to attempt to control their practices. The anxiety produced by ongoing negotiations of medical authority and power also helped to produce the very self-promotional texts by Héroard and Bourgeois that have been the focus here.

Women and men responded to the shifting definitions of medical authority produced by communities in and outside the royal court in differing ways, dependent on their life experiences, networks and opportunities. Despite the increasing interest in and publication of child-care texts by both the medical and wider community, the women chosen to oversee the health and wellbeing of the royal children were not selected for any medical expertise recognised by the universities as such. The role of patronage and court politics in the selection of individual women cannot be ignored. Governesses were chosen largely for their family connections and because they were themselves mothers, and wetnurses selected for their own physical health. In this respect, royal child-carers were not dissimilar to the carers of poor and foundling children. Even at the turn of the seventeenth century, women's claims to practical child-care expertise as mothers themselves held sway. However, what was changing over the century was the increasing authority of court physicians and surgeons to impose their views on the daily care of royal children in the nursery.

Notes

1 C. A. E. Wickersheimer, *Dictionnaire biographique des médecins en France au moyen âge* (Paris, 1936) ed. Guy Beaujouan. vol. 1 (Geneva: Droz, 1979), p. 267.
2 For comparative cases of mothering at the elite and royal level in the medieval period, see John Carmi Parsons and Bonnie Wheeler (eds), *Medieval Mothering* (New York: Garland, 1996).
3 Emile Aron, *Louis XI et ses guérisseurs* (Chambray: CLD, 1983), p. 107 and Louis XI, *Lettres choisies*, ed. Henri Dubois (Paris: Livre de Poche, 1996), p. 443.

4 See Foisil's view of the governess Montglat as somewhat severe compared to Héroard in the upbringing of Louis XIII. Introduction to *Journal de Jean Héroard*, ed. Madeleine Foisil, vol. 1 (Paris: Fayard, 1989).
5 (BN ms fr. 8459, fol. 5) Le Roux de Lincy, *Vie de la reine Anne de Bretagne*, vol. 1 (Paris: L. Curmer, 1860), pp. 117–18.
6 *Ibid.*, p. 132.
7 *Ibid.*, pp. 132–3.
8 Le Roux de Lincy, *Vie de la reine Anne de Bretagne*, vol. 4, p. 203.
9 Le Roux de Lincy, *Vie de la reine Anne de Bretagne*, vol. 1, p. 135.
10 (Ms fonds Bethune 8465, fol. 52r) in Le Roux de Lincy, *Vie de la reine Anne de Bretagne*, vol. 3, pp. 29–30.
11 Le Roux de Lincy, *Vie de la reine Anne de Bretagne*, vol. 3, pp. 29–30.
12 *Ibid.*, pp. 29–30.
13 (Bethune, 8457, fol. 5) in *ibid.*, p. 40.
14 See letters of 17 June, 1 July, 26 July and again in 1507.
15 Janine Bertier, 'Un traité scolastique de medicine des enfants: Le Pedenemicon de Gabriel Miron', *Santé, médecine et assistance au moyen âge* (Actes du 110e congrès national des sociétés savantes, Montpellier, 1985) (Paris: Editions du CTHS, 1987), pp. 9–22, p. 21.
16 *Ibid.*, p. 14.
17 *Ibid.*, p. 14.
18 *Ibid.*, pp. 13–14.
19 *Ibid.*, pp. 13–14.
20 *Ibid.*, p. 13.
21 Diane de Poitiers, *Lettres inédites*, ed. Georges Guiffrey (Paris, 1866) (Geneva: Slatkine, 1970), p. 11, n. 1.
22 *Lettres de Catherine de Medici*, vol. 1, ed. H. de la Ferrière (Paris: Imprimerie Nationale, 1880), p. 18.
23 *Livre de la nature et utilité des moys des femmes, & de la curation des maladies qui en surviennent*, trans. Guillaume Chrestian (Paris: Guillaume Morel, 1559), p. 107.
24 Diane de Poitiers, *Lettres inédites*, p. 15, n. 1.
25 *Lettres de Catherine de Medici*, vol. 1, p. 32.
26 *Ibid.*, p. 40.
27 Mémoires de Vieilleville, livre III, chap 17, in Diane de Poytiers, *Lettres inédites*, p. 87.
28 Diane de Poitiers, *Lettres inédites*, p. 85.
29 *Ibid.*, p. 85.
30 *Lettres de Catherine de Medici*, vol. 1, p. 41.
31 *Ibid.*, pp. 41–2.
32 Diane de Poitiers, *Lettres inédites*, pp. 87–8.
33 *Ibid.*, p. 73.
34 *Lettres de Catherine de Medici*, vol. 1, pp. 23–4.
35 *Ibid.*, p. 41.
36 *Ibid.*, pp. 57–8.
37 Diane de Poitiers, *Lettres inédites*, pp. 15–16.
38 *Lettres de Catherine de Medici*, vol. 1, p. 70.

39 *Ibid.*, pp. 23–4.
40 *Ibid.*, p. 70.
41 Poitiers, *Lettres inédites*, pp. 15–16.
42 *Ibid.*, p. 91.
43 *Ibid.*, pp. 83–4.
44 *Ibid.*, pp. 85–6.
45 *Ibid.*, p. 105.
46 See Catherine's use of the same strategy in another context, in Chapter 8.
47 Louise Boursier, *Récit véritable de la naissance de Messeigneurs et Dames les Enfans de France, instruction à ma fille et autres textes*, eds Francois Rouget and Colette H. Winn (Geneva: Droz, 2000), p. 79.
48 *Journal de Jean Héroard*, vol. 1, p. 81.
49 *Ibid.*, p. 81.
50 *Recueil des lettres missives de Henri IV*, vol. 7 (Paris: Imprimerie Royale, 1858), p. 500.
51 *Journal de Jean Héroard*, vol. 1, p. 375.
52 *Ibid.*, p. 379.
53 *Ibid.*, p. 383.
54 *Ibid.*, p. 387.
55 *Ibid.*, p. 615.
56 *Ibid.*, p. 1321.
57 *Ibid.*, p. 835.
58 Louis Batiffol, *La Vie intime d'une reine de France au XVIIe siècle* (Paris: Calmann-Levy, [1906]), p. 261.
59 *Journal de Jean Héroard*, vol. 1, p. 86.
60 *Recueil des lettres missives de Henri IV*, vol. 7, p. 385.
61 Madeleine Foisil, *L'Enfant Louis XIII: l'éducation d'un roi, 1601–1617* (Paris: Perrin, 1996), p. 91.
62 *Journal de Jean Héroard*, vol. 2, p. 1738.
63 *Journal de Jean Héroard*, vol. 1, p. 82.
64 *Ibid.*, p. 459.
65 *Ibid.*, p. 606.
66 Jacques Guillemeau *De l'heureux accouchement des femmes où il est traicté du gouvernement de leur grossesse, de leur travail naturel et contre nature, du traictement estant accouchées et de leurs maladies* (Paris: Nicolas Buon, 1609), p. 232.
67 Jacques du Val, *Des Hermaphrodits, accouchemens des femmes, et traitement qui est requis pour les relever en santé, & bien élever leurs enfans* (Rouen: David Geuffroy, 1612), p. 200.
68 Françoise Lehoux, *Le Cadre de vie des médecins parisiens aux XVIe et XVIIe siècles* (Paris: A. and J. Picard, 1976), p. 23.
69 Louise Bourgeois, *Observations diverses sur la sterilité, perte de fruicts, foecondité, accouchemens, et maladies des femmes et enfants nouveaux naiz* (1609) (Paris: Abraham Saugrain, 1617), p. 110.
70 Allen G. Debus, *The French Paracelsians: The Chemical Challenge to Medical and Scientific Tradition in Early Modern France* (Cambridge: Cambridge University Press, 1991), p. 48. For an understanding of Paracelsus and his theories, see Walter Pagel, *Paracelsus: An Introduction to Philosophical Medicine in the Era of the*

Renaissance, 2nd edn (Basel: Karger, 1982). For an overview of Paracelsianism and court politics see, Hugh Trevor-Roper, 'The court physician and paracelsianism', in Vivian Nutton (ed.), *Medicine at the Courts of Europe, 1500–1837* (London: Routledge, 1990), pp. 79–94, p. 86.

71 Andrew Wear, 'Medicine in Early Modern Europe, 1500–1700', in Lawrence I. Conrad, Michael Neve, Vivan Nutton, Roy Porter and Andrew Wear (eds), *The Western Medical Tradition 800BC to AD 1800* (Cambridge: Cambridge University Press, 1995), p. 322.

72 Debus, *The French Paracelsians*, pp. 49–50.

73 *Ibid.*, p. 50.

74 Wendy Perkins's article provides a more detailed summary of Bourgeois's arguments than can be discussed here. 'Midwives versus doctors: the case of Louise Bourgeois', *The Seventeenth Century* (1988), pp. 135–57.

75 Louise Bourgeois, *Apologie de Louyse Bourgeois dite Bourcier sage femme de la Royne Mere du Roy, & de feu Madame. Contre le Rapport des Medecins* (Paris: Melchior Mondiere, 1627), p. 3.

76 *Ibid.*, p. 4.

77 *Ibid.*, p. 4.

78 *Ibid.*, pp. 5–6.

79 *Ibid.*, pp. 12–13.

80 *Ibid.*, pp. 13–14.

81 *Ibid.*, p. 8.

82 *Ibid.*, pp. 9–10.

83 *Ibid.*, p. 15.

84 *Ibid.*, pp. 17–18.

85 *Ibid.*, pp. 18–19.

86 *Ibid.*, p. 19.

87 *Ibid.*, p. 9.

88 Charles Guillemeau, *Remonstrance à Madame Bourcier, touchant son Apologie, contre le Rapport que les medecins ont fait, de ce qui a causé la mort deplorable de Madame* (Paris: Julian Jacquin, 1627), p. 14.

89 *Ibid.*, p. 14.

90 *Ibid.*, fol. Aviir.

91 *Ibid.*, fol. Av.

92 *Ibid.*, fol. Ar.

93 *Ibid.*, fol. Av.

8

French women and reproductive knowledge at the Spanish court

WE HAVE SEEN in the previous chapter how women of differing social status, from queens to rural wetnurses, negotiated medical authority over child care at the French royal court during the sixteenth century. How did these same women fare when they attempted to establish their authority at the foreign courts to which they were sent as consorts and as part of the royal entourage? This chapter examines the intersections between university medicine and the reproductive knowledge of court women across sixteenth-century France and Spain. It explores their discussions of menstruation, pregnancy and childbirth in the correspondence surrounding the reign of Elisabeth de Valois as Queen of Spain between 1559 and 1568. Elisabeth, the eldest daughter of Henri II and Catherine de Medici, married Philip II of Spain in 1559 when she was not yet fourteen. Discrete discussion of Elisabeth's menstrual regularity and childbearing capacity passed between France and Spain in letters written by her mother, attendant ladies-in-waiting and the French ambassadors in Spain. How were women able to discuss their reproductive knowledge and, furthermore, what opportunities did they have to speak authoritatively on matters of female health? While Elisabeth de Valois was queen in Spain, women's reproductive knowledge became one area in which Franco-Spanish power was contested, articulating anxieties about boundaries of male and female authority in gynaecological and obstetrical matters. During her short life, she would suffer at least three clear miscarriages, bear two healthy girls and ultimately die in childbirth at the age of 23. This chapter demonstrates how the pubescent and parturient body of Elisabeth de Valois became a region of cultural confrontation and compromise, and a place of entry for female authority in French medicine.

Elite women not only developed their own knowledge and practices about reproductive health that they shared with friends or family, but they could also participate in a wider arena, alongside physicians, midwives and other medical practitioners. This chapter will examine the areas to which elite and royal women at court could contribute and the strategies they employed to justify their knowledge. In sixteenth-century France, few royal women discussed their reproductive knowledge, particularly with husbands or male relatives, in their private correspondence. Catherine de Bourbon, sister of the king Henri IV, showed her unwillingness to admit reproductive or sexual knowledge to him. She wrote modestly that Henri would produce an heir before her, since he knew 'already how one must make them, and me, . . . so ignorant in all that'.[1] Catherine's comments suggest that she felt it was inappropriate to discuss her reproductive affairs in detail with him: 'This style is very different from that of a year ago [before her marriage] . . . when one is with men, one learns to speak thus'.[2]

Given this reticence to discuss matters reproductive, the few texts *between* women which allude to their understanding of their own bodies are invaluable and highly significant. Women's letters to other women sometimes provided advice and recipes of their own for reproductive complaints. The Medici correspondence is an unusually abundant and exciting resource in this regard. Elisabeth de Valois's reproductive activity was her primary role as a royal consort, particularly to produce male heirs. Her reproductive health was carefully scrutinised by her attendant ladies-in-waiting and questioned by her mother, Catherine de Medici. Monarch's and consort's body and health were always heavily surveilled and were perceived to have political consequences. Indeed, as Melzer and Norberg have argued, the body and health of the monarch or consort had ramifications for the royal lineage and for foreign politics. A monarch's fertility could be seen to represent the fertility and future of the whole country.[3] But the fact that Elisabeth was living in Spain while Catherine remained at the French court means that we have detailed extant records and written discussion of her reproductive life, which might otherwise have occurred by word of mouth. By comparison, there is virtually no extant written correspondence by Catherine about another daughter, Claude, who remained in France once married. Since Catherine could not oversee Elisabeth's pregnancies for herself, she requested enormously detailed information regarding her health from her male ambassadors and Elisabeth's attendant ladies.

The carriers of female reproductive knowledge and their contributions

Firstly who were the participants in the sections of the Medici correspondence that concerned Elisabeth's reproductive health, and what were the matters about which they could communicate? The relatively small amount of attention that reproductive issues received in the overall Medici correspondence suggests that women's knowledge was typically transmitted verbally. The English translator of Jacques Guillemeau's handbook for surgeons and midwives apologised if he had 'been Offensiue to Women, in prostituting and divulging that, which they would not have come to open light'.[4] Of all female health issues, menstruation seems the least discussed by early modern women themselves. As Patricia Crawford has observed in her study of early modern Englishwomen's discussion of menstruation, 'it is clear that women viewed menstruation as a private matter'.[5] Nevertheless, the unusual circumstances and extreme importance of Elisabeth's reproductive capacity as reigning queen of the most powerful monarch in Europe reveals unusually frank discussion of menstruation in sixteenth-century women's correspondence. When Elisabeth left France to join Philip in Spain in mid-December 1559, she was thirteen and it seems likely that her menstrual cycle was not yet regular. This was a key concern, not only as to her ability to conceive, but also to establish whether the royal couple could commence regular sexual relations. Many of the attending women's early letters to Catherine seek to assure her of the regularity of Elisabeth's 'besongnes', a term which can be approximately translated as her monthly 'needs'.

Catherine was kept well informed of the regularity of Elisabeth's menstruation by her daughter's French ladies-in-waiting, whom Catherine required to 'write as soon as her needs come to her'.[6] It was the task of Louise de Clermont to inform Catherine that 'she has not yet any appearance of her needs: I will not fail to let you know' and later remarked upon Elisabeth's pubescent puppy fat in her letters to Catherine as a hopeful sign of impending menstruation. She reported that she had become 'rather fat ... which everyone approves very well'.[7] She dutifully reported back to Catherine in detail on Elisabeth's irregular menstrual cycle and the attendant physicians' remedies: 'They are making her bathe ... to bring on her needs. The time that we had marked, which was the ninth of the month, passed without us seeing anything'.[8] Hot baths continued to be recommended as an ever popular treatment for all manner of gynaecological complaints.

Elisabeth's menstrual cycle appears to have stabilised after 1560 (given the subsequent lack of discussion surrounding this matter), and so attention turned to the issue of her conceiving. Catherine herself was not unfamiliar with the difficulties of falling pregnant. Her own marriage had been fraught by problems of infertility for the first eleven years. 'She does not hesitate to take by mouth all the medicines that could help her to bear children', the Venetian ambassador had once reported home about Catherine,[9] and it was not until 1543 that she could write happily 'of the hope I have of being pregnant... which is the beginning of my wellbeing and happiness'.[10] As Claude de Vineulx, one of Elisabeth's attendants, indicated to Catherine in August 1560, 'I hope that God will give us the grace that in ten months she will have a child, ... seeing as her needs have come very well since being here, which they had not done before, ... she is so big and well formed'.[11] In May 1562, Claude de Vineulx wrote to Catherine that she would be

> so happy to be able to send you the news which you desire of the Queen your daughter; but, for the moment, I have seen no signs to suggest she is pregnant; I have thought so sometimes for many reasons; but, among other things, I think that the desire to see her thus makes me believe it. She is always well and her needs are very regular every month, if they are late, it is only by three or four days, for which reason it seems to me that she cannot long delay from becoming so, and ... I am assured, Madame, that she will be soon, for her humeral temperament is very good and that of the King her husband also.[12]

However, Catherine also had other sources of knowledge from which to ascertain the state of her daughter's reproductive health. When she arrived in Spain, Elisabeth brought with her a considerable retinue, including two chief ladies of her bedchamber, eight ladies-in-waiting, four chamberwomen, kitchen staff, as well her physician Burgensis, surgeon Dunoir and two apothecaries.[13] Several of her ladies, including Louise de Clermont, had attended Elisabeth since her birth, knew well her constitution and fed back regular reports to Catherine. Further to this, Catherine also received letters from Elisabeth's medical retinue and from the French ambassadors in Spain. The latter served as intermediaries for Catherine, reporting back on Elisabeth's health from a distinctly different, male perspective. Notably, Catherine asked her ambassadors for different types of information from that which she demanded from Elisabeth's ladies-in-waiting. While Catherine regularly requested information from her male ambassadors about Elisabeth's general and even reproductive wellbeing, detailed discussion of her menstrual cycle occurred almost entirely in letters between Catherine and the ladies-in-waiting.

Even the terminology that men and women used to discuss menstruation varied. The French ambassador, the Baron de Fourquevaux, chose the delicate term 'the flowers' on the rare occasions when he mentioned 'what concerns women's little secrets'.[14] This, and 'the months' were the terms used most frequently by medical authors in the sixteenth century.[15] The word used by women in their correspondence to each other is 'besongnes', or monthly 'needs'. I am told that a similar phrase, *il bisogno mensile*, can still be occasionally heard among older women in the Italian countryside.[16] This term has not yet been recorded as meaning menses, to my knowledge. Neither Cotgrave, compiler of the famous seventeenth-century French–English dictionary, nor Huguet, composer of the modern sixteenth-century French dictionary, give a meaning of menses to the word *besongnes*, a term usually translated by contemporaries as 'tasks'. It seems likely that since Cotgrave supervised a male editorial collective, and Huguet drew his meanings largely from male-authored texts, neither had come across the term in the sense that sixteenth-century women used it among themselves. However, it may also be simply a term Catherine de Medici (by birth Italian) used as a translation of the Italian equivalent, and which her female correspondents adopted from her use of it.

As observers in Spain, French ambassadors could only be of limited use to Catherine in matters of female health. Indeed, the Bishop of Limoges, one of the first French ambassadors while Elisabeth was queen, clearly differentiated between the realms of access and knowledge of men and women around the queen, writing home to Catherine about Claude de Vineulx, one of Elisabeth's ladies-in-waiting, that 'she told me ... that she knew all the secrets of the queen' that remained a mystery to him.[17] The ambassador Fourquevaux was not privy to Elisabeth's private comments about her pregnancy, nor could he observe her as closely as her attendant doctors and ladies were able to. 'I assure you, Madame, that her doctor, M. Vincens, and her apothecary, and La Cousture and others hold for certain that she is pregnant since she was bathed. But Her Majesty dares not assure me of it, for fear that she is not'.[18] He was forced to wait for confirmation of the happy event, determined by the quickening, from Elisabeth herself. Therefore, he could only be at most a secondhand source of information, and was unlikely to be the first to hear the news: 'your daughter confessed to me of late that she has felt the fruit that she carries two or three times, which is the reason that La Cousture, one of her ladies-in-waiting, left immediately to carry the certain good news to Your Majesties'.[19] By his own admission, Fourquevaux knew his information would not be the first to reach Catherine.

French ambassadors to Spain occupied a difficult and ambiguous position as purveyors of female knowledge among women and to men. Besides corresponding directly with her daughter, Catherine also frequently directed her ambassadors to pass on important recipes and female secrets to her daughter. This placed them in the awkward position of imposing on the intimate female cultural space of women's reproductive knowledge. When it seemed that Elisabeth might have conceived, in October 1560, Catherine instructed her ambassador Limoges to advise Elisabeth on appropriate conduct while pregnant:

> if she is so, by fortune, she will be more healthy and her child will be better, when she does a little exercise, provided that it is not violent and that she does not go about in a coach or on horse; to go in her litter, she will not hurt herself... the thing that I desire most in the world is to see her with child.

Since Elisabeth was already surrounded by Spanish and French medical practitioners, the French ambassadors served as mediators of Catherine's advice concerning female health, treatment and care. Much of this appears to stem largely from her own experiences and conduct while pregnant:

> tell her that she must not refrain from doing a little exercise, and she has seen me pregnant, being so ill that I could not walk, and much older than she is, and with all that I still forced myself to have two people support me so as to not loll about in bed.[20]

Just as difficult for the French ambassadors were the negotiations that they had to undertake for Catherine with the physicians about the correct treatment of her daughter. Catherine sent remedies to the French physician via the intermediary of the ambassador Limoges: 'I am sending you a recipe that you will pass on to the physician of the Queen my daughter, which I found useful for having children, so that he might make her use it'.[21] Later she commanded another ambassador, Fourquevaux, 'to carry the letters that I have written to the doctor of the Queen my daughter, which are full of recipes that she might need'.[22] Generally, female medical advice was not welcomed by the university-trained practitioners. Catherine's ambassadors encountered some difficulty trying to intercede and influence the physicians with her counsel.

Furthermore, Catherine also expected her ambassadors to promote her superior reproductive knowledge to King Philip II himself. If intervention with the attendant physicians failed, ambassadors were to act as mediators of her female wisdom to the king who ultimately held the power to override their actions. When correspondents in Spain wrote hopefully of a pregnancy in October 1560, Catherine was doubtful. 'I pray you speak to the King my son-in-law that, for the desire he has to see her pregnant, he does not hesitate to command the doctors that they do not confine her to bed, for, if she is not, I fear that this would keep her from it and prevent nature from doing what it must.'[23] Catherine also wrote directly to Philip herself where she felt the concern and 'love of a mother' might convince him to follow her course of action on matters of childbearing. Catherine's antenatal advice extended to the matter of Elisabeth's diet, considered an important aspect of humeral balance. Women were frequently warned against eating spicy foods and alcohol, which might upset their *naturel* or constitution. Catherine, who claimed to know 'her constitution better than anyone', sent the King a personalised dietary regime for Elisabeth, recommending the following modest fare in October 1568:

> having heard that the queen your wife is ill and from what I can see from what they write to me about it, it is from ... retaining too many humours and not doing enough exercise, something that I feared in the end would bring some difficulty to her and her child, it is the reason that I want to beg Your Majesty to please command her not live in such a fashion and to eat only two meals and between them eat only bread, if she cannot wait until *souper* or dinner.[24]

Franco-Spanish medical rivalry

The rivalries between the French and Spanish carers (practitioners and attendants) resulted in a context where women could be contributors to accepted medical knowledge and were even encouraged by their university-trained compatriots. My object here is, rather than following a chronological analysis of Elisabeth's reproductive history, to highlight the types of contexts which allowed women to participate. Although in many circumstances French physicians were reluctant to accept female superiority in gynaecological and obstetrical matters, concepts of medical authority could display volatility in moments of crisis. As the queen of one of the most powerful rulers in Europe, Elisabeth's reproductive capacity was a concern of international importance and she was attended in reproductive matters by four distinct groups: French physicians, French women, Spanish physicians and Spanish women. As becomes clear from the correspondence, Elisabeth's health and treatment became an issue around which a minor power struggle, reflective of international Franco-Spanish politics, developed. Indeed, even in Elisabeth's first year in Spain, there had been such dissension among the ladies of France and Spain that most of her French ladies-in-waiting had been sent back to France. Such a moment allows us to chart the complexities of boundaries between male and female reproductive knowledge and to view the contexts in which women could be seen as healers, participants and contributors to medical knowledge.

Unlike other European countries, little has been written recently on the relationship of physicians and the court in Spain during the early modern period. Neither of the edited collections of Vivian Nutton or Bruce T. Moran concerning science and medicine at the royal courts of Europe contains chapters on Spanish medicine and the court.[25] It is clear, though, from contemporary sources that, because of the rigidity of its practices, the quality of Spanish medicine did not enjoy a high reputation elsewhere in Europe. University medicine in Spain was particularly associated with Jewish and Muslim traditions, and renowned for its strict adherence to conservative Galenism. It was the Galenic schools in the faculties that provided physicians for the court and who formed the powerful *protomedicato* which controlled medical regulation across Spain. Andreas Vesalius, whom Philip II had brought back from Brussels as his personal physician, was known to have had great difficulty working with his Spanish colleagues.[26] One contemporary Tuscan ambassador once reported home in regard to Spanish medical practices, 'Who hasn't seen it can't believe it'.[27] French and Spanish physicians appear, from a reading of the French correspondence, to have clashed over their theories of bodily health generally, although I shall focus on their conflicts about reproductive medicine here.

From the time of the arrival of Elisabeth and her retinue in Spain, Spanish physicians (who remain an anonymous entity 'the Spanish physicians' in most of the French correspondence) took little account of the knowledge and cures offered by Elisabeth's French ladies-in-waiting. Claude de Vineulx complained bitterly to the Bishop of Limoges about her treatment, that even though she served Elisabeth 'so intimately at night, the Spanish held her in little respect'.[28] Louise de Clermont related to Catherine both her own and the attendant doctors' alternative composition of enemas, or clysters as they were known, for one occasion of constipation. After the medical practitioners created 'clysters to which she wasn't accustomed, . . . [it] did her ill to force herself so much, without being able to go, which did great ill to her fundament and caused swelling, which made me think, Madame, that it was haemorrhoids.'²⁹ Clermont then explains how she deftly 'steamed her with milk and saffron, and was forced to give her a clyster myself, which relieved her of her affairs without trouble, and since she has been quite well, for before she could not move'.³⁰ Clermont subtly implied that her more intimate knowledge of Elisabeth's constitution allowed her to select a more appropriate choice of herbs and physick to make up her clyster.

Catherine's recipes and dietary advice for Elisabeth also proved a source of conflict, showing the precariously balanced relationship between a woman's reproductive advice and that of male physicians. Indeed, under other circumstances, French physicians longed for the more strictly regulated situation of medical authority which Spain had implemented and did not appreciate the contributions of women who suggested their experiences constituted a valid medical opinion. As previous chapters have shown, French physicians such as André du Breil lamented the situation of medical regulation in France, where they claimed physicians lacked authority and any could claim to practise medicine. Although John Tate Lanning has provided an important corrective to the view that the strength of the Spanish *protomedicato* provided a unified medical system (indeed in Philip's own reign, there were complaints that the kingdom was full of unlicensed practitioners),³¹ nonetheless, outside contemporaries such as Laurent Joubert perceived Spain as a model of formal medical practice and regulation.³² However, when Catherine sent a parcel of letters written to Elisabeth's French doctor, 'full of recipes which she might need',³³ the French ambassadors and physician supported Catherine's authority to treat her daughter over that of their Spanish medical counterparts. Fourquevaux explained how the Spanish physicians had approached drying-up her milk after the birth,

> To resolve the milk, the physicians did not dare apply the suitable remedies... I have advised the [French] physician Montguion, to render an account to Your Majesty of the state of the illness without forgetting to say which of your recipes they applied and which not. For I understand that these Spanish doctors have distrusted the majority of them, like the fat beasts that they are, having nothing but presumption and arrogance among them.³⁴

As Elisabeth prepared for the return of Philip from abroad, her French physician, Vincent, attempted to employ one of Catherine's remedies to ensure she was ripe for childbearing. This too caused conflict with the Spanish physicians as Fourquevaux reported back to Catherine:

the Queen, your daughter, agreed, last Thursday, with Master Vincent, her doctor, to take a bath according to the recipe that you, Madame, had given her some time ago. But having communicated this fact to the Countess of Ureigna, who, making as though she found it the best thing in the world, the old woman made it known to Juan Manrique, who forbade her doctor and his apothecary to bathe her or do anything, not even touch a hair on her head, without first consulting the Spanish physicians residing at the court.[35]

The evident competition between the French and Spanish physicians for control of Elisabeth's reproductive health was duly noted by the French in their letters home. 'Your recipe was consulted by the Spanish doctors, who, despite their ignorance, approved it as good and suitable.' Fourquevaux could not resist adding that Catherine's recipes were efficacious and that she should instruct her daughter that, in what concerned her gynaecological health, a mother knew best, thereby asserting the right of the French to supervise Elisabeth's reproductive health. 'The preparation served as you desired . . . I think that there would be no harm if Your Majesty wrote to her daughter my lady not always to heed the Countess nor Don Juan in what concerns women's little secrets'.[36]

Significantly, the French strove to create a context in which a mother's natural role as a carer, and a woman's natural role as healer, could outweigh the learned medical theories of physicians. Catherine de Medici argued that, as Elisabeth's mother, she had special and intimate knowledge of her daughter's constitution, 'whose humour I know better than anyone'. This was an important strategy which Catherine had used many times to justify her 'interference' as a woman in Elisabeth's medical matters and one which her French ambassadors and French physicians in Spain supported. Almost every letter bears witness to this technique of creating authority, arguing that she knew 'better than anyone her constitution'. Like Louise de Clermont, Catherine sought to impose her knowledge on the basis of intimacy and empathy, but also because of her maternal relationship. Catherine's strategy of calling upon her status as a mother to intercede was not new to the sixteenth century: indeed, it was a well-worn path. In contemporary print-published women's writings, female authors commonly exploited contemporary constructions of familial relationships and duties to negotiate textual space in publications.[37] Advice books and conduct manuals for women were one area of writing in which the difficulties of presenting a female didactic voice could be lessened. Sixteenth-century Frenchwomen produced a number of comportment and educational manuals for daughters and daughter-like figures, and one contemporary mother–daughter enterprise produced France's first text on child-rearing from a female perspective.³⁸ Thus the maternal role could be a powerful female identity for women in a patriarchal society and could serve as a legitimate area of female knowledge which allowed women to construct an authoritative voice. When it came to her right to speak out on female health, Catherine de Medici reverted to arguments which invoked authority related primarily to her sex, not her powerful social status.

There can be little doubt that Catherine was sincerely a concerned mother, to which this example, just one of many in her letters, attests: 'I scarcely know how to keep myself from worrying so much that I send this courier immediately in extreme diligence to her, to know more certain news of her'. However, Catherine also employed conventional expectations of women, invoking the *topos* of the 'good mother' to convince Philip and his Spanish physicians. It is significant to note how Catherine gained authority to speak as a mother only with age, experience and circumstances. The previous chapter has explored how, as a much younger mother who was overshadowed by her husband's influential mistress, Catherine's opinions had often been overlooked when it came to decisions about the care of her young children. Now, as an older and experienced 'good mother', independent of her husband and Diane de Poitiers, Catherine argued that it was her duty to oversee her daughter's wellbeing. Since she could not be present in person, it was only proper that she select the finest French women to represent her knowledge in Spain. Indeed, Catherine implied, she would be negligent in her duties to do otherwise. During Elisabeth's first pregnancy, Catherine wrote to her ambassador, Saint-Sulpice, of her concerns that Elisabeth be attended by French midwives:

> I send this courier immediately... to make the said Prince of Eboly approve that I send down two women that they call wise here, most experienced and useful to a pregnant woman³⁹

The issue of the nationality of Elisabeth's midwives inevitably caused conflict in Spain as Elisabeth had already explained to Fourquevaux on an earlier occasion: 'I asked my lady that if she would like to have some French midwife chosen by your hand, to advise Your Majesty of it in good time. She replied to me that she had no need, for she had a Spanish woman very experienced and sufficient in such business, as well as that Spain would look badly upon it and not allow one to come from abroad.'⁴⁰ Catherine pleaded her case further to Philip that her French midwives would be carefully chosen with a mother's knowledge of her daughter's specific needs:

as the mother such as you know me to be, to give her in this place all
the aid, service and comfort that I can, not being near to her, and
knowing better than anyone her constitution, I thought it necessary
to send her two women that they call wise, who I have had served me
and found to be good in such necessities, to take care of her and to
advise her according to the situation, knowing very well that, when it
comes to first children, they cannot be experienced enough.[41]

Notwithstanding the long labour associated with first pregnancies, the
choice of such women was highly important because it was commonly
believed that the experience of the first birth would determine future
pregnancy and childbirth experiences.[42] This then placed great importance on the choice of women who would guide and assist the pregnant
woman through this significant moment in her life. So much more
significant, therefore, was the birth experience of a royal consort whose
successful reproductive capacity was of primary importance. Catherine
worried so much that she sent the Sieur de Villeroy to intercede on her
behalf to Elisabeth and then to Philip. The king was forced to send a
letter to appease the concerns of his mother-in-law, in which he thanked
her for her offer to send midwives, but explained that his wife already
had at her disposal a good number of women to help her, and who were
already familiar to her, and that to have more still would only lead to
confusion in a delicate and tense situation such as childbirth.[43]

The divergent advice of antenatal care offered by Catherine and her
Spanish ladies-in-waiting resulted in similar difficulties. When Catherine
advocated that Elisabeth take regular exercise during her pregnancies,
this brought her into conflict with Elisabeth's Spanish attendants, who
preferred her to remain in bed. Fourquevaux's letters back to Catherine
show the difference in their views:

> It will be good, Madame, that it please you to write a word to the
> Duchess of Alva to recommend to her the person and health of the
> queen your daughter, and to make her do some exercise, for these
> people here do not want her to ever make a step if not in her litter, or
> carried in her chaise.[44]

Catherine again responded by appealing to Philip 'to commend to the
queen . . . to look after herself better than the other times and that she
takes more exercise principally in her ninth month, so that God gives
us the grace to see her give birth happily'.[45] Catherine's advice about
Elisabeth's post-natal recovery was equally distrusted by the Spanish. As
Saint-Sulpice explained to Catherine, he had been forced to intercede
with the king to enable Elisabeth to carry out her mother's wishes.

The Queen your daughter has already so well begun to carry out the regime that you have sent her that not a day passes that she does not go to the field at dinner or after dinner, to which the Countess of Ureigna and Don Juan Manrique are opposed strongly for not having been accustomed to it, if I do not cease to solicit the king her husband to let her continue and she to have the desire to do it, knowing well that on it depends the conservation of her good health.[46]

Frequently, things went wrong during pregnancies, and in this Elisabeth was no exception. Here too, Catherine could also demonstrate learned medical knowledge to participate in the process of her daughter's treatment. Catherine disagreed entirely with their eager application of phlebotomy after Elisabeth's miscarriages, a practice which only seemed to enfeeble her. When, in 1564, Elisabeth fell ill while pregnant, her physicians bled her at the arm and temple. This course of action seems to have so upset Elisabeth, who had never been bled before arriving in Spain, that she miscarried. Blisters were then applied to her feet and hands but Elisabeth grew progressively weaker.[47] The Spanish physicians declared that they could do no more and advised her to prepare her will.

It was not until then that French physicians were permitted to intercede and apply their remedies. Montguyon concocted a brew of agarick and other stimulants which succeeded in reviving the dying patient.[48] Catherine wrote to her ambassador Saint-Sulpice to draw a lesson from this drama and to recommend to her daughter 'when she is sick, that she no longer allows herself to be bled as much'.[49] Spanish doctors generally were not well regarded throughout Europe for their eager application of phlebotomy as a panacea and certainly as a way of purging women's evil humours. Henry Kamen has argued that even Philip was critical of his physicians' resort to bleeding which he thought 'may do more harm than good'. He preferred, like Catherine, to maintain his health through exercise and an abundance of fresh air.[50] Elisabeth, who always feared phlebotomy, had called upon the king to hold her hand to calm her the first time she was required to be bled.[51] The psychological effect alone seems to have been to her detriment.

Strategies of authority

Catherine was well aware of the divisions between Spanish and French medical practice, especially their divergent views on the efficacy of phlebotomy, as her letter to Saint-Sulpice demonstrated. 'I've written quite a harsh letter about it to Monsieur Vincent, her [French] doctor, even though I know well that it is against his opinion, . . . it is only to be able to show it to the other physicians, if he sees that he needs to'.[52] This time, she chose to argue that there were specific national differences between Spanish and French constitutions. As she explained, 'bodies born in France (as is the said queen my daughter, whose humour I know better than anyone) cannot be more injured than by so many bleedings.'[53] This certainly accorded with contemporary theory of the humours which explained warmer climates led women to have warmer blood and menstruate at earlier ages than women in the colder, damp climates of northern Europe, who had colder constitutions and first menstruated later.[54] Even medieval treatises such as that of Lanfrank of Milan particularly warned against the practice of phlebotomy on those with cold temperaments.[55] Catherine argued accepted medical logic of the day that her daughter's French constitution was less able to stand the loss of blood than those whose natural constitution was that of the warmer climate of Spain. Besides maternal topoi, Catherine attempted to draw upon learned discourse to negotiate an authoritative argument within contemporary medical knowledge.

And yet it was her claim to innate maternal knowledge of the intimate health and wellbeing of her daughter that appears to have conferred upon Catherine some authority.[56] Philip was especially inclined to accept her advice as a mother. He appears to have been convinced of the power of the maternal connection to the extent that, after Elisabeth's first miscarriage in 1564, he inquired of the French ambassadors the history of Catherine's own pregnancies. The ambassador, Saint-Sulpice, recounting the event to Catherine, indicated that he had replied that he knew the Queen Mother had had all her children without difficulty. Whereupon Philip responded that his wife should henceforth follow the example of her mother and obey all the advice that the daughter could receive.[57] Madame La Cousture, one of Elisabeth's French chamberwomen, was thus sent to Catherine with the express purpose of reporting to her in detail on the various aspects of Elisabeth's pregnancies. On her return to Spain, she brought with her a multitude of messages from Catherine, including an account for the French physician Montguyon, containing a list of French and Italian recipes to help Elisabeth during labour.[58] Fourquevaux related to Catherine that 'after the worst contractions, he [the King] gave her with his own hand the brew which you, Madame, had ordered: this had such force that the said Lady was delivered straightaway afterwards, without feeling the slightest pain'.[59] Catherine remained convinced that the reproductive difficulties of her daughter stemmed for the most part from the incompetence of the Spanish physicians. Significantly, for Elisabeth's next pregnancy in 1566, Philip appointed one Spanish physician, Olivarez, and two French, Vincent and Montguyon, to oversee her care.[60]

There can be no denying the strong nationalist rivalries over Elisabeth's reproductive health and treatment. What is so significant about this political context is how, as a result, the rhetoric of gynaecological and obstetrical authority could be altered to suit political objectives. In this instance, French ambassadors and physicians supported women's knowledge and helped to fashion a maternal–filial context in which women's inherent reproductive wisdom and superior childbirth knowledge could be more highly valued than that of male academic learning. Equally, Elisabeth's Spanish ladies-in-waiting prioritised the academic learned knowledge of their countrymen. It was after all women, the Duchess of Alva, who opposed Catherine's orders of diet and frequent exercise and the Countess of Ureigna who previously reported the use of Catherine's recipes by French doctors to the Spanish physicians.

Despite what we might imagine, given the importance of her reproductive responsibilities, it seems that Elisabeth was the most powerless participant in the treatment of her own body. Ulinka Rublack has argued convincingly that pregnancy and the lying-in time were a socially recognised period of danger in which a woman needed to be protected and a time when her whims were to be obeyed.[61] Although documents in Spain that circulated after her death suggested Elisabeth had held the prescriptions of her Spanish doctors in scant regard,[62] the Medici correspondence gives little sense of Elisabeth's opinions at all. She appears as a blank slate upon which the medical will of physicians, or the community of matrons, can be written. Male physicians devalued her corporeal sensations as subjective and unreliable, arguing that their medical knowledge and techniques enabled them to read the female body in pregnancy objectively (even though they too used their sensory powers for their determinations). Elisabeth's mother, Catherine de Medici, and her ladies-in-waiting seem to have ignored Elisabeth as too young and too inexperienced to understand her own body as they did. Catherine herself had experienced a similar powerless situation as a young wife and mother trying to establish some authority in the royal nursery. Both men and women surrounding Elisabeth saw her as unable to articulate her bodily signs in either appropriate medical or traditional female discourse.

The Medici correspondence shows us much about the intersections and conflict between male medical learning and women's own thoughts about their bodies as well as the variety of power relations at play in the reproductive context. The letters expose strategies that drew upon contemporary understandings of the duties of a good mother and her symbiotic, empathetic bond to her children to enable Catherine de Medici to participate in the medical prescription and cures of her daughter Elisabeth. Furthermore, they testify to the substantial role played by supporting figures such as ladies-in-waiting and ambassadors, as mediators of female knowledge to men. Elisabeth's reign in Spain represents a moment of short-lived divergence within the academic medical world of men, where national identity led physicians to privilege women's knowledge and to respect their contributions as healers. The specific national rivalry that pervades the Medici correspondence allows us to see the strategies that contemporaries could use to overcome women being dismissed as valid contributors to, and serious purveyors of, important medical knowledge. The pubescent, pregnant and parturient body of Elisabeth de Valois became a place for confrontation that exposes particularly well the complexities of women's medical authority in sixteenth-century Europe. Furthermore, and importantly, Catherine de Medici relied on strategies that conferred authority based not on her exceptional social status, but rather on her sex. It is clear that maternal authority could not serve consistently as a powerful platform to voice the medical opinions of women in all circumstances. Catherine's history in these two chapters shows how she emerged from the young wife and mother in the shadow of her husband's mistress to establish herself as an independent and experienced maternal authority on medical matters. Nonetheless we should note that Catherine herself chose to emphasise that it was not her powerful political position which gave her the right to instruct on female health in this instance, but rather her claim that a mother knew best.

Notes

1 E. Freville de Lorme (ed.), 'Lettres inédites de Catherine de Bourbon', *Bibliothèque de l'Ecole des Chartes*, 18 (1857), p. 338.
2 *Ibid.*, p. 338.
3 S. E. Melzer and K. Norberg (eds), *From the Royal to the Republican Body: Incorporating the Political in Seventeenth- and Eighteenth-Century France* (Berkeley: University of California Press, 1998), p. 2.
4 Jacques Guillemeau, Translator's Preface, *Child-Birth or, The Happy Delivery of Women* (London: A. Hatfield, 1612), fol. 2v.
5 P. Crawford, 'Menstruation in seventeenth-century England', *Past and Present*, 91 (1981), p. 68.

6 *Lettres de Catherine de Médicis*, vol. 1, ed. H. de la Ferrière (Paris: Imprimerie Nationale, 1880), p. 566.
7 *Négociations, lettres et pièces diverses rélatives au règne de François II*, ed. L. Paris (Paris: Imprimerie Nationale, 1841), pp. 719–20.
8 *Ibid.*, pp. 810–12.
9 Relation de Matteo Dandalo, fin de l'annee 1542, *Recueil d'Alberi*, vol. 4, pp. 47–8 in Eugène Defrance, *Catherine de Médicis, ses astrologues et ses magiciens envoûteurs* (Paris: Mercure de France, 1911), pp. 35–7.
10 *Lettres de Catherine de Médicis*, vol. 1, p. 6.
11 *Négociations, lettres et pièces diverses*, p. 461.
12 *Lettres de Catherine de Médicis*, vol. 10, ed. Baguenault de Puchesse (Paris: Imprimerie Nationale, 1899), pp. 543–4.
13 M. Walker Freer, *Elizabeth de Valois, Queen of Spain and the Court of Philip II*, vol. 1 (London: Hurst and Blackett, 1857), p. 77.
14 *Dépêches de M. de Fourquevaux, Ambassadeur du Roi, Charles IX en Espagne, 1565–1572*, ed. C. Douais, vol. 1 (Paris: Ernest Leroux, 1896), p. 14.
15 See contemporary works by Laurent Joubert, Guillaume Chrestian and, later, Louise Bourgeois.
16 Many thanks to Catherine Kovesi-Killerby for her advice on this reference.
17 *Négociations, lettres et pièces diverses*, p. 708.
18 *Dépêches de Fourquevaux*, p. 23.
19 *Ibid.*, p. 58.
20 *Lettres de Catherine de Médicis*, vol. 1, pp. 565–6.
21 *Ibid.*, p. 320.
22 *Lettres de Catherine de Médicis*, vol. 2 (Paris: Imprimerie Nationale, 1885), p. 375.
23 *Négociations, lettres et pièces diverses*, p. 611.
24 *Lettres de Catherine de Médicis*, vol. 3 (Paris: Imprimerie Nationale, 1887), p. 193.
25 Vivian Nutton (ed.), *Medicine at the Court of Europe, 1500–1837* (London: Routledge, 1990). See also B. T. Moran (ed.), *Patronage and Institutions: Science, Technology, and Medicine at the European Court 1500–1750* (Woodbridge: Boydell Press, 1991).
26 P. Pierson, *Philip II of Spain* (London: Thames and Hudson, 1975), p. 61.
27 C. D. O'Malley, *Don Carlos of Spain, A Medical Portrait* (Berkeley, 1969), p. 9 cited in *ibid.*, p. 61.
28 *Négociations, lettres et pièces diverses*, p. 708.
29 *Ibid.*, pp. 810–11.
30 *Ibid.*, p. 811.
31 J. T. Lanning, *The Royal Protomedicato: The Regulation of the Medical Professions in the Spanish Empire* (Durham: Duke University Press, 1985), pp. 14–20.
32 Laurence Brockliss and Colin Jones, *The Medical World of Early Modern France* (Oxford: Clarendon Press, 1997), p. 278.
33 *Lettres de Catherine de Médicis*, vol. 2, p. 375.
34 *Ibid.*, p. 383.
35 *Dépêches de Fourquevaux*, p. 14.
36 *Ibid.*, p. 14.
37 See my *Women and the Book Trade in Sixteenth-Century France* (Aldershot: Ashgate, 2002).

38 See Anne de Beaujeu, *A la requeste de treshaulte et puissante ma dame Susanne de Bourbon* (Lyons: [Pierre de Sainte Lucie, 1534]) and Mesdames du Verger, *Le Verger fertile des vertus* (Paris: François Jacquin, 1595). For commentary on women's conduct manuals, see C. H. Winn, '"De mères en filles": Les manuels d'éducation sous l'Ancien Régime', *Atlantis*, 19:1 (1993), pp. 23–30 and my 'Savoir féminin puériculteur: *Le Verger Fertile des Vertus* des Mesdames du Verger', *Mots Pluriels*, 11 (1999), www.arts.uwa.edu.au/MotsPluriels/MP1199sb.html.
39 *Lettres de Catherine de Médicis*, vol. 10, p. 139.
40 *Dépêches de Fourquevaux*, p. 45.
41 *Lettres de Catherine de Médicis*, vol. 10, p. 140.
42 Wendy Perkins, *Midwifery and Medicine in Early Modern France: Louise Bourgeois* (Exeter: University of Exeter Press, 1996), p. 33.
43 Walker Freer, *Elisabeth de Valois*, vol. 2 (London: Thames and Hudson, 1857), p. 171.
44 *Lettres de Catherine de Médicis*, vol. 3, p. 25.
45 *Ibid.*, p. 34.
46 *Lettres de Catherine de Médicis*, vol. 2, p. 237n.
47 Walker Freer, *Elisabeth de Valois*, vol. 2, p. 4.
48 *Ibid.*, pp. 6–7.
49 *Lettres de Catherine de Médicis*, vol. 10, p. 144.
50 H. Kamen, *Philip of Spain* (New Haven: Yale University Press, 1997), p. 209.
51 Walker Freer, *Elisabeth de Valois*, vol. 2, p. 193.
52 *Lettres de Catherine de Médicis*, vol. 10, p. 143.
53 *Ibid.*, p. 143.
54 J. Gélis, *History of Childbirth: Fertility, Pregnancy and Birth in Early Modern Europe*, trans. Rosemary Morris (Cambridge: Polity Press, 1991), p. 12.
55 Lanfrank's 'Science of cirurgie', 18–19, cited in C. Rawcliffe, *Medicine and Society in Later Medieval England* (Stroud: Sutton Publishing, 1995, re-published 1997), p. 65.
56 For other contemporary uses of the trope of maternal authority, see the collection of essays in Naomi J. Miller and Naomi Yavneh (eds), *Maternal Measures: Figuring Caregiving in the Early Modern Period* (Aldershot: Ashgate, 2000).
57 Walker Freer, *Elisabeth de Valois*, vol. 2, pp. 13–14.
58 *Ibid.*, p. 185.
59 *Dépêches de Fourquevaux*, vol. 1, p. 111.
60 Walker Freer, *Elisabeth de Valois*, vol. 2, p. 162.
61 See U. Rublack, 'Pregnancy, childbirth and the female body in early modern Germany', *Past and Present*, 150 (1996), pp. 84–110.
62 See W. Prescott, *History of the Reign of Philip the Second, King of Spain*, vol. 2 (New York: Crowell, [1855]), p. 237.

9

Elite women and reproductive knowledge: the Nassau sisters

IN JULY 1611, Elisabeth de Nassau, duchesse de Bouillon, wrote to her sister Charlotte-Brabantine, duchesse de La Trémoille, 'if it is possible, good sister, ... make my husband trust my calculations more than his'. Elisabeth expected to give birth around the beginning of August, at which point she believed herself to be ten months pregnant. In fact, it would not be before 11 September that her son was born. What does such evidence indicate about how elite women understood gestation, and how they determined when it began? Was gynaecological and obstetrical knowledge purely the domain of the experienced midwife and physician, or did women have different perceptions of their bodies? Even if we cannot access the voice of Elisabeth de Valois on her own reproductive health, examples exist of other elite women's views of their bodies during and after pregnancy. This chapter assesses what elite women understood about their bodies, how they obtained this knowledge and how, confronted with other medical epistemologies, women justified their knowledge of their own bodies as valid.

University medical interest in pregnancy

As we saw in Chapter 5, after the introduction of print in Europe, medical texts for the general population as well as the university-trained learned community became an important source of material for publishers. This transmission of learned medical knowledge in the vernacular included texts concerned primarily with the health of women. However, this discourse was limited and hindered in ways unlike other medical disciplines. Physicians saw problems not just associated with the transmission of learned medical knowledge to the masses, but also the transmission of 'female secrets' that could be construed as libidinous. Worse still, such knowledge might be used by women to trick men about their virginity or pregnancy. Andre Le Fournier's 1530 work on women's cosmetics and embellishment, *La Decoration dhumaine nature, et aornement des dames*, demonstrates physicians' unwillingness to reveal all about women's bodies to the general reader. Although instructions for recipes of pimples, wrinkles and the like were in French, he limited instruction about most gynaecological issues to those who knew Latin.[1] Perhaps Le Fournier did so as a precaution. When, some 40 years later, the surgeon Ambroise Paré published his *De la generation de l'homme et maniere d'extraire les enfants du ventre de leur mère* in 1573, the Faculty of Medicine in Paris accused him of immorality, though of course being a surgeon and Protestant were probably also determining factors.[2]

When Laurent Joubert, the chancellor of the medical faculty of Montpellier, published his *Erreurs populaires* in 1578, which discussed among other issues gynaecological and obstetrical beliefs ('errors') in the general community, the extensive justifications he provided give some idea of the pressure on physicians not to reveal such 'secrets' publicly. Dominique Reulin in his *Contredicts aux 'Erreurs populaires' de Laurent Joubert* (Montauban, 1580), complained that Joubert was divulging professional secrets and inadvertently causing social problems.[3] As Joubert summarised in his defence, these criticisms were:

> writing about conception, generation, pregnancy and birth ... all of which would have been better in Latin than French, for two reasons: one that these remarks do not sound as bad in a foreign language as in the vulgar; and so that women and girls who are not instructed in it, cannot have knowledge of it.[4]

Joubert argued in his defence that his work did no more than Liébault in *L'Agriculture, et Maison rustique* or Vallambert for child health-care in *De la maniere de nourrir et gouverner les enfants des leur naissance*, both of which were written in French.[5] Liébault certainly offered similar instruction in his medical contributions to the *L'Agriculture, et Maison rustique*.[6]
Joubert asked,

> And where is it, I pray, that I have written dishonest and scandalous remarks, inciting women and girls to do otherwise than honour and virtue require of them? If I deal with here a work of the flesh, it is from a husband to a wife, by conjugal love and in marriage, concerning conception and pregnancy, or birth and delivery, where if I touch upon some lewdness, it is in detesting it, as severely as a theologian could do.[7]

Some in the medical community were prepared to support Joubert publicly. Barthélemy Cabrol, a master surgeon at the Montpellier faculty and surgeon to the king, came to Joubert's defence after the outcry after the publication of the first book. Beyond the wrath of the medical faculty, there were of course other authoritative bodies to consider. The Catholic Church now produced an index of forbidden books which included both the works of Protestant physicians and those medical texts which might have a dangerous influence on moral standards.

But how were physicians to understand and explain the functions of a body that was not their own? How could they describe the experiences and sensations of pregnancy, for example? If women were positioned in society in part by their biological differences from men, how could medical men then find commonality through which to understand those very features?

Early modern gynaecological knowledge presented difficulties for physicians, which we can find displayed in the work of physician and author François Rabelais. Even using a typically comic grotesque style that exploited exaggeration and hyperbole, Rabelais's depiction of female genitalia reproduced contemporary medical perceptions which constructed female reproductive organs as fearsome and 'other'. Gynaecology remained largely the construction of classical theory, as one area where Rabelais was unable to question the authority of the ancients or women with his personal experience.

The clearest reference to Rabelais's understanding of gynaecology can be found in the *Tiers Livre*, in the passages concerning Doctor Rondibilis. His discussion of gynaecology was limited to recycling classical theory. However, gynaecology posed a mystery that no amount of classical knowledge could overcome and was a constant reminder of the limitations of learned male experience in the search for new knowledge. The frustration of physicians unable to comprehend gynaecology by personal experience and observation, rather than the authority of the ancients, manifests itself in Rabelais's work in an abhorrence of the vagina. Françoise Charpentier notes that it is called a wound as, for example, in the tale of the old lady, the lion and the fox.[8] The lion, seeing the vagina of the woman, says:

> O poor woman, who has wounded you thus? ... my old friend, this gammer has been very grievously wounded between the legs, and there is manifest solution of continuity. Look how big the wound is.[9]

In this passage, the vagina is considered as a fault, a poorly healed scar, one that periodically seeps blood. Here, it appears that the scar symbolises the absence of the penis, that which has been cut off, leaving behind the ugly and faulty wound.

Rabelais's depictions of the vagina are surprisingly similar and unambiguous, considering the multiple readings he is at pains to present elsewhere. The vagina always resembles a horrible, unnatural and monstrous entity. He uses, without exception, exaggeration for the size of the female genitalia, typical of his frequent comic grotesque style, describing them thus: 'Look how big the wound is: five and half span ... What the devil! This wound is deep: you could get in over two cartloads of moss'.[10] As Elizabeth Chesney Zegura observes, the genital organs symbolise a nothingness in a world which detests void.[11] Rabelais's text symbolises the fear of this unknown and unknowable (to men) quantity, and the functions of the female reproductive system, which cannot be personally observed by men but must be accepted on the authority of the ancients or of women. Unlike other images of the comic grotesque body, the void that is the vagina symbolises a black hole of knowledge in a medical world unwilling to accept limitations to its power to discover. Thus Rabelais's representation of medical opinion in regard to gynaecology relied upon classical and scholarly works, the very ancients whose authority sixteenth-century humanists sought to question and whose lacunae were a reminder of the limitations in the quest for knowledge.[12]

Over 60 years later, a surgeon, Jacques Guillemeau, was still able to argue that the 'silence' about women's bodies had led him to offer his own *De l'heureux accouchement des femmes où il est traicté du gouvernement de leur grossesse, de leur travail naturel et contre nature, du traictement estant accouchées et de leurs maladies* in 1609. As he explained, 'necessity, the mistress of arts, constrained women, to learn and practise Medicine: finding themselves afflicted by several illnesses in their shameful parts, being destitute of any remedies'.[13] But where medical men saw silence, there was indeed a wealth of knowledge, but not from sources that they admitted as authoritative.

Other physicians, like Hippocrates before them, had begun to look beyond the university for knowledge about the female body: they approached women themselves.[14] Laurent Joubert both critiqued the *Erreurs populaires* of women, and used them as sources to prove his understanding of gynaecology. As mentioned in Chapter 1, Joubert published depositions by midwives. His exposition of their nomenclature, Alison Klairmont Lingo argues, may reveal 'a unique chance to examine an otherwise obscure vocabulary for the body and to piece together a partial picture of spoken, popular body language'.[15] In his discussion about whether a woman could conceive without menstruating, he backed up his claims, with sources drawn from 'Madame la Maréschale de

Montluc who says she has a neighbour like this'.[16] He investigated stories he had heard. Discussing the age at which women could bear children, Joubert indicated 'After having written this, I was at Lectore, where I saw the woman who had given birth at nine, and spoke to her about it',[17] as if the tale's veracity was proved by his hearing the words himself.

Of course, Joubert did not take women's words at face value. There were, to begin with, good and bad women. The latter were those who thought they knew more than the doctors themselves: 'The presumption of some women is such that they think they understand better all illnesses peculiar to women (like suffocation of the womb, abortion and birth) than the most accomplished physician'.[18] Good women, like 'the good village women around Montpellier', were those whose evidence fitted with what Joubert already understood, who could be cited authoritatively and who acknowledged physicians' superior knowledge. For an author whose dedicated aim was to expose popular 'errors', Joubert frequently supported his 'learned truths' with evidence drawn from the people.

Even if Joubert looked for views which supported his own medical beliefs, nevertheless his *Erreurs populaires* provide the historian with some basis for understanding how women of a variety of social levels perceived their bodies and how they explained their corporeal experiences. Joubert's work can be used by the historian in the same ways that Barbara Duden has argued for the works of the physician Storch in Eisenach: 'though mediated through a male doctor, [they provide] a privileged access to the dialogue between popular belief and learned interpretation' of the medical.[19]

Reproductive knowledge of learned men

Beyond the medical faculties, educated men also exhibited knowledge about the female body that can be seen in their writings. This evidence is significant to our study here because it demonstrates that in contrast to a good number of physicians, men of the lay non-medical elite did not hesitate to respect female understandings about their own reproductive system. Negative reactions towards female reproductive knowledge may have been strongest at the level of the medical faculties, and did not apply more generally to learned men.

The correspondence of the urban lawyer, Jean de Coras, with his wife indicated his reliance on a variety of sources of medical advice. Coras sought opinions on his wife's reproductive difficulties from the elite women with whom he mixed, such as 'Madame la Seneschale, one of the foremost and most Christian women of Europe [Jeanne de Quiqueron de Beaujeu] who has at times been afflicted with your illness and has promised me something which will help your recovery'.[20] Yet this was interspersed with the advice to consult her physicians, 'if the physicians find it suitable'.[21] When Coras obtained information that might have aided his wife as he did in 1566,

> I educate myself from all those to whom I speak of remedies, and having discovered some things, that I am sending you, I talked of them to people who understand them and have seen them trialed, even a lady from Avignon, who was not only cured, but had a lovely child within a year.

yet he advised her always to confirm such remedies with the physicians: 'however, do not undertake anything without informing the physicians of it, and say, as is true, that it is the ladies of Nîmes who have researched this old remedy, having seen it tried out and afterwards sent it to you'.[22]

Although women wrote different things in correspondence to women and men, men's letters showed that reproductive discussion was not limited to women alone. As children, boys could enjoy games with their sisters which created notions about reproduction. Henri de La Trémoille wrote a childhood letter to his mother in 1606 about his and his siblings' celebrations at the delivery and lying-in of his sister's doll.[23] The Nassau sisters also passed information through their husbands to their most trusted physician, François Louis. In 1598, Elisabeth wrote to her sister, Charlotte-Brabantine:

> mon^{sr} Louis who is the physician whom you wanted to speak to, writes ... that Monsieur my husband told him that you were feeling some discomfort in your nipples, being very hard, so he sent him some useful remedies if the symptom does not pass soon.[24]

Such evidence suggests that men were not excluded from discussion of female health issues. Men also corresponded with each other about their wives' pregnancies. Louis de Brézé, Diane de Poitiers' husband, wrote to Montmorency in 1518 that his wife 'has a stomach so large that I think she cannot carry it much longer, for she is in her ninth month'.[25] These documents suggest that female reproductive health may not have been the secretive discourse that physicians claimed in their work. In fact, outside of the medical faculties, men and women spoke more openly of issues which concerned them both than elite physicians were willing to present publicly.

The foundations of female gynaecological and obstetrical knowledge

This chapter focuses on the writings of women themselves. It is often much more difficult to go beyond the learned physician's textbook to discover the views of women. The Nassau letters offer the historian a rare opportunity to see how women perceived their own bodies. Guillaume de Nassau, Prince of Orange, and his third wife, the French Charlotte de Bourbon-Montpensier, had six daughters: Louise-Julienne, the Electrice Palatine; Elisabeth, duchesse de Bouillon; Catherine Belgia (who does not feature in the correspondence); Flandrine, a nun at Poitiers, then abbess at Jouarre; Charlotte-Brabantine, duchesse de La Trémoille (to whom most of these letters are addressed); and Amelie de Nassau. The sisters married into France and the German states but they maintained a constant correspondence with each other as well as with their other step-siblings and their stepmother, Guillaume's fourth wife, Louise de Coligny. Their correspondence provides an exceptional exchange of reproductive knowledge among the sisters.[26] Where possible, I have included evidence from other women, some illiterate, to reveal similarities and differences between women's reproductive understanding at different social levels.

However, before examining what the sisters discussed in their letters, it is necessary to understand the foundations of their obstetrical knowledge. Women did not write about 'innate and natural' sensations in their bodies. Women's perceptions of their bodies and understanding of what they experienced were constructed by established contemporary boundaries about what was possible behaviour for the body. Their descriptions of their sensory perceptions were as socially coded by contemporary discourses as were those of the learned physicians of the medical faculty, even if the discourses themselves were different. It would be simplistic to suggest that physicians drew their notions on the female body, about its function and reactions from medical texts, while women of all social levels drew theirs from 'authentic' observation of their bodies.

Elite women had exposure to a number of different sources of information from which to form ideas about their bodies. Women could access the most formal type of university-created medical information through medical texts. However, while many elite women were literate in the vernacular, many medical treatises continued to be composed in Latin. As we have seen in Chapter 5, French women did not typically hold medical books in their libraries. Moreover, obstetrical and gynaecological texts, written primarily for the benefit of other physicians, tended to discuss 'abnormal' or emergency birthing situations, which necessitated the intervention of the physician.[27] The range of typical birth experiences was less discussed and presumably thought to be within the capability of the midwife, and therefore not knowledge needed by the physician. Even less attention was given to discussion of the normal course of pregnancy.

Laurent Joubert even argued (in defence of claims of indecency) that women could not learn anything from his writings: 'Girls can learn nothing either good or bad, if they have not already learnt it elsewhere, as (unfortunately) the majority know only too much. But it was never by my words, private or public (and even less my writings) that they might learn something'.[28] Joubert's publisher, Simon de Millanges, also stepped in to clarify Joubert's honourable intentions and clarify the work's intended audience as married men:

> Because M. Joubert, speaking in the last four books of the first part of conception, generation, birth, and knowledge of virginity, has often been constrained in revealing the errors that are made in such acts, to use words which seem somewhat obscene, it will be good that only married men read the useful advice which is made for them in the books.[29]

As we have seen in previous chapters, during the sixteenth century, increasing numbers of texts were dedicated to elite women as patrons, in which their medical interests were acknowledged. Guillaume Chrestian, physician to the royal children, translated Jacques du Bois's *Livre de la nature et utilité des moys des femmes* dedicating it to Diane de Poitiers, saying:

> I know truly that you take great pleasure to understand such secrets, which are not commonly known to all, to aid and give help charitably to women so fainthearted and fearful that it seems to compromise their honour, or offend their modesty if they reveal their serious passions to learned and experienced physicians.[30]

Jacques du Val's defence of his discussion of female genitalia, and the criticism it addressed, assumed at least some of his readers would be female: 'Some say it is a shameful and dirty thing to treat such matters and that reading such a book could induce some libidinous desire in the thoughts of those women who read it'.[31] Gervais de La Tousche's diatribe against midwives was essentially directed at all women, in order to encourage them to take responsibility for their own bodies during birth, albeit because he believed that birth, a natural part of the animal lifecycle, could be achieved without intervention by anyone. As he argued, 'they can give birth naturally without trouble, as do the other animals on the earth, and without the help of anyone'.[32] Consequently, apart from recommending that they avoid the services of midwives, La Tousche did not instruct women on how to manage pregnancy or birth.

Elite women were also likely to consult medical professionals far more than other women. Many used the services of apothecaries and physicians to treat their illnesses. Louise de Coligny shows the ease with which elite women mixed in the company of medical men in one letter to Charlotte-Brabantine de Nassau in 1606.

> I'm sending you a box of tablets that Mme la Garde des Sceaux gave me to send to you. She says that her apothecary has the recipe for them, whom she didn't want to name to me, and says that when you would like some that you write to her; but I've said to Sieur de Bourron that he ask for the recipe from M de la Violette [one of the king's doctors].[33]

Thus the medical views of elite women were more likely to represent a mix between personal observations and their physicians' explanations of their bodily functions.

A further source of knowledge and discussion of the female body that elite women could draw upon was the oral discourse they had with women around them. There were special occasions such as attending the birth of a friend's or relative's child in which women might discuss their understandings of childbirth to reassure the expectant mother. Although elite women probably attended births less frequently than women of more modest social origins, certainly the Nassau sisters made efforts to attend their sisters in childbed. Women would also observe the actions of the midwife and perhaps hear her explanations about the female body in labour.[34] Yet the midwife did not help women to distinguish abnormal signs during pregnancy, since her role was largely restricted to the delivery. She did not provide advice step by step during the pregnancy, to reassure the pregnant woman about the transformations her body underwent. Elite women probably shared here in discussion of their bodies with women within their household, especially domestic staff.

To these multiple sources, an alternative and important source for the transmission of knowledge particularly among elite women was through letters. Women's private correspondence contains rich and varied examples of how women understood their own bodies. Their letters are full of discussion of the day-to-day aches and pains that they or those in their household experienced. Migraines, toothaches and colds are among the more mundane illness that women reported on at length to male and female correspondents. Women also exchanged a wealth of information about their reproductive bodies in letters. They described the changes they experienced in their bodies during pregnancy and compared their experiences to those of other women. Furthermore, women also exchanged treatments and provided recipes of their own. Amelie de Nassau requested her sister to 'send me the recipes for the powders that we had in Holland of rosehip, and the quantity, for madame the Electrice'.[35] For sore breasts, Elisabeth reassured her sister Charlotte-Brabantine with the advice of her physicians, at the same time promising to send her personal remedies: 'I will send them to you straightaway ... I know that he made me use rosewater'.[36]

However, discussions of maternity are not to be found in all female correspondence. Letters to women who had not borne children often seem like those addressed to men. Flandrine de Nassau, a nun, does not enter into detailed reproductive discussion with her sisters nor offer advice to them, although like their husbands she followed the course of each pregnancy with interest. This suggests that women did not offer advice because they felt that they shared innate female reproductive knowledge but rather because of their personal experience of pregnancy. They did not understand their experiences as universal but rather in ways that suggest they were historically, culturally and personally constructed. The letters they passed among themselves were in fact their means to understanding the female body by building upon the knowledge each offered through her own experience.

The norms of pregnancy

Women offered comfort and support in their letters for what pregnant women were undergoing and related their own experiences to reassure them. This functioned as an important method of verification about what was 'normal' bodily behaviour during pregnancy, and gave women some assurance. Correspondence of women became a producer of corporal norms. Elisabeth de Nassau seems to have suffered in most of her pregnancies. To her sister Charlotte-Brabantine she complained: 'my great belly hinders me greatly ... as I am in my eighth month ... being reasonably healthy, except that I cannot move about as I am so heavy and the oppression of my stomach with this thing that I carry about like a sack'.[37] Several years later, she remarked to her 'the closer one reaches to the end, the more inconvenient it is'.[38] Louise de Coligny related her observations of a young Marie de Medici's vigorous exercise regime in pregnancy to an also pregnant Charlotte-Brabantine.

> When I see the Queen and the discomforts she suffers, I think of you and of those that you suffer. It is true that you are not as big as she, for she is in her eighth month, but that does not stop her from acts that no other woman would take; for the King makes her take walks each day which makes us all ill and so annoyed that we can't stand it any longer, but Her Majesty seems to feel no discomfort in all that.[39]

The French monarch recommended a physically active pregnancy, much as in the previous chapter we saw Catherine de Medici had advised for her daughter Elisabeth in the 1560s. This information on the state of health and experience of other women was designed to comfort Charlotte-Brabantine. The collection of other women's similar experiences allowed women to create their own ideas about their body's behaviour.

Inevitably, things went wrong during pregnancies.[40] Catherine de Bourbon wrote unhappily to Henri IV of her miscarriage: 'Two days ago I realised that it was only a false pregnancy, from which I have been ill and have hardly the strength to finish this letter.'[41] 'The truth is that I lost it, they dared not tell my husband, I have cried so much about it.'[42] Women speculated about the causes of their miscarriages. Travelling on horseback or by coach was commonly considered to be harmful to a foetus. Charlotte Arbaleste bore stillborn twins during a particularly dangerous birth in which she was so convinced she would perish that she made her final religious declaration as a Huguenot. She concluded that her babies had died as a result of a long coach trip she undertook while heavily pregnant: 'I was of the opinion that the work of this journey on the cobblestones ruined my pregnancy. As in fact, some time after, with an incredible danger to my life, . . . I was delivered in Rouen of two sons that I had retained dead for some time in my belly'.[43] Women clearly knew such violent movement as bumpy road travel could be dangerous to both women and their unborn children.

When in 1526 a pregnant Guillelme Delprat was pushed to the ground in a fight to resist a tax collector at Fronton, near Toulouse, she gave birth prematurely to a baby girl who died soon after. Several days later she delivered more body parts, perhaps those of a second child, and it looked as though she would die herself. The ensuing court case provides a testimonial record of how contemporaries perceived the course of Guillelme's pregnancy, and how the violent action affected it. Guillelme's mother, Astruga Descampes, testified about the birth of the first child, that the girl 'had the left arm broken, all black and putrid, and also her back, from the waist to the fundament, broken, black and putrid ... and the said Guillelme was so ill that she feared she would die of the birth as well.'⁴⁴ When Guillelme was interviewed by the notary, she gave her version of events: 'that since she had given birth, Tuesday morning, she had had no rest as she felt broken in her kidneys and belly, and today, as her mother Astruga Descampes and Leurta Malberta had seen, she had given birth to another fruit, she knew not what, but the said Descampes and Leurta had gathered it up.' She speculated that 'she must have been pregnant with two creatures and that one of the two was killed when she fell in the room against the table when the sergeant pushed her. The said dead creature must have rotted in her belly so that she could only be delivered of it in pieces'.⁴⁵ The notary later examined 'in a lid of a broken pot, what they [Descampes and Malberta] affirmed under oath, to have found in the bed from between the thighs of the said Guillelme del Prat.' In their presence and also that of Jehanne Pailhera, 'expert and deliverer of children', the remains were examined. A group of neighbours, bystanders and investigators all testified that this was indeed the head and shoulders of a second child.⁴⁶

Women advocated that situations causing emotional stress were also to be avoided. 'They say that one must be happy to have one', wrote Catherine de Bourbon.⁴⁷ The female biographer of the Huguenot noblewoman Léonor de Condé concluded that the premature birth of stillborn twin boys and Léonor's death had been caused both by travel and the violent mob who had frightened her: 'This fury and popular rage moved this good Lady in such a way, that being at the end of her eighth month, she gave birth the same day to two sons by fright and before term ... without having the leisure to reach any of her houses.'⁴⁸ Emotional disturbances were commonly believed to have dangerous impact on the pregnant woman's body, as Ulinka Rublack's research on early modern Germany has demonstrated.⁴⁹ Similarly, Catherine de Medici was concerned that her daughter not be disturbed emotionally during her pregnancy, writing angrily back to reports that Spanish courtiers were concerned with making Elisabeth de Valois write her final testament: 'I am pained by what you have written me of the testament and it seems to me that these are things which one must not afflict and destroy the spirit of a young woman, being in the state of madame my daughter.'⁵⁰

The timing of birth

One of the most difficult issues to determine was when exactly a woman was to give birth. Although most people expected that gestation lasted nine months, they did not deny the possibility of both longer and shorter terms. Rabelais made Gargantua's gestation eleven months, highlighting the debate still underway within the medical faculties. Part of the problem was no one wanted to refute the ancients such as Hippocrates and Aristotle who, in his *Generation of Animals*, had argued that children could be born at seven months, eight months or at nine months, and as an extreme at ten months. He argued that there were even some examples of births at eleven months.[51] Laurent Joubert like others found the most plausible solution was to suggest that the ancients had been calculating according to lunar not solar months, which would account for the longer terms. Jurists too were involved, since it was necessary to determine whether children born of seven- or eleven-month terms were entitled to inherit from the paternal line.[52]

Women assumed that most pregnancies would last nine months, though they knew that they could end earlier. In November 1608, Elisabeth de Nassau's rapidly growing belly made her distrust her own calculations and believe she would give birth sooner. She composed a letter to her sister in order to obtain her advice: 'I should give birth on the fifth or sixth of the month of January to go to nine full months and yet I'm of the opinion that I will not make it past December'.[53] It is clear that Elisabeth had difficulty determining how long she had been pregnant, and frequently asked her sister Charlotte-Brabantine's opinion. In 1608 she thought she was 'in my eighth month, if I am not mistaken, since eight days ago'.[54] It mattered because she wanted to return to her house to give birth, call her husband to be near her and to choose a midwife as she explained in 1600 to Charlotte-Brabantine: 'I wish to be there before my eighth month for fear of any accidents that I could have in this pregnancy'.[55]

Pregnancy raised another question: how to determine when a woman fell pregnant, so as to calculate precisely at what stage of pregnancy she was? The case of Elisabeth de Nassau demonstrates that women had difficulty determining when pregnancy began.[56] Neither women nor physicians suggested the cessation of menstruation as a definitive sign of pregnancy. Yet it does not seem possible that they were unfamiliar with the connection between menstruation and pregnancy. One may suggest perhaps that women of the era experienced menstruation as an irregular event due to frequent pregnancies and therefore as a poor sign of conception. Physicians based the beginning of gestation from other indications. The royal physician, Jean Fernel, interpreted the reaction of a mixture of white wine and urine.[57] Later physicians were critical of the efficacy of urine, as was Guillemeau: 'such signs are by no means certain'.⁵⁸ Jacques du Val criticised impatient women who, 'curious to know if they had conceived', called upon midwives who pressed so hard as to produce a miscarriage.⁵⁹ He listed a number of symptoms that might indicate conception, including 'a compression and tightening of the mouth of the womb', 'some little pain around the navel', 'a little chill at the neck, heaviness of the tongue, so the woman is seen to stutter in speaking'.⁶⁰ In 1470, Marie de Valois wrote hopefully to her husband about her observations of her swelling belly 'for since your departure my belly has grown and I am sure it is a son for I have not slept at all.'⁶¹

The most certain sign that women (and Du Val) relied upon was the quickening occurring usually in the third or fourth month. Louise de Coligny hesitated to announce to Charlotte-Brabantine de Nassau the pregnancy of a friend who 'thinks to be in the same state as you, although she has not felt the child move'.⁶² Charlotte-Brabantine wrote to her husband of her hesitation to announce her first pregnancy in July 1598:

> Two or three days ago I thought I felt it move a little, but yesterday in the evening madamoiselle d'Averly felt it move perfectly so she said. She did not want, nor me either, to leave it any longer without sharing with you a thing which has brought me so much happiness and that I know, Monsieur, will bring no less to you.⁶³

Even when Charlotte-Brabantine felt the child move, she did not know whether this was the sign that she had heard spoken of. She had to wait for confirmation of her sensations by a more experienced woman. The letters of Elisabeth de Nassau suggest that she judged her state by looking at her belly. In May 1605, she announced to Charlotte-Brabantine that her pregnancy was not 'as my other pregnancies, when I grew large, for I am astonished with how little this one is and often I wonder if I will feel it at all, were I close to the time when I should feel it'.⁶⁴

If the most certain sign was the quickening, which occurred around the third or fourth month, this left almost a month or two either way. If women used the quickening to confirm that they were pregnant, they did not start their counting from that point onwards. Both women and men talked of gestation as typical nine months in length, and at quickening, expected the birth in approximately five to six months time. Therefore, when in December 1541 Perrette Postolle, a servant and chambermaid at Saint Marcel, assumed herself pregnant and entered negotiations with the father of her unborn child Claude Mymy, to protect the child's future, she stated in the notarial act that 'she says that she is at present pregnant with a child of three months'.⁶⁵ In March 1542, when a second agreement was passed between them, she confirmed her counting of the gestation 'she says that she is pregnant with a child of six months or about that'.[66] In the court case that followed Guillelme Delprat's premature delivery and death of twins in 1526, Leurta Malberta, a neighbour who had been present through the deliveries, was asked to provide her opinion on the matter. She argued that Delprat 'was not at full term, it was not more than six or seven weeks since she had begun to feel life in the creature or creatures, and she thus had more than three months before giving birth'.[67]

The women of the Nassau family speculated among themselves about the exact date that they had fallen pregnant. Louise de Coligny wrote to Charlotte-Brabantine at the time of her first pregnancy in 1598: 'Truly you have the advantage over all your sisters to have begun so well and so quickly. What, ten days after being married? For certain, I think it was the very day that we ate so well on your bed'.[68] The Nassau letters talk constantly of the date of the birth, often because they hoped their sisters might be with them during the birth. Louise de Coligny, stepmother of Charlotte-Brabantine, wrote disappointedly to her in 1598: 'Dear daughter, I am so disappointed not to be at the birth which I think will be in eight days... No, it is certain that I will not pardon your husband for a long time for being the cause that I should not be near to you, at the hour when I think I might have render you a great deal of service'.[69] In the absence of dates in their letters, Louise sought elsewhere among her friends for information: 'I am waiting to see Madame de Givry, to learn particularly of your news and the date when you should have the baby.'[70]

Elisabeth seems to have had many difficulties in following the progress of her pregnancies and consequently the date of childbirth. Even before the example cited at the beginning of the chapter, she had already made errors in her timing. In January 1609, her husband 'arrived home Friday in good health, and found me still with my great belly, against my opinion which was to give birth at the end of the last month, and yet I keep rolling on'.[71] So when, in 1611, she sought to recall her husband to await the delivery, he was sceptical. She then wrote a long letter to her sister in July to send her explanations and justifications for her calculations in order to confirm her logic and knowledge:

> me close to three or four days into my ninth month, have always hoped to see it arrive at the beginning of this month and, for all the consolation that you say, my dear, that I will have it on the fourth or fifth of this coming month, you would have me live with this thing which kills me, such a long term and which carries such heavy

weight... I tell you this to comfort me, my dear, and so that you change your calculations which destroy me.[72]

It is significant that women conferred authority upon other women to help determine the time of birth. Elisabeth sought the opinion of Charlotte-Brabantine, an experienced mother, to help her to determine her delivery date and, furthermore, to convince her husband of the validity of her calculations.

> If it is possible, good sister, in the name of God, deliver me from this and make my husband trust more in my calculations than his own, and that he does not judge it a longer term than the end of August. I fear that being once mistaken in my count of the pregnancy of my little plain Jane, he does not want to make a presumption and draws the conclusion that I could be ready even now, but that will not happen if one gives birth at the end of nine months and it is extraordinary to go ten, but usual to not go further than nine. For two or three of my children, I gave birth five or six days sooner than my count.[73]

Since all calculations depended on when a woman had recognised her pregnancy, it is probable that women knew of experiences where women had seemingly had gestations of ten or eleven months.

Even ten years later, in 1622, Elisabeth could again write to her sister of her doubts about the timing of her daughter's confinement: 'She thinks she will enter her seventh month at the beginning of this coming month. That would be to give birth at the end of February or beginning of March, according to her count; but she was so mistaken in her first pregnancy that I fear that she does the same in this second one'.[74] The state of pregnancy and consequently its duration was a persistent problem that confronted generations of women.[75] What is so significant about this discussion of gestation is at no point did Elisabeth or Charlotte-Brabantine mention consulting their favoured physician, François Louis, even though they frequently asked his advice on other reproductive issues. By contrast, Elisabeth consults her sister alone for her advice and assumes that her opinion will be authoritative to her husband.

The experience of birth

Evelyne Berriot-Salvadore has observed that women rarely spoke of their experiences in birth.[76] Generally this is true: women did not go into to detail about what happened to their bodies during this time, perhaps because they thought women already understood what birth entailed.

What was important was not the experience of the birth itself but the end result: the sex of the child and the health of the mother and child. Louise-Julienne, the Electrice Palatine, wrote to her younger sister Charlotte-Brabantine:

> I can't wait to know your news to hear how you behaved in your delivery and how my little nephew whom I love with all my heart is. I've also given you a little niece whom I gave birth to on the 26 of this past month, she and I are both well, thanks be to God, I have to say, dear sister that you have won the prize over us all to have a son first.[77]

The Nassau letters frequently contained information of births within the family or among their immediate friends. Louise-Julienne expressed her concerns for the Countess of Hanau: 'I wait each day for news of the confinement of my sister the Countess of Hanau ... my aunt ... is near her for this, God be so good as to give her a healthy son'.[78]

Often it was a husband or relative who announced the birth to family and friends. As Elisabeth wrote to her sister Charlotte-Brabantine after a birth in 1602: 'I will say nothing to you particularly of all that I did in labour and during the birth, having been sent all that in detail both by my dear Monsieur and by Mademoiselle d'Oserqueque'.[79] Women were thus amazed if the recovering mother took the trouble to take up the pen herself: 'I admire that you've written to me so soon after your great pains, and so well',[80] wrote Louise de Coligny to her step-daughter Charlotte-Brabantine after the birth of her son in 1598. Just over a year later, she was again surprised when Charlotte-Brabantine wrote to her husband herself: 'So you have given me a little girl! My God, I imagine she is pretty and you so brave to have written so soon, after such pains, to your dear husband'.[81]

As the last remark indicated, all recognised the birth experience as a treacherous one. 'Madame de Monceaux [Gabrielle d'Estrées] thought she would die in her confinement; her child is dead',[82] wrote Elisabeth to Charlotte-Brabantine in 1595. Amelie de Nassau wrote to her elder sister Charlotte-Brabantine about Louise-Julienne's delivery in 1601:

> Madame the Electrice had a lovely little prince on Thursday ... but God moderated our joy for she was extremely ill and then as the child was born he was in such a pitiful state that he was judged more dead than alive. The Lord showed us his grace however and fortified him in such a fashion that two or three hours after he regained his natural colour.[83]

Elisabeth de Nassau in particular was known in her family to have particular difficulties in childbirth, as she put it, 'the extreme pains which are usual to me in all my deliveries'.[84] Even their friends discussed the births, as did Philippe Duplessis-Mornay who wrote to his wife Charlotte Arbaleste in 1597 of Elisabeth's unhappy delivery:

> Madame his wife was twenty-two days in extremity with a continual fever; she is out of danger now but her husband is in great pain for they hid the death of the son from her and now she demands to see him.[85]

Amelie discussed one of Elisabeth's recent deliveries with Charlotte-Brabantine: 'she was very ill from what her husband sent Louise both before and after the birth, . . . I pray God with all my heart to strengthen her and to ease her pains'.[86]

Yet although they too had experienced childbirth, frequently the Nassau sisters and their stepmother asked for more detail about what had occurred during the birth. Louise de Coligny wrote to Charlotte-Brabantine in 1598: 'I would like to have seen you and heard what you said in your pains'.[87] In 1603 she wrote again to Charlotte-Brabantine, this time to obtain information about Elisabeth's delivery:

> I am sending, my daughter, this porter on purpose, to report to me the details of Madame de Bouillon. I think her, by this time, to have given birth, and I don't doubt that it will give her infinite happiness to have you close to her, and to you to be able to bring her some comfort, in all her pains, which I know are not small.[88]

Elisabeth's child died shortly after birth. Women did not hide their physical suffering during childbirth. Amelie de Nassau was frank to Charlotte-Brabantine of her pain both during and after the birth of her son in 1622: 'the pains which I suffered were so great . . . the birth was very painful having no rest in either my body or spirit to regain my strength'.[89]

It is also in their advice to their sisters preparing for a birth that we understand how the Nassau women experienced their deliveries. Elisabeth and Charlotte-Brabantine exchanged remedies to make the birth smoother. In particular, both placed confidence in the eagle stone.[90] The stone, believed to help the delivery, was known by contemporary physicians although they were unsure of its efficacy. Du Val was ambiguous in his approval for such remedies, advising that:

> You will tie the eagle stone . . . to the inside of the thigh . . . the skin of a snake around the stomach. And if she can have a belt made of leather from the beast that is called an elk, she will also tie that around

her thigh. But as soon as she is delivered, they must all be removed, because these remedies which have an occult ability to draw the womb lower could be dangerous.'[91]

Although these treatments did not form part of university medicine, physicians were unwillingly to discount the possibility that they assisted women in childbirth. The Parisian physician Charles Huart recorded possession of such a preciously guarded stone in his inventory, described thus: 'a little white box on the lid of which is written these words: "Stone called Diadu which is proved to help hasten the delivery of women" in which is found the said piece attached to a green taffeta'.[92]

Elisabeth and Charlotte-Brabantine also exchanged other advice, recipes and remedies for smooth deliveries. In 1602, Elisabeth advised her sister: 'I advise you to give birth standing, the labour is much shorter'. Elisabeth also offered remedies for contractions: 'I send you these remedies which I used for the contractions, which did not torment me at all'.[93] In 1596, Elisabeth recovered from one birth with the assistance of both domestic and university medicine, as she wrote to Charlotte-Brabantine: 'I have not left my room yet, even though I am well, having been well looked after by M. Louis the physician. This is not without using lots of recipes'.[94] Elisabeth also sought the advice of Louis her physician, but it was the fact that she had already tried the remedies of her doctor and her recommendations that gave them authority. 'I will send you my remedies which you can use lacking any better ones; but I found them very good and desire you to do the same.'[95]

Similarly, when Charlotte-Brabantine suffered a miscarriage in 1605, Elisabeth sought the opinion of her physician, Louis:

> I wanted to have that of M. Louis the physician on the report that you had sent me, he thinks, that . . . there is some melancolic humour . . . he approves of a bleeding of the foot . . . the best is that which I fear you find the most difficult: leeches, but I was ready to use them on my hæmorrhoids from which I suffered after my deliveries, without which I should still be in great pain.'[96]

To attest to the validity of Louis's theories, Elisabeth reported her own experience of the remedies, suggesting that her experience was a valid claim for medical authority. To the theoretical knowledge of the physicians, Elisabeth also added her own seal of approval to her sister: 'by the advice of the physicians, . . . you must not become pregnant soon and you must recover completely first. I approve their advice'.[97] Here, between women, it was the mother who approved the advice of male physicians, and not the reverse.

This chapter has examined female knowledge during the various stages of pregnancy and childbirth and has examined the sources of this female knowledge. What was the system of values and criteria of medical validity that elite women followed in what concerned their bodies in pregnancy? Although women used university knowledge to understand their bodily function in part, it would be too simple to suggest that their approach to the body was entirely determined by this discourse.[98] It is true that the understanding that women in the Nassau family had of their body was specific to their historical context. Michel Foucault pursues the idea that it is these historically specific regimes of power that determine the discourses defining the meaning and understanding of the body.[99] It seems that, in this case, one of those discourses in the sixteenth century, outside of the medical community, was that of women's own experiences, the lived experiences of their bodies. The Nassau sisters did not accept without question what they could read in medical texts or what their physicians explained to them.

On the contrary, their knowledge derived in large part from the perceptions of their bodies, as they understood them.[100] A phenomenological approach like that of Maurice Merleau-Ponty could help to specify female notions of the body and their system of criteria for corporeal knowledge. Merleau-Ponty highlights the importance of the lived experience and the perceptions that stem from them in establishing valid criteria for bodily knowledge. Women in the sixteenth century seem to have used their perceptions to judge the pertinence of a more theoretical university medicine. His emphasis on the interrelatedness of mind and body reflects the pre-Cartesian manner in which women appear to have understood bodily experiences during pregnancy. For Merleau-Ponty the body is not an object, it is the condition and context through which one is able to have a relation to objects; it is immanent and transcendent. In his approach, he sees experience as a constructed, synthetic nature of experience, simultaneously passive and active, and attributes an incontestable importance to this experience in the inscription and subversion of socio-political values. These two concepts seem aligned to the axiological system of sixteenth-century women's bodily knowledge. As Toril Moi writes of Merleau-Ponty's notion, 'the human body is fundamentally *ambiguous*: it is subject at once to natural laws and to the human production of meaning, and it can never be reduced to either one of these elements'.[101]

The Nassau sisters' system of knowledge was not entirely exterior to their bodies, but linked to what they could feel through their bodies. They did absorb and accept certain aspects of obstetrical and gynaecological knowledge from the faculties, but also rejected other aspects, so as to create their own understandings based on their personal experiences and notions of their bodies. However, female knowledge of pregnancy was by no means innate, even if it relied on sensory perceptions of the body. These sensations were socially coded. Indeed, a young Charlotte-Brabantine had to call upon a mature older woman to confirm whether the movements she felt within her were indeed those of a child. From this perspective, the collection of other female experiences during pregnancy and childbirth, their transmission by word of mouth and for elite women through letters, provided women with an idea of what was normal for their body, and what they could expect. This exchange of information, stories and reassuring words gave women the means and basis that allowed them to formulate and justify a bodily knowledge of their own – one that was both individual to the particular experiences (bodily or otherwise) of the woman concerned, and shared elements with experiences and ideas of other women. The menstruating, pregnant and parturient bodies of these women influenced how they develop both subjectivity and reproductive theory, and in turn how those around them – husbands, physicians and so on – perceived these women and the validity of their bodily ideas and the legitimacy of their experiences.

Notes

1 *La Decoration dhumaine nature, et aornement des dames. Complie & extraict des tresexcellens docteurs & plus expers medicins, tant anciens que modernes, par maistre Andre Le Fournier, docteur regent en la faculte de medicine, en luniversite de paris, nouvelleme-t corrigee & Imprimee* (Lyon: Gilles & Iacques Huguetan, 1541) (Paris: Klincksieck, 1992), fols 28r–30v. See here Alison Klairmont Lingo, 'Santé et beauté féminines dans la France de la Renaissance', *Proceedings of the 110e Congrès national des sociétés savantes*, Section d'Histoire Moderne et Contemporaine (Le Corps et la Santé), 1 (1985), pp. 191–9.
2 J. Guiart, *Histoire de la médecine française: son passé, son présent, son avenir* (Paris: Nagel, 1947), p. 119.
3 Alison Klairmont Lingo, 'The fate of popular terms for female anatomy in the age of print', *French Historical Studies*, 22:3 (1999), pp. 335–49, p. 342.
4 Laurent Joubert, *La Médecine et le régime de santé, des erreurs populaires et propos vulgaires*, Livres 2, 3, 4, 5 (Bordeaux: Simon Millanges, 1578) ed. Madeleine Tiollais, vol. 2 (Paris: L'Harmattan, 1997), p. 25.
5 Joubert, *La Médecine et le régime de santé*, vol. 1, p. 29.
6 *L'Agriculture, et maison rustique de M. M. Charles Estienne, & Iean Liebault, Docteurs en Medecine* (Paris: Nicolas de la Vigne, 1640), p. 162.

7 Joubert, *La Médecine et le régime de santé*, vol. 2, p. 56.
8 F. Charpentier, 'Un royaume qui perdure sans femmes', in R. La Charité (ed.), *Rabelais's Incomparable Book: Essays on his Art* (Lexington, Kentucky: French Forum Publishers, 1986), p. 207.
9 *The Complete Works of François Rabelais*, trans. D. Frame (Berkeley: University of California Press, 1991), p. 184.
10 *Ibid.*, pp. 184–5.
11 E. Chesney Zegura, 'Toward a feminist reading of Rabelais', *Journal of Medieval and Renaissance Studies*, 15:1 (1985), p. 129.
12 See my paper, 'Rabelais, the pursuit of knowledge, and early modern gynaecology', *Limina: A Journal of Historical and Cultural Studies*, 4 (1998), pp. 24–34.
13 Jacques Guillemeau, *De l'heureux accouchement des femmes où il est traicté du gouvernement de leur grossesse, de leur travail naturel et contre nature, du traictement estant accouchées et de leurs maladies* (Paris: Nicolas Buon, 1609), p. 143.
14 Lesley Dean-Jones, 'Autopsia, historia and what women know: the authority of women in Hippocratic gynaecology', in Don Bates (ed.), *Knowledge and the Scholarly Medical Traditions* (Cambridge: Cambridge University Press, 1995), pp. 41–58.
15 Klairmont Lingo, 'The fate of popular terms for female anatomy', p. 338.
16 Joubert, *La Médecine et le régime de santé*, vol. 2, p. 46.
17 *Ibid.*, p. 50.
18 *Ibid.*, p. 167.
19 Barbara Duden, *The Woman Beneath the Skin: A Doctor's Patients in Eighteenth-Century Germany*, trans. Thomas Dunlap (Cambridge, Mass.: Harvard University Press, 1991), pp. 32–3.
20 *Lettres de Coras, de sa femme, de son fils & de ses amis*, ed. Charles Pradel (Albi: G.-M. Nouguiès, 1880), p. 5.
21 *Ibid.*, p. 5.
22 *Ibid.*, p. 6.
23 (Archives nationales (AN), Chartrier de Thouars, 1 AP 393, no 21) Evelyne Berriot-Salvadore, *Les Femmes dans la société française de la Renaissance* (Geneva: Droz, 1990), p. 484.
24 AN, Chartrier de Thouars, 1 AP 333, 1 October 1598.
25 H. de la Ferrière (ed.) *Les Chasses de François Ier racontées par Louis de Brézé*, Paris 1869, in Ivan Cloulas, *Diane de Poitiers* (Paris: Fayard, 1997), p. 374.
26 See my discussion of the sisters' letters in 'Lettres de Louise-Julienne de Nassau, d'Elisabeth de Nassau, et d'Amélie de Nassau à Charlotte-Brabantine de Nassau (1595–1601)' in *Lettres de Femmes (XVIe–XVIIIe siècle)*, eds Elizabeth Goldsmith and Colette H. Winn, forthcoming.
27 Laurence Brockliss and Colin Jones, *The Medical World of Early Modern France* (Oxford: Clarendon Press, 1997), p. 263.
28 Joubert, *La Médecine et le régime de santé*, vol. 1, p. 56.
29 'S. Millanges au lecteur' Bordeaux, 1579, in Joubert, *La Médecine et le régime de santé*, vol. 1, p. 60.
30 Jacques Sylvius, *Livre de la nature et utilité des moys des femmes, & de la curation des maladies qui en surviennent*, trans. Guillaume Christian (Paris: Guillaume Morel, 1559), pp. 104–5.

31 Jacques du Val, *Des Hermaphrodits, accouchemens des femmes, et traitement qui est requis pour les relever en santé, & bien élever leurs enfans* (Rouen: David Geuffroy, 1612), p. [53].

32 Gervais de La Tousche, *La Tres-Haute et Tres-Souveraine Science de l'art et industrie naturelle d'enfanter. Contre la maudicte et perverse impericie des femmes que l'on appelle saiges-femmes ou belles meres, lesquelles par leur ignorance font iournellement perir une infinité de femmes & d'enfans à l'enfantement. Adce que desormais toutes femmes enfantent heureusement, & sans aucun peril ny destourbier, tant d'elles que de leurs enfans, estant toutes saiges & perites en icelle science* (Paris: D. Millot, 1587), fol. 5v.

33 *Lettres de Louise de Coligny, Princesse d'Orange à sa belle-fille Charlotte-Brabantine de Nassau, Duchesse de la Trémoille*, ed. Paul Marchegay (Les Roches-Baritaud, Vendée: L. Gasté, 1872), p. 45. Where letters among the Nassau family are available in a printed edition, I have referenced citations to these works.

34 For discussion of a seventeenth-century birthing environment in England, see Adrian Wilson, 'Participant or patient? Seventeenth century childbirth from the mother's point of view', in Roy Porter (ed.), *Patients and Practitioners: Lay Perceptions of Medicine in Pre-Industrial Society* (Cambridge: Cambridge University Press, 1985), pp. 129–44, and 'The ceremony of childbirth and its interpretation', in Valerie A. Fildes (ed.), *Women as Mothers in Pre-Industrial England: Essays in Memory of Dorothy McLaren* (London: Routledge, 1990), pp. 68–107.

35 AN, Chartrier de Thouars, 1 AP 340, 22 August [1597].

36 AN, Chartrier de Thouars, 1 AP 333, 1 October 1598.

37 *Lettres d'Elisabeth de Nassau, Duchesse de Bouillon, à sa sœur Charlotte-Brabantine de Nassau, Duchesse de La Trémoille 1595–1628*, ed. Paul Marchegay (Les Roches-Baritaud, Vendée: L. Gasté, 1875), pp. 76–7.

38 Ibid., p. 89.

39 *Lettres de Louise de Coligny*, pp. 27–8.

40 See also Linda A. Pollock, 'Embarking on a rough passage: the experience of pregnancy in early modern society', in Fildes (ed.), *Women as Mothers in Pre-Industrial England*, pp. 39–67.

41 'Lettres inédites de Catherine de Bourbon', *Bibliothèque de l'Ecole des Chartes*, ed. E. Freville de Lorme, 18 (1857), p. 339.

42 'Lettres inédites de Catherine de Bourbon', p. 326.

43 *Mémoires et correspondance de Duplessis-Mornay*, vol. 1 (Paris: Treuttel et Würtz, 1824), p. 144.

44 Annie Charnay, *Paroles de voleurs: gens de sac et de corde en pays toulousain au début du XVIe siècle* (Paris: Champion, 1998), p. 319.

45 Ibid., p. 325.

46 Ibid., p. 325.

47 'Lettres inédites de Catherine de Bourbon', p. 338.

48 Anon., *Epistre d'une damoiselle françoise* (n.p. 1564), fol. Aiii r.

49 See Ulinka Rublack, 'Pregnancy, childbirth and the female body in early modern Germany', *Past and Present*, 150 (1996), pp. 84–110.

50 *Lettres de Catherine de Médicis*, vol. 2, ed. H. de la Ferrière (Paris: Imprimerie nationale, 1885), p. 362.

51 Aristotle, *Generation of Animals*, iv, 4.
52 Roland Antonioli, *Rabelais et la médecine*, Etudes Rabelaisiennes 12 (Geneva: Droz, 1976), p. 162.
53 AN, Chartrier de Thouars, 1 AP 333, 10 November 1608.
54 *Lettres d'Elisabeth de Nassau*, p. 76.
55 AN, Chartrier de Thouars, 1 AP 333, 5 October 1600.
56 On the difficulties of reading the female body in pregnancy, see Cathy McClive, 'The hidden truths of the belly: the uncertainties of pregnancy in early modern Europe', *Social History of Medicine*, 15:2 (2002), pp. 209–27.
57 Roger Bouissou, *Histoire de la médecine* (Paris: Larousse, 1967), p. 119.
58 Guillemeau, *De l'heureux accouchement des femmes*, pp. 9–10.
59 Du Val, *Des Hermaphrodits, accouchemens des femmes*, pp. 112–13.
60 *Ibid.*, p. 113.
61 *Lettres de Marie de Valois, fille de Charles VII et d'Agnès Sorel, à Olivier de Coetivy, sgr de Taillebourg, son mari 1458–1472*, ed. Paul Marchegay (Les Roches-Baritaud, Vendée: L. Gasté, 1875), p. 24.
62 *Lettres de Louise de Coligny*, p. 18.
63 Berriot-Salvadore, *Les Femmes dans la société française de la Renaissance*, p. 145.
64 AN, Chartrier de Thouars, 1 AP 333, 2 May 1605.
65 No 2161, *Recueil d'actes notariés relatifs à l'histoire de Paris et de ses environs au XVIe siècle, 1498–1545*, ed. E. Coyecque, vol. 1 (Paris: Imprimerie nationale, 1905), p. 406.
66 No 2237, *Ibid.*, p. 421.
67 Charnay, *Paroles de voleurs*, p. 335.
68 *Lettres de Louise de Coligny*, p. 4.
69 J. Delaborde, *Louise de Coligny, Princesse d'Orange*, vol. 1 (Geneva: Slatkine, 1970), p. 384.
70 Delaborde, *Louise de Coligny*, vol. 2, p. 12.
71 *Lettres d'Elisabeth de Nassau*, p. 89.
72 *Ibid.*, p. 92.
73 *Ibid.*, pp. 92–3.
74 *Ibid.*, p. 115.
75 See discussion of late births by the medical and legal communities of the seventeenth and eighteenth centuries in Lindsay Wilson, *Women and Medicine in the French Enlightenment: The Debate over* Maladies des femmes (Baltimore: The Johns Hopkins University Press, 1993).
76 Evelyne Berriot-Salvadore, *Un Corps, un destin: La femme dans la médecine de la Renaissance* (Paris: H. Champion, 1993), p. 143.
77 AN, Chartrier de Thouars, 1 AP 337, January 1594.
78 AN, Chartrier de Thouars, 1 AP 337, 16 August 1597.
79 AN, Chartrier de Thouars, 1 AP 333, 2 February 1602.
80 Delaborde, *Louise de Coligny*, vol. 1, p. 387.
81 *Ibid.*, p. 412.
82 Paul Marchegay, *Les Deux Duchesses, lettres de Madame de Bouillon à Madame de La Tremoille (1621–22), lettres du duc et de la duchesse de Bouillon à Charlotte-Brabantine de Nassau, 1595–1597* (Paris: Meyrueis, 1866), p. 28.
83 AN, Chartrier de Thouars, 1 AP 340, 30 September 1601.

84 AN, Chartrier de Thouars, 1 AP 333, 20 August [1604].
85 Delaborde, *Louise de Coligny*, p. 360.
86 AN, Chartrier de Thouars, 1 AP 340 2 January 1609.
87 *Lettres de Louise de Coligny*, p. 4.
88 Delaborde, *Louise de Coligny*, vol. 2, p. 58.
89 AN, Chartrier de Thouars, 1 AP 341, 30 August 1622.
90 *Lettres d'Elisabeth de Nassau*, p. 72.
91 Du Val, *Des Hermaphrodits, accouchemens des femmes*, p. 189.
92 Françoise Lehoux, *Le Cadre de vie des médecins parisiens aux XVIe et XVIIe siècles* (Paris: A. and J. Picard, 1976), p. 447.
93 AN, Chartrier de Thouars, 1 AP 333, 2 February 1602.
94 Delaborde, *Louise de Coligny*, vol. 1, pp. 343–4.
95 *Lettres d'Elisabeth de Nassau*, pp. 57–8.
96 Chartrier de Thouars, 1 AP 333, 7 February 1605.
97 AN, Chartrier de Thouars, 1 AP 333, 1601.
98 See a feminist critique of theories on the female bodies by Elizabeth Grosz, *Volatile Bodies: Toward a Corporeal Feminism* (Sydney: Allen and Unwin, 1994).
99 For discussion of Foucault's theories in the medical context, see Colin Jones and Roy Porter (eds), *Reassessing Foucault: Power, Medicine and the Body* (London: Routledge, 1994).
100 M. Merleau-Ponty, *Phénoménologie de la perception* (Paris: Gallimard, 1945), see *Première partie: le corps*. See also commentary and critique of Merleau-Ponty in Grosz, *Volatile Bodies*, p. 86.
101 Emphasis in the original. Toril Moi, *What is a Woman? And Other Essays* (Oxford: Oxford University Press, 1999), p. 69.

Afterword

The period 1460–1630, roughly speaking the sixteenth century, marked a point of evolution and innovation in the status of women's medical knowledge and practices, a transformation which combined both progress and regression.

One of the evolutions occurring in medicine at this period was the guild incorporation and encroachment into the domain of the university of particular medical services. This process conferred new status and recognition by the university and crown on certain groups of medical providers. For example, midwifery became a field of medical work accredited and supervised by the university medical body, which permitted the development of an occupational female medical identity in the vein of surgeons and apothecaries. However, incorporation did not provide midwives with status nor access to university medical knowledge equal to their licensed and faculty-approved male counterparts. Moreover, the effects of incorporation also reduced women's access to these other medical occupations, such as surgery and pharmacy.

The era saw the emergence of print as an instrument of rapid dissemination of medical ideas and practices. The press provoked new questioning about the transmission of knowledge among members of different groups, both within communities and to the whole population. In the medical context, the diffusion of texts exposed certain healthcare theories and practices to literate women, and brought recognition to particular female authors such as the midwife Louise Bourgeois. The press also brought to light female medical practices and knowledge not through women writers, but as they were observed and discussed by physicians such as Laurent Joubert and Jean Liébault, with mixed consequences for women's subsequent application of these medical theories.

As the moral and physical wellbeing of children was scrutinised ever closer in the period by moralists and medical authors alike, those who cared for children experienced transformations to their status and practices. The poor women who nursed orphan and foundling children saw their remuneration increase as substantial child-care programmes were implemented and endorsed by town councils across France. For those women who nursed and supervised the daily welfare of the royal children, though, a re-evaluation of the child brought new competitors into the nursery. Physicians made use of the new medium of print to transmit their notions of paediatric health, discipline and daily care to elite women. The household of the royal children served a site for patronage and advancement among varied providers of child care, and as a locus for measuring the legitimacy between those who appointed, supervised, or served. Maternal authority could provide some women with compelling authority in certain contexts and to particular communities, but by no means uniformly or universally.

Religious experiences and choices are key to developments in medicine during the period. The politics of Huguenot and Catholic healthcare providers led to the creation of sites of religiously segregated medical power between the court and faculties, as well as focus on particular medical research priorities such as Paracelsianism. The decision of the crown to assume control of hospital administration saw religious communities struggle to maintain traditional services and practices. Female nursing work provided continuity in the period against changes to hospital personnel in some areas from nuns to female servants and townswomen. Furthermore, spiritual healing beliefs were re-defined by the Council of Trent in ways that saw some women revered as saintly healers and others investigated for witchcraft. Medical practice and authority were thus both negotiable and always changeable according to the specific context of the moment.

A focus on women as practitioners can help to examine this phenomenon. The evidence and arguments presented here do not suggest that women were universally condemned for medical work because they were women, nor that a neat division of gender struggle existed between male and female practitioners. Women performed a wide range of medical work with a positive perception from a variety of different early modern communities. The villagers gave their support to the health services that Jeanne Lescallier provided for them; Lescallier's lawyer mobilised local support to defend her health-care work, which benefited the rural community, against the opposition of the local university faculty. The barber Jehan Estevent prepared the way for his divorced wife to continue his trade. At the highest level of society, female authors such as Marguerite de Navarre projected an image of women proud of their medical expertise. Learned men, such as the jurists René Choppin and Jean Coras, recognised the importance of female medical aid. Elite men like Olivier de Serres and the husbands of noblewomen encouraged and conferred authority upon their herbal and bodily knowledge. The king of Spain, Philip II, privileged the intimate maternal knowledge of Catherine de Medici, and placed it above that of his court physicians. Within the university medical community itself, the practices and knowledge of women were supported, though not without limitations. Women's botanical practices were approved in Liébault's work and discussion of female bodily knowledge in that of Laurent Joubert often amounts to accreditation of their expertise in that domain. The French physicians preferred to promote the reproductive knowledge of their French compatriots than that of their Spanish university counterparts. The divisions between medical service providers reflect myriad social differences and community identifications, whether religious, social level, regional, urban, linguistic, occupational or otherwise.

Gender then would seem to operate immensely flexibly. It does not appear to have an immutable effect as a social factor in early modern medicine. It was one of many factors, conditions and identities, like those mentioned above, that could influence how individual women experienced medical work in particular contexts in France during this period. Catherine de Medici serves as an example of how complex such factors could be. Although she was able to establish legitimacy for her reproductive knowledge to Philip in Spain as Elisabeth's mother, within the context of the French court, maternal authority provided little help in enabling her to contribute to child care in the royal nursery. Gender was one of many factors that produced this difference in medical situations in which women (or men) could participate. Contemporaries perceived Catherine through many different lens, of which being a woman was only one or a part: as a foreigner, as representative of the interests of France (by those in Spain), as a queen, as a widow, as a politician, as a young woman or experienced mother, and so on. The evidence of this study appears to support Toril Moi's argument that gender behaves in a relational way.[1] Clearly, gender was not always the most relevant element in some medical contexts for women. However, gender is certainly always in play at some level, and if this is the case, there can be little justification to ignore the rich possibilities offered by gender as an analytical tool in the production of histories of medicine: 'insofar as gender is implicated in all other social fields, it is always in principle a relevant factor in all social analysis'.[2]

This work has also sought particularly to re-define terminology used in histories of French medicine to be more inclusive of a wider medical framework. Here the term 'medicine' has been used to reflect both preventative and restorative health-care work and such terms as 'qualified', 'trained' and 'authorised' have been employed with precision of the legitimising community meant in that context. In doing so, the nature and perception of the medical work that was performed by many women, with approval from early modern communities, has been brought to prominence. For a majority of the population in early modern France, women were vital and dominant providers of medical services and care.

Re-defining medical work and its providers is by no means an issue only for historical debate. Modern Western medical arenas continue to define certain medical activities and their practitioners as 'official', 'professional', 'para-medical', 'alternative' or 'domestic', for example. Some of these demarcations in medical activities follow frameworks established at least as early as the early modern era. By discovering and highlighting methods developed in the past that defined some technologies and knowledge as valid in particular contexts from other modes of learning and knowledge, research into European medical systems of the past can be key to an understanding of the ongoing privileging of certain health science domains today, of the way we recognise and value certain skills, practices and knowledge as medical. Historical studies can offer some explanations not only for the ongoing gendering of medical tasks, but also the acceptance (including recognition and funding) accorded to some medical service providers and their practices (for example, those produced within the university domain) over others (such as aged and child care-giving health work performed in the household forum). Historical research of this kind can encourage the development of flexible new methodologies to assess and incorporate work in so-called 'alternative and para-medical fields' in past societies. These methodologies might also prove beneficial today, by helping us to recognise and value innovative knowledge and technology from varied communities into the future.

Notes

1 Toril Moi, *What is a Woman? And Other Essays* (Oxford: Oxford University Press, 1999), p. 288.
2 *Ibid.*, p. 291.

Select bibliography

Manuscript sources

ARCHIVES NATIONALES
(Chartrier de Thouars)
1 AP 251 Lettres et documents concernant Anne de Laval
1 AP 255 Lettres missives de Charlotte, religieuse à Fontevrault et Jacqueline, comtesse de Sancerre
1 AP 330 et 331 Lettres de Charlotte-Brabantine de Nassau Lettres à son mari, à son fils
1 AP 333 (1595–1609), 334 (1610–18), 335 (1619–22) et 336 (1623–28) Lettres d'Elisabeth de Nassau à Charlotte-Brabantine de Nassau
1 AP 337 et 338 (1597–1628) Lettres de Louise-Julienne de Nassau, électrice palatine à Claude et Charlotte-Brabantine de Tremoille
1 AP 339 (1602–35) Lettres de Flandrine de Nassau à Charlotte-Brabantine
1 AP 340 (1601–35) et 341 (1613–28) Lettres d'Amélie de Nassau à Charlotte-Brabantine
1 AP 342 Lettres de Louise de Coligy à Charlotte-Brabantine
1 AP 566 Lettres de Marie de Valois, femme d'Olivier de Coétigny

BIBLIOTHÈQUE NATIONALE
BN Ms Baluze 222 Playdr de M. Matras et Marion sur une femme qui exercoit la Medecine en lannee 1573, fols 1–11.
BN Ms Fr. 21737 18 avril 1578, Arrest notable qui defend a une femme d'Anjou d'exercer la medecine, fols 302–309.

ARCHIVES DÉPARTEMENTALES D'INDRE ET LOIRE
H dépôt 1/23 Amboise Hôtel-Dieu, livres de comptes 1470–1565
H dépôt 4/88 Tours Charité, Délibérations du bureau, 1563–67
H dépôt 4/89 Tours Charité, Délibérations du bureau, 1564–68
H dépôt 4/167 Tours Charité, Comptes du receveur, 1554–55
H dépôt 4/218 Tours Hôtel-Dieu, Comptes du receveur, 1583
1 J 1165 *Les déclarations faites à la chapelle de Sainte Catherine de Fierbois, près de Sainte-Maure en Touraine, de 245 miracles arrivés de 1375 à 1536*

ARCHIVES MUNICIPALES DE TOURS
GG 2–8 Documents des hospices, hôpitaux, aumônes de Tours 1560–1600
GG 20 Documents de Sanitas 1563–99

BIBLIOTHÈQUE MUNICIPALE DE REIMS
MS 1081, liasse 4, Procès contre Isabelle Estevent, fols. 7–13, 69v, 115v.

Printed sources

Chartularium Universitatis Parisiensis, ed. H. Denifle, 4 vols (1891–99) (Brussels: Culture et Civilisation, 1964).

Commentaires de la Faculté de Médecine de l'Université de Paris (1395–1516), vol. 1 ed. C. A. E. Wickersheimer (Paris: Imprimerie Nationale, 1915), vol. 2 (1516–1560) ed. Marie Concasty (Paris: Imprimerie Nationale, 1964).

Epistre d'une damoiselle françoise (n.p., 1564).

Le Grand Calendrier et compost des bergers (Troyes: 1494).

Le Grand Kalendrier et compost des bergiers (Paris, Alain Lotrian, [15??]).

Index Chronologicus Chartarum pertinentium ad historiam Universitatis Parisiensis ad ejus originibus ad finem decimi sexti sæculi, ed. C. Jourdain (Paris, 1862) (Brussels: Culture et Civilisation, 1966).

Livre des miracles de Sainte-Catherine-de-Fierbois, ed. Yves Chauvin, vol. 60 (Poitiers: Société des Archives historiques de Poitou, 1976).

Le Mesnagier de Paris, eds Georgina E. Brereton and Janet M. Ferrier (trans) Karin Ueltschi (Paris: Livre de Poche, 1994).

Négociations, lettres et pièces diverses relatives au règne de François II, ed. L. Paris (Paris: Imprimerie Nationale, 1841).

Vie et miracles de la bienheureuse Philippe de Chantemilan, ed. Ulysse Chevalier (Valence: Jules Céas, 1894).

Arbaleste, Charlotte, *et al.*, *Mémoires et correspondance de Duplessis-Mornay* (Paris: Treuttel et Wurtz, 1824).

Beaujeu, Anne de, *A la requeste de treshaulte et puissante ma dame Susanne de Bourbon* (Lyons: [Pierre de Sainte Lucie, 1534]).

Beaujeu, Anne de, *Les Enseignements d'Anne de France Duchesse de Bourbonnois et d'Auverge à sa fille Susanne de Bourbon*, ed. A-M. Chazaud (Moulins: C. Desrosiers, 1878) (Marseille: Lafitte, 1978).

Bodin, Jean, *De la démonomanie des sorciers* (1580) (Paris: Jacques du Puys, 1587).

Bouchet, Guillaume, *Les Serées*, Premier Livre (1584) ed. C. E. Roybet, 6 vols (Paris: Alphonse Lemerre, 1873–82).

Bourbon, Catherine de, 'Lettres inédites', ed. E. Freville de Lorme, *Bibliothèque de l'Ecole des Chartes*, 18 (1857), 127–52, 325–45.

Bourgeois, Louise, *Observations diverses sur la sterilité, perte de fruicts, foecondité, accouchemens, et maladies des femmes et enfants nouveaux naiz* (1609) (Paris: Abraham Saugrain, 1617).

—— *Observations diverses sur la sterilité perte de fruict foecondité accouchements et Maladies des femmes et enfants nouveaux naiz. Amplement traictees et heureusement praticquées par L. Bourgeois dite Boursier Sage Femme de la Roine* (Paris: Jean Dehoury, 1710).

—— *Recueil de secrets choisis et eprouvez pour diverses maladies, principalement celles des Femmes, & pour leur embellissement, Louïse Bourgeois, dite Boursier,*

Sage-femme de la Reyne Marie de Medicis (1635) (Paris: Laurent d'Houry, 1710).

—— *Apologie de Louyse Bourgeois dite Bourcier sage femme de la Royne Mere du Roy, & de feu Madame. Contre le Rapport des Medecins* (Paris: Melchior Mondiere, 1627).

—— *Récit véritable de la naissance de Messeigneurs et Dames les enfans de France, Instruction à ma fille et autres textes*, eds Francois Rouget and Colette H. Winn (Geneva: Droz, 2000).

Choppin, René, *Traicte des privileges des personnes vivans aux champs* in *Les Oeuvres de Me René Choppin* (Paris: P. Ménard, 1663).

Colbert, Charles, *Rapport sur l'Anjou*, in *Archives d'Anjou: Recueil de documents et memoires inédits sur cette province*, ed. Paul Marchegay, vol. 1 (Angers: Charles Labussière, 1843).

Coligny, Louise de, *Lettres de Louise de Coligny, Princesse d'Orange à sa belle-fille Charlotte-Brabantine de Nassau, Duchesse de la Trémoille*, ed. Paul Marchegay (Les Roches-Baritaud, Vendée: L. Gasté, 1872).

Colin, Sébastien, *Lordre et regime qu'on doit garder et tenir en la cure des fievres* (Poitiers: Enguilbert de Marnef, 1558).

Coras, Jean de, et al., *Lettres de Coras, de sa femme, de son fils & de ses amis*, ed. Charles Pradel (Albi, G-M. Nouguiès, 1880).

Crespin, Jean, *Histoire des martyrs persecutez pour la verité de l'évangile, depuis le temps des apostres jusques a present* (1619) 3 vols (Toulouse: Société des Livres religieux, 1885, 1887, 1889).

des Roches, Mesdames, *Les Oeuvres* (1578) ed. A. Larsen (Geneva: Droz, 1993).

—— *Les Secondes Oeuvres de Mes-dames des Roches de Poictiers, Mere et Fille* (Poitiers: Nicolas Courtoys, 1583).

du Bois, Jacques, Guillaume Chrestian (trans.) *Livre de la nature et utilité des moys des femmes, & de la curation des maladies qui en surviennent* (Paris: Guillaume Morel, 1559).

du Breil, André, *La Police de l'art et science de medecine, contenant la refutation des erreurs, & insignes abus, qui s'y commettent pour le iourd'huy* (Paris: Leon Cavellat, 1580).

du Laurens, Jeanne, *Genealogie de Messieurs du Laurens descrite par moy Jeanne du laurens veufve a Monsieur Gleyse et couchée nayvement en ces termes*, ed. Charles de Ribbe, *Une famille au XVIe siècle* (Paris: Joseph Albanel, 1868).

du Val, Jacques, *Des hermaphrodits, accouchemens des femmes, et traitement qui est requis pour les relever en santé, & bien élever leurs enfans* (Rouen: David Geuffroy, 1612).

du Verger, Mesdames, *Le Verger fertile des vertus* (Paris: François Jacquin, 1595).

Estienne, Nicole, *Misères et grandeur de la femme au XVIe siècle*, ed. I. Zinguer (Geneva: Slatkine, 1982).

Fourquevaux, Raymond de Beccarie de Pavie, Bon de, *Dépêches de M. de Fourquevaux, ambassadeur du roi, Charles IX en Espagne, 1565–1572*, ed. C. Douais, vol. 1 (Paris: Ernest Leroux, 1896).

Galen, *De L'usage des parties du corps humains Livres XVII, escriptes par Claude Galien, & traduicts fidellement du Grec en François*, trans. Claude Dalechamps (Lyon: Guillaume Roville, 1566).

Glanville, Barthélemy de, *La Grand Proprietaire de toutes choses. Tresutile et profitable pour tenir le corps humain en santé. Contenant plusieurs diverses maladies, & dont ilz procedent, & aussi le remedes preservatifz*, trans. Jean Corbichon (Paris: Jean Ruelle, 1556).

[Guillemeau, Charles], *Remonstrance à Madame Bourcier, touchant son Apologie, contre le Rapport que les medecins ont fait, de ce qui a causé la mort deplorable de Madame* (Paris: Julian Jacquin, 1627).

Guillemeau, Jacques, *De l'heureux accouchement des femmes où il est traicté du gouvernement de leur grossesse, de leur travail naturel et contre nature, du traictement estant accouchées et de leurs maladies* (Paris: Nicolas Buon, 1609).

—— *Les Oeuvres de chirurgie* (1612) (Rouen: Jean Viret, François Vaultier, Clement Malassis, Jacques Besongne, 1649).

—— *Child-Birth or, The Happy Delivery of Women* (London: A. Hatfield, 1612).

Henri IV, *Recueil des lettres missives de Henri IV*, ed. M Berger de Xivrey, 7 vols (Paris: Imprimerie Royale, 1843–58).

Héroard, Jean, *Journal de Jean Héroard*, ed. Madeleine Foisil, 2 vols (Paris: Fayard, 1989).

Joubert, Laurent, *La Médecine et le régime de santé, des erreurs populaires et propos vulgaires*, Livre I (Bordeaux: Simon Millanges, 1578) ed. Madeleine Tiollais, 2 vols (Paris: L'Harmattan, 1997).

—— *Chirurgie de M. Gui de Chauliac* (Lyon: Estienne Michel, 1580).

La Brosse, Guy de, *De la nature, vertu, et utilité des plantes* (Paris: Rollin Baragnès, 1628).

La Tousche, Gervais de, *La Tres-Haute et Tres-Souveraine Science de l'art et industrie naturelle d'enfanter. Contre la Maudicte et Perverse impericie des femmes que l'on appelle saiges-femmes ou belles meres, lesquelles par leur ignorance font iournellement perir une infinité de femmes & d'enfans à l'enfantement. Adce que desormais toutes femmes enfantent heureusement, & sans aucun peril ny destourbier, tant d'elles que de leurs enfans, estant toutes saiges & perites en icelle science* (Paris: Didier Millot, 1587).

Le Caron, Louis, *De la Tranquilité d'Esprit, Livre Singulier, plus un discours sur le procès criminel faict à une sorcière condamnée à mort par Arrest de la Court de Parlement* (Paris: Jacques Du Puy, 1588).

Le Fournier, André, *La Decoration dhumaine nature, et aornement des dames. Compilé & extrait des tresexcellens docteurs & plus expers medicins, tant anciens que modernes, par maistre Andre Le Fournier, docteur regent en la faculte de medicine, en luniversite de paris, nouvellement corrigee & Imprimee* (Lyon: Gilles et Jacques Huguetan, 1541) (Paris: Klincksieck, 1992).

Le Prevost, Marie, et al., *Le Tombeau de feu Missire François du Parc* (n.p. Pierre Sallière, 1590).

Liébault, Jean, and Charles Estienne, *L'Agriculture, et maison rustique de M. M. Charles Estienne, & Iean Liebault, Docteurs en Medecine* (1564) (Paris: Nicolas de la Vigne, 1640).

Louis XI, *Lettres choisies*, ed. Henri Dubois (Paris: Livre de Poche, 1996).

Lyège, Jean, *Raison de vivre pour toutes fièvres, congnues premierement par leurs differences, causes, signes, & symptomes, auec les prognostiques d'icelles* (Paris: M. Vascosan, 1557).

Medici, Catherine de, *Lettres*, ed. H. de la Ferrière, 9 vols, vol. 1 (Paris: Imprimerie Nationale, 1880) vol. 2 (1885), vol. 3 (1887), vol. 10, ed. Baguenault de Puchesse (1899).

Monteux, Hierosme de, *Commentaire de la conservation de santé, et prolongation de vie*, trans. Claude Valgelas (Lyon: Jean de Tournes, 1559).

—— *Commentaire de la conservation de santé, et prolongation de vie*, trans. Claude Valgelas (Paris: Simon Calvarin, 1572).

Nassau, Elisabeth de, *Les Deux Duchesses, lettres de Madame de Bouillon à Madame de La Tremoille (1621–22), lettres du duc et de la duchesse de Bouillon à Charlotte-Brabantine de Nassau, 1595–1597*, ed. Paul Marchegay (Paris: Meyrueis, 1866).

—— *Lettres d'Elisabeth de Nassau, Duchesse de Bouillon, à sa sœur Charlotte-Brabantine de Nassau, Duchesse de La Trémoille 1595–1628*, ed. Paul Marchegay (Les Roches-Baritaud, Vendée: L. Gasté, 1875).

Navarre, Marguerite de, *Théâtre profane*, ed. Verdun L. Saulnier (Paris: Droz, 1946).

Pizan, Christine de, *Le Livre des trois vertus*, intro. Charity Cannon Willard (Text) Willard and Eric Hicks (Paris: Champion, 1989).

Platter, Thomas, *Journal of a Younger Brother: The Life of Thomas Platter as a Medical Student in Montpellier at the Close of the Sixteenth Century*, ed. Sean Jennett (London: Frederick Muller, 1963).

Poitiers, Diane de, *Lettres inédites*, ed. Georges Guiffrey (Paris, 1866) (Geneva: Slatkine, 1970).

Rabelais, François, *Oeuvres complètes*, ed. J. Boulenger (Paris: Gallimard, 1955).

—— *The Complete Works of François Rabelais*, trans. D. Frame (Berkeley: University of California Press, 1991).

Serres, Olivier de, *Théâtre d'agriculture et mesnage des champs d'Olivier de Serres, Seigneur du Pradel* (Rouen: Jean Berthelin, 1646).

Sonnet de Courval, Thomas, *Satyre contre les charlatans, et pseudomedecins empyriques* (Paris: Jean Milot, 1610).

Thou, Jacques-Auguste de, *Mémoires de Jacques-Auguste de Thou depuis 1553 jusqu'en 1601* in *Choix de chroniques et mémoires relatifs à l'histoire de France*, ed. J.-A.-C. Buchon (Orleans: H. Herluison, 1875).

Valois, Marguerite de, *Mémoires* in J.-A.-C. Buchon (ed.), *Choix de chroniques et mémoires relatifs à l'histoire de France* (Orleans: H. Herluison, 1875).

Valois, Marie de, *Lettres de Marie de Valois, fille de Charles VII et d'Agnès Sorel, à Olivier de Coetivy, sgr de Taillebourg, son mari, 1458–1472*, ed. Paul Marchegay (Les Roches-Baritaud, Vendée: L. Gasté, 1875).

Vives, Jean-Louis, *Livre de l'institution de la femme chrestienne*, trans. Pierre de Changy (Paris: Jacques Kerver, 1542) (Havre: Lemale, 1891).

Secondary sources

Albou, P., 'Histoire des Oeuvres charitables de Philibert Guybert', *Histoire des Sciences Médicales*, 32:1 (1998), pp. 11–26.

Anglo, S. (ed.), *The Damned Art: Essays in the Literature of Witchcraft* (London: Routledge, 1977).

Antonioli, R., *Rabelais et la médecine*, Etudes Rabelaisiennes 12 (Geneva: Droz, 1976).

Ariès, P., *Centuries of Childhood*, trans. R. Baldick (London: Jonathan Cape, 1962).

Aron, E., *Louis XI et ses guérisseurs* (Chambray: CLD, 1983).

Artaud, J., *Le Grand Hôtel-Dieu de Lyon* (n.p., 1898).

Bakhtin, M., *L'Oeuvre de François Rabelais et la culture populaire au moyen âge et sous la Renaissance*, trans. A. Robel (Paris: Gallimard, 1970).

Barbot, J., *Les Chroniques de la Faculté de Médecine de Toulouse du treizième au vingtième siècle*, vol. 1: *1229–1793* (Toulouse: Charles Dirion, 1905).

Bates, D. (ed.), *Knowledge and the Scholarly Medical Traditions* (Cambridge: Cambridge University Press, 1995).

Batiffol, L., *La Vie intime d'une reine de France au XVIIe siècle* (Paris: Calmann-Levy, [1906]).

Baudrier, H. and J., *Bibliographie lyonnaise: recherches sur les imprimeurs, libraires, relieurs et fondeurs de lettres de Lyon au XVIe siècle* (Lyon: 1895) vols 1–13 (Paris: F. de Noble, 1964).

Béchu, C., F. Greffe and I. Pébay (eds), *Minutier central des notaires de Paris, minutes du XVe siècle de l'étude XIX* (Paris: Archives Nationales, 1993).

Béghin, C., 'Donneuses d'ouvrages, apprenties et salariées aux XIVe et XVe siècles dans les sociétés urbaines languedociennes', *Clio. Histoire, femmes et sociétés*, 3 (1996), pp. 31–54.

Belfort, A. de, *Archives de la Maison-Dieu de Châteaudun* (Paris/Châteaudun: Pouiller-Vandegraine, 1888).

Benedict, P. (ed.), *Cities and Social Change in Early Modern France* (London: Unwin Hyman, 1989).

Bennett, J. M., ' "History that stands still": women's work in the European past', *Feminist Studies*, 14:2 (1988), pp. 269–83.

Benoiston de Châteauneuf, L. F., *Considérations sur les enfans trouvés dans les principaux états de l'Europe* (Paris: Martinet, 1824).

Berriot-Salvadore, E., *Les Femmes dans la société française de la Renaissance* (Geneva: Droz, 1990).

SELECT BIBLIOGRAPHY

—— *Un Corps, un destin: la femme dans la médecine de la Renaissance* (Paris: H. Champion, 1993).

Bloor, D., *Knowledge and Social Inquiry* (London: Routledge and Kegan Paul, 1976).

Boswell, J., *The Kindness of Strangers: The Abandonment of Children in Western Europe From Late Antiquity to the Renaissance* (New York: Pantheon Books, 1988).

Boucher, A., 'L'ancien Hôtel-Dieu de Chinon', *Bulletin de la société des amis de vieux Chinon*, 7:9 (1975), pp. 847–54.

Bouissou, R., *Histoire de la médecine* (Paris: Larousse, 1967).

Boutineau, F. E., *Un Mémoire d'apothicaire de Tours au XVIe siècle* (Tours: Tourangelle, 1900).

Bouvier, P., *Etude sur l'Hôtel-Dieu d'Orléans au moyen âge et au XVIe siècle* (Orleans: Paul Pigelet, 1914).

Bowers, T., *The Politics of Motherhood: British Writing and Culture, 1680–1760* (Cambridge: Cambridge University Press, 1996).

Brabant, H., *Médecins, malades et maladies de la Renaissance* (Brussels: La Renaissance du livre, 1966).

Briggs, R., *Communities of Belief: Cultural and Social Tension in Early Modern France* (Oxford: Clarendon Press, 1989).

—— 'Women as victims? Witches, judges, and the community', *French History*, 5 (1991), pp. 438–80.

Brissaud, J., *A History of French Public Law*, trans. James W. Garner (London: John Murray, 1915).

Brockliss, L. and C. Jones, *The Medical World of Early Modern France* (Oxford: Clarendon Press, 1997).

Broomhall, S., 'Rabelais, the pursuit of knowledge, and early modern gynaecology', *Limina: A Journal of Historical and Cultural Studies*, 4 (1998), pp. 24–34.

—— 'Savoir féminin puériculteur: Le Verger Fertile des Vertus des Mesdames du Verger', *Mots Pluriels*, 11 (1999), www.arts.uwa.edu.au/MotsPluriels/MP1199sb.html.

—— *Women and the Book Trade in Sixteenth-Century France* (Aldershot: Ashgate, 2002).

Brown, J. C., 'A women's place was in the home: women's work in Renaissance Tuscany', in Margaret W. Ferguson, Maureen Quilligan and Nancy J. Vickers (eds), *Rewriting the Renaissance: The Discourses of Sexual Difference in Early Modern Europe* (Chicago: The University of Chicago Press, 1986), pp. 206–24.

Bullough, V. L., *The Development of Medicine as a Profession: The Contribution of the Medieval University to Modern Medicine* (Basel: S. Karger, 1966).

Bushnell, R. W., *A Culture of Teaching: Early Modern Humanism in Theory and Practice* (Ithaca: Cornell University Press, 1996), pp. 73–116.

Cadden, J., *The Meanings of Sex Difference in the Middle Ages: Medicine, Science, and Culture* (Cambridge: Cambridge University Press, 1993).

Caine, B., E. Grosz and M. de Lepervanche (eds), *Crossing Boundaries: Feminism and the Critique of Knowledge* (Sydney: Allen and Unwin, 1988).

Caisso, R. 'Les aumônes et l'hôpital des enfants exposés de Tours', *Bulletin de la société archéologique de Tours*, 39 (1981), pp. 811–55.

Campbell Hurd-Mead, K., *A History of Women in Medicine from the Earliest Times to the Beginning of the Nineteenth Century* (Haddam: The Haddam Press, 1938).

Carey, J. A., *Judicial Reform in France before the Revolution of 1789* (Cambridge, Mass., Harvard University Press, 1981).

Carmi Parsons, J. and B. Wheeler (eds), *Medieval Mothering* (New York: Garland, 1996).

Carré, H., 'Quelques mots sur la sorcellerie dans les provinces de l'Ouest au XVIe et XVIIe siècle', *Bulletin de la Société des Antiquaires de l'Ouest*, 7 (1925–7), pp. 631–74.

Carrier, H., *Origines de la Maternité de Paris: les maîtresses sages-femmes et l'office des accouchées de l'ancien Hôtel-Dieu (1378–1796)* (Paris: Georges Steinhal, 1888).

Céard, J., M-M. Fontaine and J-C. Margolin (eds), *Le Corps à la Renaissance: actes du XXXe colloque de Tours, 1987* (Paris: Amateurs de Livres, 1990).

Charnay, A., *Paroles de voleurs: gens de sac et de corde en pays toulousain au début du XVIe siècle* (Paris: Champion, 1998).

Chartier, R. (ed.), *A History of Private Life*, vol. 3, *Passions of the Renaissance*, trans. A. Goldhammer (Cambridge, Mass.: The Belknap Press of the Harvard University Press, 1989).

Chevalier, A., *L'Hôtel-Dieu de Paris et les sœurs augustines (650 à 1810)* (Paris: Champion, 1901).

Clark, Stuart, 'The "gendering" of witchcraft in French demonology: misogyny or polarity?' *French History*, 5 (1991), pp. 406–37.

Cloulas, I., *Diane de Poitiers* (Paris: Fayard, 1997).

Code, L., *What Can She Know? Feminist Theory and the Construction of Knowledge* (Ithaca: Cornell University Press, 1991).

—— *Rhetorical Spaces: Essays on Gendered Locations* (New York: Routledge, 1995).

Cohen, I. B., 'History and the Philosophy of Science', in Frederick Suppe (ed.), *The Structure of Scientific Theories*, 2nd edn (Urbana and Chicago: University of Illinois Press, 1977).

Collière, M.-F., *Proumouvoir la vie* (Paris: InterEditions, 1982).

Conrad, L. I., M. Neve, V. Nutton, R. Porter and A. Wear (eds), *The Western Medical Tradition, 800BC to AD 1800* (Cambridge: Cambridge University Press, 1995).

Coursault, R., *La Médecine en Touraine du moyen-âge à nos jours* (Paris: Maisonneuve & Larose, 1991).

Coyecque, E. (ed.), *L'Hôtel-Dieu de Paris au moyen âge: histoire et documents*, vol. 1: *Documents (1316–1552)* (Paris: H. Champion, 1891); vol. 2: *Délibérations* du Chapitre de Nôtre-Dame de Paris relatives à l'Hôtel-Dieu (1326–1539) (Paris: H. Champion, 1889).

—— (ed.), Recueil d'actes notariés relatifs à l'histoire de Paris et de ses environs au XVIe siècle, 1498–1545 (Paris: Imprimerie Nationale, 1905).

Crawford, P. 'Menstruation in seventeenth-century England', Past and Present, 91 (1981), pp. 47–73.

Croze, A., 'Etudes et documents pour servir à l'histoire hospitalière lyonnaise', Revue d'histoire de Lyon (1912 and 1915).

Davis, N. Z., Society and Culture in Early Modern France (Stanford: Stanford University Press, 1975).

—— 'Women in the crafts in sixteenth-century Lyon', Feminist Studies, 8:1 (1982), pp. 47–80.

—— 'Scandale à l'Hôtel-Dieu de Lyon (1537–1543)', La France d'Ancien Régime: études réunies en l'honneur de Pierre Goubert, vol. 1 (Toulouse: Privat, 1984).

—— Fiction in the Archives: Pardon Tales and their Tellers in Sixteenth-Century France (Stanford: Stanford University Press, 1987).

—— The Gift in Sixteenth-Century France (Madison: The University of Wisconsin Press, 2000).

Debus, A. G., The French Paracelsians: The Chemical Challenge to Medical and Scientific Tradition in Early Modern France (Cambridge: Cambridge University Press, 1991).

—— (ed.), Science, Medicine and Society in the Renaissance: Essays to honor Walter Pagel, 2 vols (London: Heinemann, 1972).

Defrance, E., Catherine de Médicis, ses astrologues et ses magiciens envoûteurs (Paris: Mercure de France, 1911).

Delaborde, J., Louise de Coligny, Princesse d'Orange, 2 vols (Paris, 1890) (Geneva: Slatkine, 1970).

Delcambre, E., Les Devins-guérisseurs dans la Lorraine ducale: leur activité et leurs méthodes (Nancy: Société d'archéologie lorraine et Musée historique lorrain, 1951).

Delooz, P., 'Towards a sociological study of canonized sainthood in the Catholic Church', in S. Wilson (ed.), Saints and their Cults: Studies in Religious Sociology, Folklore and History (Cambridge: Cambridge University Press, 1983), pp. 189–216.

Demaitre, L., 'The idea of childhood and child care in medical writings of the Middle Ages', Journal of Psychohistory, 4:4 (1977), pp. 461–90.

Demars-Sion, V., 'Illégitimité et abandon d'enfant: la position des provinces du Nord (XVIe–XVIIIe)', Revue du Nord, 65:258 (1983), pp. 481–506.

Depauw, J., 'L'Assistance à Paris à la fin du XVIe siècle', Bulletin de la Société française d'histoire des hôpitaux, 59 (1989), pp. 10–24.

Desnoyers, J., 'Recherches sur le sort des enfants trouvés en France, antérieurement à saint Vincent de Paul', Bulletin du comité historique des monuments écrits de l'histoire de France, 3 (1855–56), pp. 444–74.

Dick, D., *Yesterday's Babies: A History of Babycare* (London: Bodley Head, 1987).
Diedler, J-C., *Démons et sorcières en Lorraine: le bien et le mal dans les communautés rurales de 1550 à 1660* (Paris: Messène, 1996).
Dinet-Lecomte, M.-C., 'Les religieuses hospitalières à Blois aux XVIIe et XVIIIe siècles', *Annales de Bretagne et des Pays de l'Ouest*, 96:1 (1989), pp. 15–40.
—— 'Les soeurs hospitalières au service des pauvres malades aux XVIIe et XVIIIe siècles', *Annales de démographie historique* (1994), pp. 277–92.
—— 'Les hôpitaux sous l'Ancien Régime: des entreprises difficiles à gérer?' *Histoire, économie et société*, 18:3 (1999), pp. 527–45.
Dorveaux, P., *Notice sur la vie et les œuvres de Thibault Lespleigney apothicaire à Tours (1496–1567)* (Paris: H. Welter, 1898).
Doucet, R., *Les Institutions de la France au XVIe siècle*, 2 vols (Paris: A et J. Picard, 1948).
Drivon, J., *Les Anciens Hôpitaux de Lyon: Hôpital des Passants* (Lyon: Association typographique, 1905).
—— *Miscellanées médicales et historiques: notes pour servir à l'histoire de la médecine à Lyon* (Lyon: Association typographique, 1908, 1910 and 1913).
Dubreuil-Chambardel, L., 'L'Enseignement des sages-femmes en Touraine', *Bulletin et mémoires de la société archéologique de Touraine*, 48 (1909), pp. 33–127.
Duden, B., *The Woman Beneath the Skin: A Doctor's Patients in Eighteenth-Century Germany*, trans. Thomas Dunlap (Cambridge, Mass.: Harvard University Press, 1991).
Dulieu, L., 'La diététique et la nutrition à Montpellier à travers les âges', *Monspeliensis Hippocrates* (1969), pp. 5–16.
—— *La Médecine à Montpellier*, vol. 2: *La Renaissance* (Avignon: Les Presses universelles, 1979).
Dumas, G., 'Les femmes et les pratiques de la santé dans le "Registre de plaidoiries du Parlement de Paris, 1364–1427"', *Canadian Bulletin of Medicine*, 13 (1996), pp. 13–27.
Dupoux, A., *Sur les pas de Monsieur Vincent. Trois cents ans d'histoire parisienne de l'enfance abandonnée* (Paris: Revue de l'Assistance publique à Paris, 1958).
Du Prat, A-T., *Histoire d'Elisabeth de Valois, Reine d'Espagne, 1545–1568* (Paris: Techener, 1859).
Durand, G., *Le Patrimoine foncier de l'Hôtel-Dieu de Lyon (1482–1791)* (Lyon: Centre d'histoire economique et sociale de la région lyonnaise, 1974).
Eastgate Brink, J., 'A tax loop-hole in the sixteenth century: the battle over the claim of the medical school of Montpellier to exemptions from the taille', *Proceedings of the Annual Meeting of the Western Society for French History*, 3 (1975), pp. 2–12.
Eisenstein, E. L., *The Printing Press as an Agent of Change: Communications and Cultural Transformations in Early Modern Europe* (Cambridge: Cambridge University Press, 1979).

Enfance abandonnée et société en Europe XIVe–XXe siècles (Rome, 30–31 janvier, 1987) (Rome: Ecole française de Rome, 1991).
Erasmus, C. J., 'Changing folk beliefs and the relativity of empirical knowledge', *Southwestern Journal of Anthropology*, 8 (1952), pp. 411–28.
Evenden, D., *The Midwives of Seventeenth-Century London* (Cambridge: Cambridge University Press, 2000).
Fairchilds, C. C., *Poverty and Charity in Aix-en-Provence, 1640–1789* (Baltimore: The Johns Hopkins University Press, 1976).
Favreau, R., 'La sorcellerie en Poitou à la fin du moyen âge', *Bulletin de la Société des Antiquaires de l'Ouest*, 18 (1985), pp. 133–54.
Fery-Hue, F., 'Une expertise pour viol au XVIe siècle: pratique médico-légale et vocabulaire gynécologique', *Violences et contestation au moyen âge, actes du 114e congrès national des sociétés savantes (Paris, 1989)* (Paris: Editions du Comité des travaux historiques et scientifiques, 1990), pp. 321–43.
Ffolliott, S., 'A queen's garden of power: Catherine de' Medici and the locus of female power', in M. A. Di Cesare (ed.), *Reconsidering the Renaissance* (Binghamton, NY: Medieval and Renaissance Texts and Studies, 1992), pp. 245–55.
Fildes, V. A., *Breasts, Bottles and Babies: A History of Infant Feeding* (Edinburgh: Edinburgh University Press, 1986).
—— *Wet Nursing: A History from Antiquity to the Present* (Oxford: Blackwell, 1988).
—— (ed.), *Women as Mothers in Pre-Industrial England: Essays in Memory of Dorothy McLaren* (London: Routledge, 1990).
Fishel Sargent, C., *The Cultural Context of Therapeutic Choice: Obstetrical Care Decisions Among the Bariba of Benin* (Dordrecht: D. Reidel, 1982).
Fisher, S., *Nursing Wounds: Nurse Practitioners, Doctors, Women Patients and the Negotiation of Meaning* (New Brunswick: Rutgers University Press, 1995).
Flandrin, J.-L., *Families in Former Times: Kinship, Household and Sexuality*, trans. R. Southern (Cambridge: Cambridge University Press, 1979).
—— *Le Sexe et l'Occident: évolution des attitudes et des comportements* (Paris: Seuil, 1981).
Foisil, M., *L'Enfant Louis XIII: l'éducation d'un roi, 1601–1617* (Paris: Perrin, 1996).
Fosseyeux, M., 'L'Assistance parisienne au milieu du XVIe siècle', *Mémoires de l'histoire de Paris et de l'Ile-de-France* (1916), pp. 83–128.
Foucault, M., *The Archaeology of Knowledge*, trans. A. M. Sheridan (New York: Harper, 1972).
Franklin, A., *Les Corporations ouvrières de Paris du XIIe au XVIIIe siècle* (1884) (New York: Burt Franklin, 1971).
—— *La Vie privée d'autrefois: L'enfant, la naissance, le baptême* (Paris: Plon, 1895).
Friedman, M., 'Remarks on the history of science and the history of philosophy', in P. Horwich (ed.), *World Changes: Thomas Kuhn and the Nature of Science* (Cambridge, Mass.: The MIT Press, 1993).

Furst, L. R. (ed.), *Women Healers and Physicians: Climbing a Long Hill* (Lexington: The University Press of Kentucky, 1997).
Gager, K. E., *Blood Ties and Fictive Ties: Adoption and Family Life in Early Modern France* (Princeton: Princeton University Press, 1996).
Garcia-Ballester, L., R. French, J. Arrizabalaga and A. Cunningham (eds), *Practical Medicine from Salerno to the Black Death* (Cambridge: Cambridge University Press, 1994).
Gélis, J., *L'Arbre et le fruit: la naissance dans l'Occident moderne XVIe–XIXe siècles* (Paris: Fayard, 1984).
—— *History of Childbirth: Fertility, Pregnancy and Birth in Early Modern Europe*, trans. Rosemary Morris (Cambridge: Polity Press, 1991).
Gentilcore, D., *From Bishop to Witch: The System of the Sacred in Early Modern Terra d'Otranto* (Manchester: Manchester University Press, 1992).
—— *Healers and Healing in Early Modern Italy* (Manchester: Manchester University Press, 1998).
Gerando, J. M. de, *De la bienfaisance publique* (Paris: Jules Renouard, 1839).
Geremek, B., *Poverty: A History*, trans. A. Kolakowska (Oxford: Blackwell, 1994).
Giraudet, A., 'Histoire de l'ancien Hôtel-Dieu de Tours', *Bulletin de la société archéologique de Tours*, 2 (1871–3), pp. 78–161.
Giraudet, E., *Histoire de la ville de Tours* (1873) (Brussels: Culture et Civilisations, 1976).
Glidden, H. H., *The Storyteller as Humanist: The Serées of Guillaume Bouchet*, French Forum Monograph 25 (Lexington: French Forum, 1981).
Goglin, J. L., *Les Misérables dans l'Occident médiéval* (Paris: Editions du Seuil, 1976).
Gonthier, N., 'Les hôpitaux et les pauvres à la fin du moyen âge: l'exemple de Lyon', *Le Moyen Age* (1978), pp. 279–308.
Good, B. J., *Medicine, Rationality, and Experience: An Anthropological Perspective* (Cambridge: Cambridge University Press, 1994).
Graham, H., 'Providers, negotiators, and mediators: women as the hidden carers', in Ellen Lewin and Virginia Olsen (eds), *Women, Health and Healing: Toward a new perspective* (New York: Tavistock, 1985), pp. 25–52.
Green, M. H., 'Women's medical practice and health care in medieval Europe', in J. M. Bennett, E. A. Clark, J. F. O'Barr, A. Vilen and S. Westphal-Wihl (eds), *Sisters and Workers in the Middle Ages* (Chicago: Chicago University Press, 1989), pp. 39–78.
—— *Women's Healthcare in the Medieval West: Texts and Contexts* (Aldershot: Ashgate, 2000).
—— 'Books as a source of medical education for women in the middle ages', *Dynamis*, 20 (2000), pp. 331–69.
Greenbaum, L. S., 'Science, medicine, religion: three views of health care in France in the eve of the French Revolution', *Studies in Eighteenth Century Culture*, 10 (1981), pp. 373–91.

Greffe, F., and V. Brouselles (eds), *Documents du minutier central des notaires de Paris: inventaires après décès*, vol. 2: 1547–1560 (Paris: Archives Nationales, 1997).

Grell, O. P. and A. Cunningham (eds), *Medicine and the Reformation* (London and New York: Routledge, 1993).

—— and A. Cunningham with J. Arrizabalaga (eds), *Health Care and Poor Relief in Counter-Reformation Europe* (London: Routledge, 1999).

Greyerz, K. von (ed.), *Religion and Society in Early Modern Europe, 1500–1800* (London: Allen and Unwin, 1984).

Grosz, E., *Volatile Bodies: Toward a Corporeal Feminism* (Sydney: Allen and Unwin, 1994).

Guérin, P. (ed.), *Les Petits Bollandistes vies des saints de l'Ancien et du Nouveau Testament*, 17 vols (Paris: Bloud et Barral, 1872).

Guiart, J., *Histoire de la médecine française: son passé, son présent, son avenir* (Paris: Nagel, 1947).

Gutton, J.-P., *La Société et les pauvres, l'exemple de la généralité de Lyon. 1534–1789* (Paris: les Belles Lettres, 1971).

—— *La Société et les pauvres en Europe, XVIe–XVIIIe siècles* (Paris: Presses universitaires de France, 1974).

Haase-Dubosc, D. and E. Viennot (eds), *Femmes et pouvoirs sous l'Ancien Régime* (Paris: Rivages/Histoire, 1991).

Hamy, E-T., 'Jacques Gohory et le Lycium philosophal de Saint-Marceau-lès-Paris (1571–1576)', *Nouvelles Archives du Muséum*, 4e série (1899), pp. 1–26.

Hanawalt, B. A. (ed.), *Women and Work in Preindustrial Europe* (Bloomington: Indiana University Press, 1986).

Harding, S., *Whose Science? Whose Knowledge? Thinking From Women's Lives* (Milton Keynes: Open University Press, 1991).

—— *Is Science Multicultural? Postcolonialisms, Feminisms, and Epistemologies* (Bloomington: Indiana University Press, 1998).

Hickey, D., *Local Hospitals in Ancien Régime France: Rationalization, Resistance, Renewal 1530–1789* (Montreal and Kingston: McGill-Queens University Press, 1997).

Hildesheimer, F., *Fléaux et société de la Grande Peste au choléra XIVe–XIXe siècle* (Paris: Hachette, 1993).

Hirsh, E. and Olson, G. A. (eds), *Women Writing Culture* (Albany, NY: State University of New York Press, 1995).

Hobhouse, P., *Plants in Garden History* (1992) (London: Pavilion, 1997).

Hordern, P. and R. Smith (eds), *The Locus of Care: Families, Communities, Institutions and the Provision of Welfare since Antiquity* (London: Routledge, 1998).

Huard, P. and R. Laplane, *Histoire illustrée de la puériculture: aspects diététiques, socio-culturels et ethnologique* (Paris: Les Editions Roger Dacosta, 1979).

Hufton, O., *The Poor of Eighteenth-Century France, 1750–1789* (Oxford: Clarendon Press, 1974).

―― *The Prospect Before Her: A History of Women in Western Europe*, vol. 1: *1500–1800* (London: Harper Collins, 1995).
Hughes, M. J., *Women Healers in Medieval Life and Literature* (1943) (Freeport, NY: Books for Libraries Press, 1968).
Hunter, L. and S. Hutton (eds), *Women, Science and Medicine 1500–1700* (Stroud: Sutton Publishing, 1997).
Imbert, J., *Les Hôpitaux en droit canonique* (Paris: J. Vrin, 1947).
―― 'L'église et l'état face au problème hospitalier au XVIe siècle', *Etudes d'Histoire du Droit Canonique dédiées à Gabriel Le Bras*, vol. 1 (Paris: Sirey, 1965), pp. 577–92.
―― 'Les prescriptions hospitalières du Concile de Trente et leur diffusion en France', *Revue d'histoire de l'Eglise de France*, 42 (1965), pp. 5–28.
―― *Le Droit hospitalier de l'ancien régime* (Paris: Presses universitaires de France, 1993).
―― (ed.), *Histoire des hôpitaux en France* (Toulouse, Privat, 1982).
Inventaire Sommaire des Archives Hospitalieres: Hospices de Sillé-Le-Guillaume, Archives départementales de Sarthe (Le Mans: Monnoyer, 1931).
Jacquart, D., *Le Milieu médical en France du XIIe au XVe siècle* (Geneva: Droz, 1981).
Jones, C., *Charity and Bienfaisance: The Treatment of the Poor in the Montpellier Region, 1740–1815* (Cambridge: Cambridge University Press, 1982).
―― *The Charitable Imperative: Hospitals and Nursing in Ancien Regime and Revolutionary France* (London: Routledge, 1989).
―― and R. Porter (eds), *Reassessing Foucault: Power, Medicine and the Body* (London: Routledge, 1994).
Jordanova, L., *Sexual Visions: Images of Gender in Science and Medicine between the Eighteenth and the Twentieth Centuries* (London: Harvester Wheatsheaf, 1989).
―― 'Gender and the historiography of science', *British Journal for the History of Science*, 26 (1993), pp. 469–83.
―― 'The social construction of medical knowledge', *Social History of Medicine*, 8:3 (1995), pp. 361–81.
Jorland, G., *La Science dans la philosophie. Les recherches épistemologiques d'Alexandre Koyré* (Paris: Gallimard, 1981).
Jurgens, M. (ed.), *Documents du minutier central des notaires de Paris: inventaires après décès*, vol. 1: *1483–1547* (Paris: Archives Nationales, 1982).
Kamen, H., *Philip of Spain* (New Haven, Yale University Press, 1997).
Kibre, P., 'The Faculty of Medicine at Paris, charlatanism, and unlicensed medical practices in the later middle ages', *Bulletin of the History of Medicine*, 27:1 (1953), pp. 8–11.
―― *Scholarly Privileges in the Middle Ages: The Rights, Privileges and Immunities of Scholars and Universities at Bologna, Padua, Paris and Oxford* (Cambridge, Mass.: Medieval Academy of America, 1962).

Kieckhefer, R., 'The holy and the unholy: sainthood, witchcraft and magic in late medieval Europe', *Journal of Medieval and Renaissance Studies* (1994), pp. 355-85.

Klairmont Lingo, A., *The Rise of Medical Practitioners in Sixteenth-Century France: the Case of Lyon and Montpellier* (PhD, University of California-Berkeley, 1980).

—— 'Santé et beauté féminines dans la France de la Renaissance', *Proceedings of the 110e Congrès national des Sociétés savantes*, Section d'Histoire Moderne et Contemporaine (Le Corps et la Santé) 1 (1985), pp. 191-9.

—— 'Empirics and charlatans in early modern France: the genesis of the classification of the "Other" in medical practice', *Journal of Social History*, 19 (1985-86), pp. 583-603.

—— 'Print's role in the politics of women's health care in early modern France', in Barbara B. Diefendorf and Carla Hesse (eds), *Culture and Identity in Early Modern Europe (1500-1800): Essays in Honor of Natalie Zemon Davis* (Ann Arbor: The University of Michigan Press, 1993).

—— 'The fate of popular terms for female anatomy in the age of print', *French Historical Studies*, 22:3 (1999), pp. 335-49.

—— 'Women healers and the medical marketplace of sixteenth-century Lyon', *Dynamis*, 19 (1999), pp. 79-94.

Kleinberg, A. M., *Prophets in their Own Country: Living Saints and the Making of Sainthood in the Later Middle Ages* (Chicago: The University of Chicago Press, 1992).

Knibiehler, Y. and C. Fouquet, *La Femme et les médecins* (Paris: Hachette, 1983).

Kuhn, T. S., *The Structure of Scientific Revolutions* (3rd edn) (Chicago: The University of Chicago Press, 1996).

La Charité, R. (ed.), *Rabelais's Incomparable Book: Essays on his Art* (Lexington: French Forum Publishers, 1986).

La Fons, A. de, Bon de Mélicocq (ed.), 'Dépenses faites par la ville de Lille pour les enfants trouvés', *Bulletin du comité historique des monuments écrits de l'histoire de France*, 3 (1855-56), pp. 475-80.

Laignel-Lavastine, M. (ed.), *Histoire générale de la médecine, de la pharmacie, de l'art dentaire et de l'art vétérinaire*, 3 vols (Paris: Albin Michel, 1936, 1938, 1949).

Lallemand, L., *Histoire des enfants abandonés et délaissés: Etudes sur la protection de l'enfance aux diverses époques de la civilisation* (Paris: A. Picard, 1885).

Langlois, F., 'Les enfants abandonnés à Caen, 1661-1820', *Histoire, économie, et société*, 6:3 (1987), pp. 307-28.

Lanning, J. T., *The Royal Protomedicato: The Regulation of the Medical Professions in the Spanish Empire* (Durham: Duke University Press, 1985).

La Trémoille, L. de (ed.), *Inventaire de François de La Trémoille, 1542, et comptes d'Anne de Laval* (Nantes: E. Grimaud, 1888).

—— (ed.), *Les La Trémoille pendant cinq siècles*. vol. 2. *Louis I, Louis II, Jean et Jacques, 1431–1525* (Nantes: E. Grimaud, 1892); vol. 3: *Charles, François et Louis III, 1485–1577* (1894).

Laval, V., *Histoire de la Faculté de Médecine d'Avignon: ses origines, son organisation et son enseignement (1303–1791)*, vol. 1 (Paris: E. Lechevalier, 1889).

Lebrun, F., *Se soigner autrefois: médecins, saints et sorciers aux XVIIe et XVIIIe siècles* (Paris: Temps Actuel, 1983).

Lecourt, D., *L'Epistémologie historique de G. Bachelard* (Paris: Vrin, 1969).

Le Grand, L., *Statuts d'Hôtels-Dieu et de léproseries: recueil de textes du XIIe au XIVe siècles* (Paris: A. Picard, 1901).

Lehoux, F., *Le Cadre de vie des médecins parisiens aux XVIe et XVIIe siècles* (Paris: A. et J. Picard, 1976).

Le Roux de Lincy, *Vie de la reine Anne de Bretagne*, 4 vols (Paris: L. Curmer, 1860).

Lespinasse, R. (ed.), *Les Métiers et corporations de la ville de Paris XIVe–XVIIIe siècles*, vols 1 and 3 (Paris: Imprimerie Nationale, 1886 and 1898).

Lipinska, M., *Des femmes médecins depuis l'antiquité jusqu'à nos jours* (Paris: G. Jacques, 1900).

—— *Les Femmes et le progrès des sciences médicales* (Paris: Masson, 1930).

Loux, F. and P. Richard, *Sagesse du corps: la santé et la maladie dans les proverbes français* (Paris: G-P. Maisonneuve et Larose, 1978).

McClive, C., 'The hidden truths of the belly: the uncertainties of pregnancy in early modern Europe', *Social History of Medicine*, 15:2 (2002), pp. 209–27.

McTavish, L., 'On display: portraits of seventeenth-century French men-midwives', *Social History of Medicine*, 14:3 (2001), pp. 389–415.

Mandrou, R., *Magistrats et sorciers en France au XVIIe siècle: une analyse de psychologie historique* (Paris: Plon, 1968).

—— (ed.), *Sorciers, demonologues, magistrats, théologiens et médecins aux XVIe et XVIIe siècles* (microfiche collection) (Paris: Microeditions Hachette, 1975).

Margolin, J-C. and R. Sauzet (eds), *Pratiques et discours alimentaires à la Renaissance: actes du colloque de Tours de mars 1979* (Paris: Maisonneuve et Larose, 1982).

Marland, H. (ed.), *The Art of Midwifery: Early Modern Midwives in Europe* (London: Routledge, 1993).

—— and M. Pelling (eds), *The Task of Healing: Medicine, Religion and Gender in England and the Netherlands, 1450–1800* (Rotterdam: Erasmus Publishing, 1996).

Martin, O., *Les Manuscrits de Simon Marion, et la coutume de Paris au XVIe siècle* (Rennes: Imprimeries Oberthur, 1922).

Martin, X., 'La part du corps de ville dans la gestion de l'Hôtel-Dieu d'Angers à la fin du XVIe siècle', *Annales de Bretagne et des pays de l'Ouest*, 82 (1975), pp. 149–62.

—— 'Aspects de la sorcellerie en Anjou, 1570–1640', *Histoire des faits de la Sorcellerie* (Angers: Presses de l'Université d'Angers, 1985), pp. 71–110.

Melzer, S. E. and K. Norberg (eds), *From the Royal to the Republican Body: Incorporating the Political in Seventeenth- and Eighteenth-Century France* (Berkeley: University of California Press, 1998).

Mercier, R., *Histoire de la médecine en Touraine* (Tours: Arrault, 1936).

Merleau-Ponty, M., *Phénoménologie de la perception* (Paris: Gallimard, 1945).

Messing, K., 'Hospital Trash: Cleaners Speak of their Role in Disease Prevention', *Medical Anthropology Quarterly*, 12:2 (1998), pp. 168–87.

Miles, A., *Women, Health and Medicine* (Milton Keynes: Open Press University, 1991).

Miller, N. J. and N. Yavneh (eds), *Maternal Measures: Figuring Caregiving in the Early Modern Period* (Aldershot: Ashgate, 2000).

Moi, T., *What is a Woman? And Other Essays* (Oxford: Oxford University Press, 1999).

Mollat, M., *Les Pauvres au moyen âge, étude sociale* (Paris: Hachette, 1978).

Monter, E. William, *Witchcraft in France and Switzerland: The Borderlands During the Reformation* (Ithaca: Cornell University Press, 1976).

Moran, B. T. (ed.), *Patronage and Institutions: Science, Technology, and Medicine at the European Court 1500–1750* (Woodbridge: Boydell Press, 1991).

Mowery Andrews, R., *Law, Magistracy and Crime in Old Regime Paris, 1735–1789*, vol. 1: *The System of Criminal Justice* (Cambridge: Cambridge University Press, 1994).

Muchembled, R., *Sorcières: justice et société aux 16e et 17e siècles* (Paris: Imago, 1982).

Numbers, R. L. and D. W. Amundsen (eds), *Caring and Curing: Health and Medicine in the Western Religious Traditions* (New York: Macmillan, 1986).

Nutton, V. (ed.), *Medicine at the Courts of Europe, 1500–1837* (London: Routledge, 1990).

O'Boyle, C., *The Art of Medicine: Medical Teaching at the University of Paris, 1250–1400* (Leiden: Brill, 1998).

O'Day, R., *The Family and Family Relationships, 1500–1900; England, France & the United States of America* (Houndmills, Basingstoke: Macmillan, 1994).

Olivier-Martin, F., *L'Organisation corporative de la France d'ancien régime* (Paris: Sirey, 1938).

—— *Précis d'Histoire du droit français* (3rd edn) (Paris: Librairie Dalloz, 1938).

Ouin-LaCroix, C., *Histoire des anciennes corporations d'arts et métiers et des confréries religieuses de la capitale de la Normandie* (Rouen: Lacointe Freres, 1850).

Pagel, W., *Paracelsus: An Introduction to Philosophical Medicine in the Era of the Renaissance* (2nd edn) (Basel: Karger, 1982).

Panel, G. (ed.), *Documents concernant les pauvres de Rouen*, vol. 1: *1224 to 1630* (Paris: Picard, 1917).

Pelling, M., 'Child health as a social value in early modern England', *Social History of Medicine*, 1:2 (1988), pp. 135–64.

—— 'The women of the family? Speculations around early modern British physicians', *Social History of Medicine*, 8:3 (1995), pp. 383–401.

—— *The Common Lot: Sickness, Medical Occupations and the Urban Poor in Early Modern England* (London: Longman, 1998).

Perkins, W., 'Midwives versus doctors: the case of Louise Bourgeois', *The Seventeenth Century* (1988), pp. 135–57.

—— 'The relationship between midwife and client in the works of Louise Bourgeois', *Seventeenth-Century French Studies* (1989), pp. 28–45.

—— *Midwifery and Medicine in Early Modern France: Louise Bourgeois* (Exeter: University of Exeter Press, 1996).

Perkinson, M. A., 'Socialization to the family caregiving role within a continuing care retirement community', *Medical Anthropology*, 16 (1995), pp. 249–67.

Petrelli, R. L., 'The Regulation of French midwifery during the Ancien Régime', *Journal of the History of Medicine* (1971), pp. 276–92.

Pierson, P., *Philip II of Spain* (London: Thames and Hudson, 1975).

Plumwood, V., *Feminism and the Mastery of Nature* (London: Routledge, 1993).

Porter, R. (ed.), *Patients and Practitioners: Lay Perceptions of Medicine in Preindustrial Society* (Cambridge: Cambridge University Press, 1985).

Prescott, W., *History of the Reign of Philip the Second, King of Spain*, vol. 2 (New York: Crowell, [1855]).

Pringle, R., *Sex and Medicine: Gender, Power and Authority in the Medical Profession* (Cambridge: Cambridge University Press, 1998).

Pullan, B., *Orphans and Foundlings in Early Modern Europe* (Berkshire: University of Reading, 1989).

Rambaud, P., 'Le Rôle des femmes au point de vue de l'assistance publique à Poitiers', *Mémoires de la Société des Antiquaires de l'Ouest*, 3 (1909), pp. xix–lii.

Ramsey, M., *Professional and Popular Medicine in France, 1770–1830: The Social World of Medical Practice* (Cambridge: Cambridge University Press, 1988).

Rawcliffe, C., *Medicine and Society in Later Medieval England* (Stroud: Sutton, 1997).

—— 'Hospital nurses and their work', in R. Britnell (ed.), *Daily Life in the Late Middle Ages* (Stroud: Sutton, 1998), pp. 43–64.

Remâcle, B-B., *Des Hospices des enfans trouvés en Europe, et principalement en France* (Paris: Treuttel et Wurtz, 1838).

Reutter de Rosemont, L., *Histoire de la pharmacie à travers les âges*, vol. 1 (Paris: Peyronnet, 1931).

Robillard de Beaurepaire, C. de, 'Notes extraites des premières registres de l'Hôtel-Dieu de Rouen', *Extrait du précis des travaux de l'Académie des Sciences, Belles-Lettres et Arts de Rouen* (Rouen: H. Boissel, [1870]), pp. 1–29.

Robin, I. and A. Walch, 'Géographie des enfants trouvés de Paris aux XVIIe et XVIIIe siècles', *Histoire, économie, et société* 6:3 (1987), pp. 343–60.

Roger, J., *Pour une histoire des sciences à part entière* (Paris: Albin Michel, 1995).

Rose, H., 'Women's work: women's knowledge' in Juliet Mitchell and Ann Oakley (eds), *What is Feminism?* (Oxford: Basil Blackwell, 1986), pp. 161–83.
Rossi, P. *La Naissance de la science moderne en Europe*, trans. Patrick Vighetti (Paris: Seuil, 1999).
Rouget, F., 'De la sage-femme à la femme sage: réflexion et réflexivité dans les *Observations* de Louise Boursier', *Papers on French Seventeenth-Century Literature*, 49 (1998), pp. 483–96.
Rublack, U., 'Pregnancy, childbirth and the female body in early modern Germany', *Past and Present*, 150 (1996), pp. 84–110.
Samaran, C., *Archives de la maison de La Tremoille* (Paris: Honoré Champion, 1928).
Santé, médecine et assistance au moyen âge (Actes du 110e congrès national des sociétés savantes, Montpellier, 1985) (Paris: Editions du CTHS, 1987).
Saulnier, A., 'De l'enfant à l'hôpital à l'hôpital pour enfants. Tentative d'analyse de l'élaboration d'une adaptation spécifique de l'hospitalisation pour l'enfant au tournant des XVe et XVIe siècles', *Annales de démographie historique* (1994), pp. 293–302.
Schiebinger, L., *The Mind Has No Sex? Women and the Origins of Modern Science* (Cambridge: Harvard University Press, 1989).
—— *Nature's Body: Gender in the Making of Modern Science* (Boston: Beacon Press, 1993).
—— *Has Feminism Changed Science?* (Cambridge: Harvard University Press, 1999).
Scott, J., 'Gender: a useful category of historical analysis', *American Historical Review*, 91 (1986), pp. 1053–75.
Scully, T., 'The sickdish in early French recipe collections', in S. Campbell, B. Hall and D. Klausner (eds), *Health, Disease and Healing in Medieval Culture* (New York: St Martin's Press, 1992), pp. 132–51.
Shapin, S. and S. Schaffer, *Leviathan and the Air-Pump: Hobbes, Boyle, and the Experimental Life* (Princeton: Princeton University Press, 1985).
Smith, L. W., 'Reassessing the role of the family: women's health care in eighteenth-century England', *Social History of Medicine*, forthcoming.
Soman, A., *Sorcellerie et justice criminelle: le Parlement de Paris (16e–18e siècles)* (Aldershot: Variorum, 1992).
Sournia, J-C., *Histoire de la médecine* (Paris: La Découverte, 1992).
Spiegeler, P. de, *Les Hôpitaux et l'Assistance à Liège (X–XVe siècles): Aspects institutionnels et sociaux*, Bibliothèque de la Faculté de Philosophie et Lettres de l'Université de Liège, Fascicule CCXLIX (Paris: Société d'Edition 'Les Belles Lettres', 1987).
Stone, H., 'The French Language in Renaissance Medicine', *Bibliothèque d'Humanisme et Renaissance*, 15 (1953), pp. 315–46.
Sussman, G., *Selling Mother's Milk: The Wet-Nursing Business in France, 1715–1914* (Urbana: University of Illinois Press, 1982).

Thierry, A. (ed.), *Recueil des monuments inédits de l'histoire du tiers état: première serie, chartes, coutumes, actes municipaux, statuts des corporations d'arts et metiers des villes et communes de France, region du nord*, vols 2 and 4 (Paris: Firmin-Didot, 1853 and 1870).

Thomas, K., *Religion and the Decline of Magic: Studies in Popular Beliefs in Sixteenth and Seventeenth Century England* (London: Weidenfeld and Nicolson, 1971).

Thorndike, L., *A History of Magic and Experimental Science*, 8 vols (New York: Columbia University Press, 1923-58).

—— *University Records and Life in the Middle Ages* (New York: Octagon Books, 1971).

Varin, P. (ed.), *Archives législatives de la ville de Reims, seconde partie: statuts*, vol. 1 (Paris: Imprimerie de Crapelet, 1844).

Vauchez, A., *La Sainteté en Occident aux derniers siècles du moyen âge: d'après les proces de canonisation et les documents hagiographiques* (Rome: Ecole française de Rome, 1981).

Verdier, M., *La Jurisprudence de la médecine en France*, 2 vols (Alençon: Malassis, 1763 and 1762).

Walker Freer, M., *Elizabeth de Valois, Queen of Spain and the Court of Philip II*, 2 vols (London: Hurst and Blackett, 1857).

Wear, A., R. K. French and I. M. Lonie (eds), *The Medical Renaissance of the Sixteenth Century* (Cambridge: Cambridge University Press, 1985).

Webster, C. (ed.), *Health, Medicine and Mortality in the Sixteenth Century* (Cambridge: Cambridge University Press, 1979).

Wickersheimer, C. A. E., *La Médecine et les médecins en France à l'époque de la Renaissance* (Paris: A. Maloine, 1906).

—— *Dictionnaire biographique des médecins en France au moyen âge* (Paris, 1936) ed. Guy Beaujouan, 2 vols (Geneva: Droz, 1979).

Wiesner-Hanks, M., *Working Women in Renaissance Germany* (New Brunswick: Rutgers University Press, 1986).

Wilson, L. *Women and Medicine in the French Enlightenment: The Debate over Maladies des femmes* (Baltimore: The Johns Hopkins University Press, 1993).

Winn, C. H., '"De mères en filles": les manuels d'éducation sous l'Ancien Régime', *Atlantis*, 19:1 (1993), pp. 23-30.

Wynne Hellwarth, J., '"Be unto me as a precious ointment": Lady Grace Mildmay, sixteenth-century female practitioner', *Dynamis*, 19 (1999), pp. 95-117.

Zegura, E. Chesney, 'Toward a feminist reading of Rabelais', *Journal of Medieval and Renaissance Studies*, 15:1 (1985), pp. 125-34.

Index

abandonment 168–73
Abbeville 28
abortion 36, 38, 54, 134
active religious life 75, 81, 84–5
Albou, Philippe 132
Alliot, Sainte, child carer 164, 166
ambassadors, French 214–31
Amboise 37, 188
Amiens 21, 30, 65, 137
anatomy 32, 57, 60–1, 136
Angers 96, 102–3, 107, 115, 121n.4
  see also medical faculty, Angers
Anne de Beaujeu 98
Anne of Brittany 167, 188–93
Antidotary see Salerno
apothecaries 3–5, 16, 20, 28–31, 38, 46–8, 51–2, 55, 62–3, 65, 75–6, 80, 100, 106–7, 128–32, 141–3, 146–8, 156, 159, 186, 217, 240, 257
apprenticeships and education 19, 25, 29, 31, 36, 55, 65, 160, 174–5, 186–7, 200
Arbaleste, Charlotte 242, 249
Aristotle 244
Arles 64
Asseline, Jeanne, Hôtel-Dieu prioress 87
asthma 146
Aubagne, Hugone, d', wetnurse 161
Aubeterre, Antoinette d' 136
Avignon 25–6, 58–9, 237

Bachelard, Gaston 3
Balzac, Robert de 85
baptism 31, 36–7
barbers 16–31, 38, 46, 48–9, 52, 55, 62, 75, 105, 130, 133, 257
  see also surgeons
Béghin, Cécile 19, 24
Bellenger, Silvine, hospital servant 159
Bergerac 160
Berriot-Salvadore, Evelyne 247
Bertier, Janine 191
Besionne, unlicensed practitioner 57
Bienassis, Paul, translator 32
Biguet, Jehan, master barber 17, 27
Bloor, David 3
Bodin, Jean, legal scholar 116–17, 119

bone-setters 21, 100, 138, 159
Bordeaux 31, 117
Boswell, John 160, 175
Bourbon, Antoinette de 99, 135
Bourbon, Catherine 215, 242–3
Bourbon, Gabrielle de 31
Bourbon-Montpensier, Charlotte de 238
Bourbon-Montpensier, Marie de 205–6
Bourdieu, Pierre 7
Bourgenymée, Geneviève, sicknurse 82
Bourgeois, Louise, midwife 9, 37, 129, 133–5, 198–9, 202–10, 257
Bourges 109–10
Boursier, Martin, surgeon 133
Boyer, Catherine, child carer 164
Braillier, Pierre, apothecary 30, 148
Breche, Jean, surgeon 128
Brémone, wetnurse 161
Brézé, Louis de 237
Bricard, Marguerite, practitioner 159
Briçonnet, Jean, Hôtel-Dieu governor 77–9
Briggs, Robin 118–19
Brockliss, Lawrence 4, 5, 8, 13n.29
Brown, Judith 25
Burke, Peter 112
Bussière, Marguerite, practitioner 159

Cabrol, Barthélemy, master surgeon 233–4
Castellan, Honoré de, medical professor 64
Castres 57–8
Catherine de Medici 192–8, 214–31, 242–3, 258–9
Challieu, Simon de, unlicensed practitioner 58
Châlons-sur-Saone 25
Chambaulde, Catherine, hospital nurse 89
Champgaillard, 'Old Woman of', unlicensed practitioner 52–3, 59
Champier, Symphorien, physician 85
chandlers 28, 30
Chantemilan, Philippe de, Blessed 110, 112
charity 10, 24, 81, 96, 98–103, 105–6, 110, 112, 120, 142–3, 168, 170, 178

INDEX

Charles, unlicensed practitioner 52
Charles V 160
Charles VII 22, 170
Charles VIII 20, 28, 188–9
Charpentier, André, unlicensed practitioner 53
Charpentier, Françoise 234
Chartier, Roger 61
chastity *see* sexuality
Chaussade, Bernard, physician 190
Chevellu, Pierre, barber-surgeon 26
childbirth 31–3, 54, 73, 75, 135, 203, 205–6, 214–15, 225–7, 237, 239–40, 242–3, 247–50
child care 1, 9–10, 52–3, 55, 58, 77–8, 156–85, 186–213, 257–9
children of Charles VII and Anne of Brittany 188–92
  see also Claude de France
children of Henri II and Catherine de Medici 194–7, 215
  see also Elisabeth de Valois
Chinon 37, 73
Choppin, René, lawyer 107, 258
Chrestian, Guillaume, physician 131, 135, 192, 239
Church, Catholic 31, 37, 102, 109–14, 234
Clauchepied, Claudette, diviner 114, 118
Claude de France 167, 189–90, 191
Clermont, Louise de, lady-in-waiting 216, 221–3
Clysters 221–2
Code, Lorraine 8
Colbert, Charles 108, 120n.3
Coligny, Louise de 238, 240–1, 245–6, 248–9
Colin, Sébastien 136, 147
competition and rivalry 20–3, 46–9, 100, 129, 133, 186, 194, 197–9, 202–3, 205, 208–9, 214–31
Condé, Léonor de 243
confectioners 28, 30
Converse, Jehanne, hospital nurse 80
Cop, Guillaume, physician 191
Coras, Jean de, lawyer 236–7, 258
corporal punishment and discipline, for children 191, 200–1, 211n.4
correspondence 11, 147, 179, 188–90, 193–8, 214–32, 236–56
Costes, Johanna de, Hôtel-Dieu sub-prioress 78–9

Couche de Nôtre-Dame 170, 177–8
Court, royal 9–10, 186–31, 258
Coyecque, Ernest 73
Crawford, Patricia 216
culinary therapy 9, 77–80, 98, 100, 130–1, 138, 140–1, 143, 146–7, 186–7, 194, 196, 220
Culotte, Françoise, hospital nurse 89

Daast, Melchior, unlicensed practitioner 53
Dabaron, Jeanne, apothecary's wife 30
Daburon, Pierre, physician 96
Dalechamps, Claude, surgeon 128, 131, 135–6
Dannemarie, Anne Lemaye, wetnurse 193
Dansezune, Louise 135–6
daughters 25–6, 45, 63
Daughters of Charity 71
Davis, Natalie Zemon 23, 85, 97, 132, 174, 177
Debus, Allen G. 49
Delcambre, Etienne 118
Delprat, Guillelme 242–3, 246
Demey, Laurence, hospital nurse 26
dentistry 59, 128
Descampes, Astruga 242–3
Desfossés, Flourentine, hospital nurse 159
Deshayes, Marguerite, sicknurse 82
Des Roches, Catherine, author 139
Diane de Poitiers 135–6, 147, 153n.53, 192–8, 224, 237, 239
dietetic medicine *see* culinary therapy
Dijon 99, 157
Dinet-Lecomte, Marie-Claude 71
Dioscorides 149
dissection *see* anatomy
distillers 29, 143
diviners 113–15, 117–19, 130
domestic medicine *see* culinary therapy; herbal medicine; household and domestic sphere
domestic staff 26–7, 30–1, 72–3, 82, 84, 110, 138, 142, 159, 173, 217, 240, 258
Dompremi, Jean de, unlicensed practitioner 54
Dorée, Barbe, diviner 113–14, 116
Douai 111
Du Bois, Jacques, physician 131, 239
Du Bouchage, Madame, governess 189–90, 202, 210

INDEX

Du Breil, André, physician 51–2, 103, 114, 132, 140, 222
Du Cluzel, Benoist, barber 26
Duden, Barbara 7, 236
Du Laurens, André, physician 64, 199
Du Laurens, Jeanne, memorialist 64
Du Laurens, Louis, physician 64
Du Luys, Guillemette, surgeoness 186
Duperon, Marie-Catherine de Pierrevive, governess 193–4, 196
Duplessis-Mornay, Philippe 249
Dupuis, Madame, midwife 202, 204
Dupuy, Albert, physician 190–1
Du Val, Jacques, physician 32–3, 239, 245, 249

eagle stone 249–50
economics, medical 18, 21, 25, 48–50, 65 102–3, 105–7, 131–2, 138, 145, 147
Elisabeth de Valois, daughter of Henri II and Catherine de Medici 196–7, 214–31, 232, 242–3, 259
emergency *see* primary medicine
Empirics 4–5, 44, 47–50, 57, 104–8, 120, 132, 141
Erasmus, Desiderius 172
Estevent, Jehan, master barber 16–18, 24–5, 27–8, 41n.59, 258
Estevent, Isabelle, master barber's wife 16–18, 24–8, 41n.59, 258
exorcists 113

Felicie, Jacqueline, unlicensed practitioner 44, 50, 52, 55
Fernel, Jean, physician 20, 197, 244
Ferrara 53, 104
Fisher, Sue 9
Foisil, Madeleine 187
Foix, Claude de 147
Fontaine, Marie-Madeleine 168
Forgue, Emile 20
Foucault, Michel 251
foundlings *see* abandonment; orphans and foundlings
Fouquet, Catherine 82
Fourquevaux, Raymond de, ambassador 218–19, 222–3, 225, 227
Franche-Comté 118
François I 22, 176, 191–2
François II 28–9

fraud and charlatanism 49, 51, 56, 117–18, 134

Galenism 128, 131, 148, 204–5, 208, 221
Gascony 104
Geipoulleau, Jehanne, child carer 164–5
Genas, Catherine de, mother of Laurent Joubert 63–4, 100
Gentilcore, David 5
Gervaise, midwife 32, 61
gestation *see* pregnancy
Gilles, Marie, hospital nurse 79
Glidden, Hope 128
Glorielle, Vincente, practitioner 178
Gorris, Pierre de, unlicensed practitioner 53
governesses 1, 10, 186–213
Gracieuse, Barbe, sicknurse 158
Gravelle, Pierre, master barber 17, 27
Greek translations 46–7, 54, 62, 128, 131, 143, 168
Green, Monica H. 1, 6, 9, 19, 52, 54–5, 136–7, 152n.51
Grenoble 190
Grevin, Martin, hospital master 87
Gruot, Claude, Hôtel-Dieu prioress 88
Guibert, Philibert, physician 61, 131–2, 148
Guichard, Jean, physician 63
Guichard, Louise, wife of Laurent Joubert 63
Guilds 2, 10–11, 16–43, 47, 51, 55, 58, 60, 64–5, 257
Guillemeau, Charles, physician 208–9
Guillemeau, Jacques, surgeon 32, 35, 100, 168, 203, 216, 235, 244
Guillemette, hospital nurse 80
Guillotine, Marion, sicknurse 82
Guyon, Anne, child carer 178

haberdashers 28
Harding, Sandra 8
Harvillier, Jeanne, diviner 116
Hassart, Germaine, midwife 35
Hélène, Perenelle, hospital nurse 74
Hémard, Urbain, surgeon 128
Henri II 192–8, 214
Henri III 22
Henri IV 117, 148, 158, 193, 198–9, 200–1, 204–5, 210, 215, 242
Henry, Jehan, Hôtel-Dieu governor 74, 76, 81

INDEX

herbal medicine, 57, 63–4, 96, 98, 105–7, 113, 119, 140–1, 146–50, 259
Héroard, Jean, physician 187, 198–203
Herpin, Guillaume, surgeon 32–3
Hickey, Daniel 77
Hippocrates 149, 207, 235, 244
Hôpital de La Trinité 170, 177
Hôpital des Enfants-Dieu 169
hospital nursing 1, 26, 71–95, 110, 161
hospitals 1, 2, 9–10, 71–96, 98–9, 156–61, 169–71, 173–7, 258
 see also individual Hôtels-Dieu
Hôtel-Dieu, Beaune 85
Hôtel-Dieu, Caen 175
Hôtel-Dieu, Chinon 73
Hôtel-Dieu, Lyon 26, 76, 85, 110
Hôtel-Dieu, Meaux 80
Hôtel-Dieu, Orléans 80, 89, 147, 175
Hôtel-Dieu, Paris 37, 71–95, 98–9, 107, 169–70, 176–7, 206
Hôtel-Dieu, Poitiers 156–8, 178, 179n.3
Hôtel-Dieu, Pontoise 81, 89
Hôtel-Dieu, Reims 81
Hôtel-Dieu, Rouen 171
Hôtel-Dieu, Tours 84–5, 158–9, 164, 173–4
Hothman, Catherine, wetnurse 200
Hotman, Pierre, La Couche accountant 178
Houël, Nicolas, apothecary 148
housecalls 62, 64, 69n.89
household and domestic sphere 1–2, 10, 24–5, 62–3, 82, 97–155
Huart, Charles, physician 250
humanism 2, 47, 160, 167, 172
humeral theory 129–30, 220, 226–7
Humières, Jean de, royal governor 192–3, 195
Humières, Madame de, Françoise de Contay governess, 192–8, 210
hygiene/cleaning work 74, 76, 95n.111, 138, 156–7

illegitimacy 37–8, 134, 168, 171
Imbert, Jean 71–3
infanticide 36–7
infertility 35, 217
innate female knowledge 34, 227, 238–41, 251–2
 see also maternal authority

Jacquart, Danielle 48
Jacquelin, Michelle, unlicensed practitioner 107
Janotine, Jeanne, hospital nurse 85
Jean II 51
Jeanne de Valois, Saint 109, 112
Jewish practitioners 47–8
Jones, Colin 4, 5, 8, 13n.29, 89
Jordanova, Ludmilla 8
Joubert, Laurent 20, 32–3, 57–8, 61, 63, 100, 132, 140, 222, 233–6, 239, 244, 257, 259
Jouve, Claude, la Calandre, unlicensed practitioner 57

Kamen, Henry 226
kidney stones 146
Klairmont Lingo, Alison 25, 32, 46, 48, 51, 57–8, 63–4, 128, 130, 157, 235
Knibiehler, Yvonne 82
Koyré, Alexandre 3
Kuhn, Thomas 3

La Bellière, Madame de, governess 187
La Brosse, Guy de, physician 149
La Cacheleuse, Jehanne, hospital nurse 84
La Calabre, unlicensed practitioner 54–5
'La Chemanière', practitioner 159
La Cour, Catherine de, plague nurse 157
La Cousture, Madame, lady-in-waiting 218, 227
La Croix, Marie de, child carer 178
ladies-in-waiting 214–31
La Gausse, unlicensed practitioner 54
La Grosse Gorge, Barbe, diviner 114, 118
La Mauvaise, Perrette, culinary therapist 147
Lancre, Pierre de, councillor 117
Lanfrank of Milan 227
Lanning, John Tate 222
La Petite, Hélène, Hôtel-Dieu prioress 78, 169, 176
La Tache, Perenelle, Hôtel-Dieu prioress 78–9, 88
Latin translations and texts 4, 20, 22, 29–30, 32, 46, 54, 62, 99, 128, 136–7, 143, 148, 168, 192, 233
La Tousche, Gervais de, author 33–4, 239–40
La Trémoille, Henri de 237
Laurent, Olivier, physician 190

INDEX

Laval, Anne de 147
La Vielzville, Jacqueline, hospital nurse 79
law 10, 17–18, 25–6, 33–5, 38, 42n.88, 44–5, 49–50, 52–3, 56–8, 96–126, 169, 244, 258
Le Barbandier, Laurent, unlicensed practitioner 50
Lebrun, François 4
Le Febvre, Marion, sicknurse 82
Le Fournier, André, physician 233
Lehoux, Françoise 46, 61–3
Lemaire, Helin, wetnurse 199–200
Le Mans 169
Leproust, Guillemette, hospital patron 157
Lescallier, Jeanne, practitioner, 96–126, 145, 258
L'Estoile, Pierre de, memorialist 133
libraries 61–2, 136–7, 152n.51, 238
Liébault, Jean, physician 140, 145–9, 233, 257, 259
Lille 38, 111, 161, 171–2, 178
Limoges, Bishop of, ambassador 218–19, 221
linen, collection and purchase 73–4, 98, 157, 173
see also hygiene/cleaning work
literacy 4, 11, 12n.12, 20, 30, 35, 49, 53–4, 56–7, 62, 100–1, 132–3, 136–8, 147, 152n.51, 174–6, 257
literature, medical 2–4, 9–10, 32, 35, 48, 99, 106, 127–55, 167–8, 172, 182n.50, 191–2, 199, 202–10, 223–4, 232–6, 238–40, 257–8
lithotomists 21, 59, 159
Loches 37
Lonie, Iain M. 44
Lorraine 118
Louis, François, physician 237, 247, 250
Louis XI 17–18, 22–3, 147, 186–7
Louis XII 109, 158, 189
Louis XIII 187, 198–203, 208
Louise de Savoie 191
Lyège, Jean, physician 99, 131, 135
Lyon 25–6, 30, 46, 58, 63, 85, 110, 157–9, 174, 188

Mabille, Jeanne, unlicensed practitioner 52
Maillé, Jeanne-Marie de, Blessed 109
Maison-Dieu, Ballon 169
Maison-Dieu, Châteaudun 73

Malberta, Leurta 243, 246
Mandrou, Robert 116, 119
Manrique, Juan 223, 226
Marche, Jehanne, wetnurse 164
Mareschal, Cecille, Hôtel-Dieu subprioress 88, 169
Mareuil, Gabrielle de 99–100
Marguerite, Jeanne, sicknurse 82
Marguerite de Navarre 86, 139–42, 169, 258
Marie de Medici 133, 198–204, 209, 242
Marillac, Louise de 89
Marion, unlicensed practitioner 52
Marion, Simon, lawyer 97, 104, 108, 114–19, 121n.5
Marland, Hilary 38
marriage patterns and practices 25–6, 63–4, 69n.89
Marseilles 160–1, 183n.85
Martin, Marie, diviner 119
maternal authority 9, 165, 190–8, 210, 214–31, 258–9
Matras, Bautru, René, sieur de, lawyer 97, 101–3, 105–6, 115, 117
McTavish, Lianne 134
medical faculties 8, 10–11, 20, 23, 31, 36, 38–9, 44–6, 108, 221, 236, 257–8
medical faculty
   Angers 96–126, 145
   Avignon 58
   Montpellier 20–1, 23, 29, 33, 45, 56–8, 63–4, 68n.71, 100, 108, 132, 148, 204, 233
   Paris 20–2, 28, 44–6, 108, 132, 148–9, 204, 208, 210, 233
Melzer, Sara E. 215
menstruation 10, 214–31, 235–6, 244
Merleau-Ponty, Maurice 251
midwives 1, 6, 9, 16, 31–9, 54–5, 60–1, 75, 129, 133–5, 156, 168, 171, 186, 202–10, 224–5, 239–40, 257
see also obstetrics
Millanges, Simon de 239
Miller, Naomi J. 165
miracles 109–14
Miron, Gabriel, physician 167–8, 190–2
miscarriage 214, 226, 242–3
Moi, Toril 7, 251, 259
Moinarde, Toinette, hospital porter 157
Monbel, Jacqueline de 135–6
Montaigne, Michel de 61

INDEX

Monter, E. William 118
Monteux, Hierosme de 131
Montglat, Madame de, Françoise de Longjoue, governess 198–202
Montmorency, Anne de 195, 237
Montpellier 23–4, 30, 32, 46, 53, 56–8, 60, 63, 76, 160–1, 181n.39, 183n.85, 204, 236
  see also medical faculty, Montpellier
Moran, Bruce T. 221
Morin, Jehanne, hospital servant 159
Morisette, Jehanne, hospital nurse 80
mortality rates, children 165–7, 184n.108, 189
Mousy, Catherine, child carer 178
Mymy, Claude 245

Nassau, Amelie de 238, 241, 249
Nassau, Charlotte-Brabantine de, duchesse de La Trémoille 232, 237–8, 240–2, 244–50, 252
Nassau, Elisabeth de, duchesse de Bouillon 232, 237–8, 241, 244–50
Nassau, Flandrine de 238, 241
Nassau, Louise-Julienne de 238, 241, 248
Nicolle, hospital nurse 80
Nîmes 237
Norberg, Kathryn 215
Nôtre-Dame, Chapter 72, 77–8, 83–4, 88, 170, 177
nuns 2, 10, 71–90, 176–7, 238, 258
Nutton, Vivian 221

O'Boyle, Cornelius 46–7
obstetrics 10, 31–9, 54–5, 58, 133–5, 167, 202–10, 232–57
O'Connell, Marvin R. 113
Oquefre, Catherine, sicknurse 82
orphanage 85, 156–85
orphans and foundlings 1, 148, 156–86, 257
Otis, Leah L. 161

Pachaude, Léonarde, master barber's wife 25
Page, Françoise, practitioner 26, 158
Pailhera, Jehanne, midwife 34, 243
papacy 45, 47, 58, 112
Paracelsianism 57, 148–9, 204–5, 258
Pardieu, Marie de, hospital nurse 89
Paré, Ambroise, surgeon 108–9, 128–9, 133, 233

Paris 9, 18–19, 21–2, 25, 28–31, 36–7, 44–58, 61–4, 71–95, 136, 149, 169–71, 174, 176–8, 203–4
  see also Hôtel-Dieu, Paris; medical faculty, Paris; Parlement, Paris;
Parius, Claudius, priest 84
Parlement, Paris 17, 29, 35, 46–8, 72, 75, 77–8, 83, 89, 97, 105, 107–8, 116, 119–20, 125n.119, 170, 177, 205
patients 5, 14n.41, 20–1, 38–9, 50, 53, 56–7, 59, 63, 78–82, 84, 86–7, 89, 97–9, 102, 110, 115, 117–20, 138, 140, 156–7
Patine, Catherine, hospital novice 89
patronage 63, 187, 192–3, 198, 200, 204–5, 209–10
  women as 98–9, 135–7, 140, 156–7, 179n.3
Paul, St Vincent de 71, 89
Pelling, Margaret 5, 69n.89
Peronne, Peretta, surgical practitioner 55–6, 59
pharmacy see apothecaries; herbal medicine
Philip II of Spain 214–15, 219–22, 224–7, 258–9
phlebotomy 18, 22, 141, 226–7
physicians 1, 3–5, 8–10, 20–9, 32–8, 44–66, 71, 75–6, 79–80, 82, 96, 99–114, 118–20, 129, 131–6, 139–49, 156, 159, 167, 179, 186–92, 194–210, 216, 220–4, 226–9, 232–9, 240–1, 244, 247, 249–50, 257–9
pilgrimage 109–11, 118, 178
Pizan, Christine de, author 98
plague 76, 84, 110, 130, 156–7, 159, 173
Platter, Thomas, medical student 21, 60
Poitiers 156–8, 178, 179n.3
Pomata, Gianna 5
poor relief 10, 21, 37, 71, 76, 111, 138, 156–85
Postolle, Perrette 245–6
Pouquelin, Jeanne, female barber 41n.57
Poztier, Jehanne, hospital nurse 85
pregnancy 1, 10, 55, 73, 75, 111, 134–5, 147, 214–56
preventative medicine 9, 138
  see also hygiene/cleaning work
primary medicine 9, 137–55
  see also herbal medicine
Protestantism 57, 60, 109, 128–9, 204–5, 233–4, 258

INDEX

Protomedicato, Spain 221–2
publishers and printers 48, 127, 129, 133, 239

quickening 218, 245

Rabelais, François 234–5, 244
Ramsey, Matthew 4, 114
rape 33, 35, 42n.88
Reformation and Counter-Reformation 2, 112–14
Reims 16–18, 24, 27, 28, 81
religious healing 2, 4–5, 8, 10, 52, 96–8 108–114, 143, 145, 147, 189, 258
Renou, Jean de, physician 100, 149–50
reproductive knowledge 10–11, 214–56, 259
Reulin, Dominique, physician 233
Richer de Belleval, Pierre, physician 148
ringworm 159, 173, 178, 183
Robert, Anne, lawyer 35
Rodillon, Marie, practitioner 158
Roeslin, Eucharius 32
Roger, Jacques 3
Rouen 19, 22, 28, 30–1, 98, 176, 242
see also Hôtel-Dieu, Rouen
Rouget, François 134
Rouille, Michelle, wetnurse 164
Rublack, Ulinka 228, 243
rural folk 51, 97, 102–4, 107, 120, 137, 142–6, 163, 188, 193, 258

Saint Esprit houses, order of 160–1, 169–70, 178, 181n.28
saints 1, 10, 109–14, 117
Saint-Sulpice, ambassador 224–7
Salerno, Nicolas of 30, 132
Salmon, unlicensed practitioner 54
Saulnier, Annie 35
Sauvoyonne, Jeanne, hospital nurse 175
Schaffer, Simon 3
Schiebinger, Londa 8
Scott, Joan 7
scurvy 178
Serres, Olivier de, author 98, 142–6, 149, 258
sexuality 83–6, 168–9, 172
sexual knowledge 215, 233–4, 239
Shapin, Steven 3
sicknursing 1, 10, 53, 58, 82, 99–100, 110, 138–9, 158
see also hospital nursing
Slack, Paul 130

social status 7, 20–3, 33, 38, 46–7, 52, 58, 82, 98–101, 112, 136–7, 146, 168, 214, 224, 257
Soman, Alfred 119
Sonnet de Courval, Thomas, physician 51, 114, 136
Spain 11, 58, 214–31, 258–9
spicers 28–30, 47, 50, 131
students 22–3, 46, 51, 60–1, 69n.89
supernatural healing 109–19, 130
see also witchcraft
surgeons 1, 3–5, 8, 10, 16–28, 33–8, 46–8, 50–1, 55–6, 58–9, 75–6, 80, 82, 100, 105–6, 128–30, 133, 138, 142, 156, 159, 179, 186, 203–4, 208–9, 233, 235, 257
see also barbers
syphilis 158–9

Tarascon 64
Tareau, midwife 37
Theophrastus 149
Theurot, Pierre, barber 25
Thibault, Jean, unlicensed practitioner 48–50
Thiebourg, Etienne, unlicensed practitioner 50
Thou, Jacques-Auguste de 99–100
Tongrelou, Jehanne de, hospital governor 157
toothache 149
Toulouse 57–8, 160
Tours 21, 32, 37, 84, 109, 158–67, 171–5, 179, 183n.85, 189, 191
see also Hôtel-Dieu, Tours
Trent, Council of 2, 77, 113, 258
Triquière, Renée de, practitioner 107
Troyes 160

uroscopy 52, 244

Valence 111
Valgelas, Claude, physician 131, 135–6
Vallambert, Simon de, physician 167–8, 191, 233
Valois, Marie de 187, 245
Vauverde, Jehanne, hospital nurse 79
Vesalius, Andreas, physician 221
Vienne 110–12
Vineulx, Claude de, lady-in-waiting 217–18, 221
virginity 35–6, 38, 110, 232–3, 239

visual representation 134
Vives, Jean-Louis 82, 138–9, 172

weaning 168, 202
Wear, Andrew 204
Webster, Charles 5
wetnurses 1, 10, 147, 160–71, 175–7, 186–214, 257

widows 17, 20, 24–8, 30–1, 37–8, 51, 62, 64–5, 137, 160, 162–3, 170, 177
witchcraft 10, 58, 106–9, 113–20, 125n.103, n.109, n.112, 141, 258
wives 24–8, 30, 37–8, 45, 51, 53, 62–3, 65, 137–50, 162–3

Zegura, Elizabeth Chesney 235

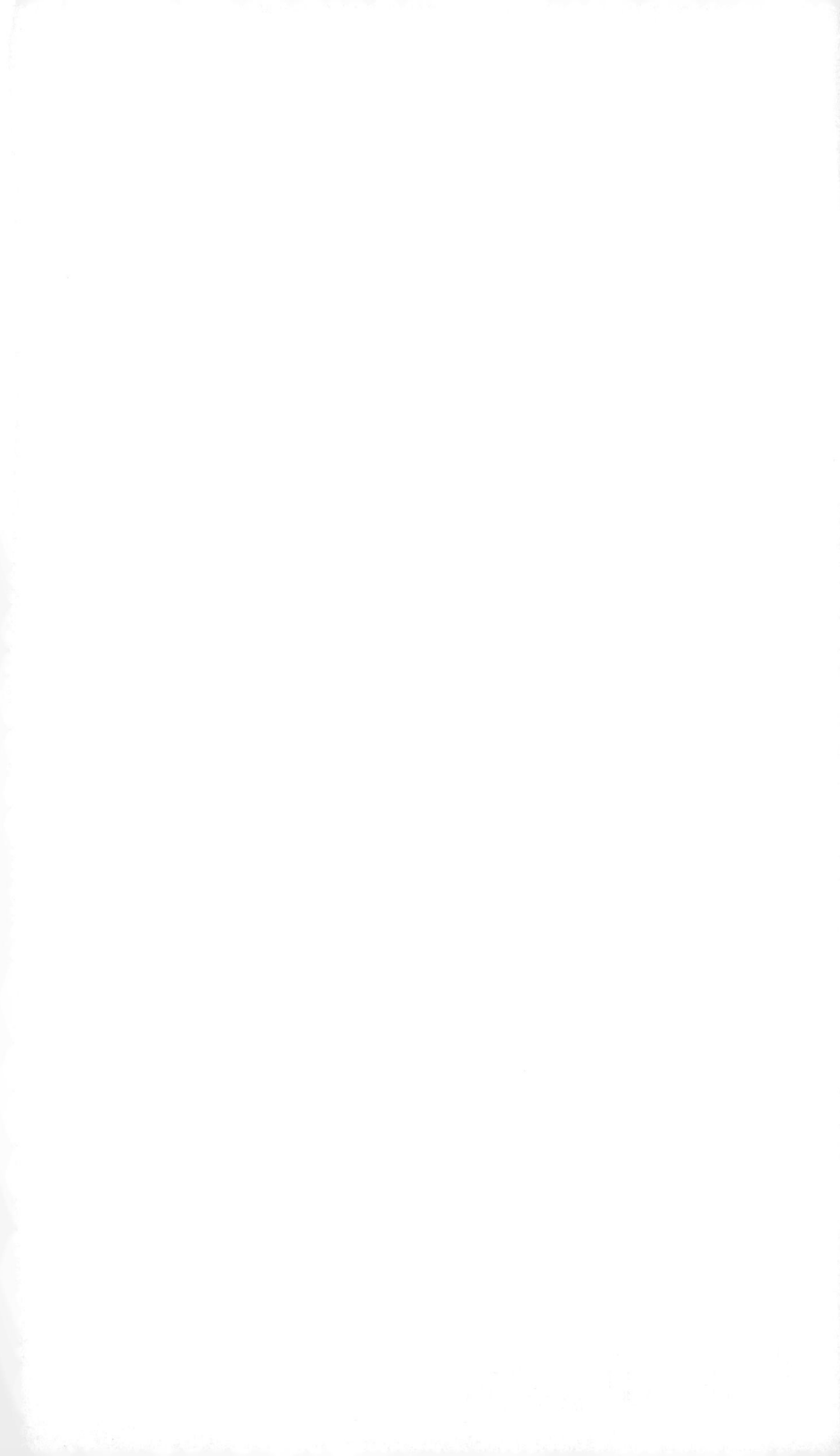

EU authorised representative for GPSR:
Easy Access System Europe, Mustamäe tee 50,
10621 Tallinn, Estonia
gpsr.requests@easproject.com

www.ingramcontent.com/pod-product-compliance
Ingram Content Group UK Ltd.
Pitfield, Milton Keynes, MK11 3LW, UK
UKHW021832140426
5217IPUK00021B/1403